Gynecologic Oncology

Ramez N. Eskander
Robert E. Bristow
Editors

Gynecologic Oncology

A Pocketbook

Springer

Editors
Ramez N. Eskander, M.D.
Assistant Professor
Division of Gynecologic Oncology
Department of Obstetrics and Gynecology
University of California, Irvine Medical Center
Orange, CA, USA

Robert E. Bristow, M.D., M.B.A.
The Philip J. DiSaia Prestigious Chair in Gynecologic Oncology
Professor and Director
Division of Gynecologic Oncology
Department of Obstetrics and Gynecology
University of California,
Irvine Medical Center
Orange, CA, USA

ISBN 978-1-4939-1975-8 ISBN 978-1-4939-1976-5 (eBook)
DOI 10.1007/978-1-4939-1976-5
Springer New York Heidelberg Dordrecht London

Library of Congress Control Number: 2014953587

Printed on acid-free paper

Springer is part of Springer Science+Business Media (www.springer.com)

Preface

It is with much enthusiasm that we introduce the first edition of "Gynecologic Oncology: A Pocketbook." Medical students, house staff, fellows, and junior faculty are required to adapt to growing responsibilities, while simultaneously expanding their knowledge base and clinical acumen. In an era of "online" medicine, health care providers are faced with a growing obligation to rapidly and effectively access, understand, and share information relating to treatment planning and patient care.

This task is difficult to accomplish using traditional textbooks, and requires a user-friendly print/electronic handbook that distills complex evaluation and management algorithms into easily accessible and understandable chapters. As an obstetrics and gynecology resident and gynecologic oncology fellow, such a source was lacking. This is what ultimately motivated the creation of this handbook.

Divided into nine chapters focusing on disease site, radiation therapy, chemotherapy, critical care, palliative care, and end-of-life care, this handbook is efficiently structured to provide a mobile source of reliable information in bullet point and table format. Each disease section details epidemiology, genetics, staging, and surgical management with a comprehensive review of key clinical trials that inform current treatment. Additionally, the radiation, chemotherapy, critical care, and palliative care chapters are analogously structured to provide essential information in a high-yield format unlike any companion handbook previously published.

Ultimately, it is our hope that this handbook will emerge as a reliable reference and educational guide, complimenting the substantial information contained in the critical textbooks that serve as the pillars of gynecologic oncology education and training.

We look forward to hearing from you, as we work to improve and build upon this first edition.

Orange, CA, USA

Ramez N. Eskander
Robert E. Bristow

Acknowledgements

This handbook is dedicated to our wives Michelle and Rachel, and our amazing children, Jackson, Chloe, Haley, Chloe, and Abigail, whose relentless support and encouragement have catalyzed our success. In addition, we would like to thank our colleagues and mentors for their guidance as well as our patients, whose courage and determination in the face of cancer are an inspirational and motivational force.

Contents

Section 1 Disease Sites

1 **Epithelial Ovarian Cancer, Low Malignant Potential, and Sex Cord Stromal Tumors of the Ovary** 3
Ramez N. Eskander and Robert E. Bristow

2 **Cervical Cancer** 55
Sara M. Jordan and Krishnansu S. Tewari

3 **Cancer of the Vulva and Vagina** 85
Lauren Krill and Leslie M. Randall

4 **Uterine Corpus Cancers** 133
Kristy K. Ward and Michael T. McHale

5 **Gestational Trophoblastic Disease** 175
Elizabeth L. Dickson and Sally A. Mullany

Section 2 Chemotherapy

6 **Chemotherapy for Gynecologic Cancer** 205
Quan Li and Jack L. Watkins

Section 3 Radiation Therapy

7 **Radiation Therapy in Gynecologic Cancer** 289
Susan G.R. McDuff and Catheryn M. Yashar

Section 4 Critical Care

8 Critical Care 337
Alexandre Buckley and Ana I. Tergas

Section 5 Palliative Care

9 Palliative Care 371
Solomon Liao, Rosene D. Pirrello,
Rebecca Liddicoat Yamarik, and Jamie Capasso

Index 415

Contributors

Robert E. Bristow, M.D., M.B.A. Division of Gynecologic Oncology, Department of Obstetrics and Gynecology, Irvine Medical Center, University of California, Orange, CA, USA

Alexandre Buckley, M.D. Division of Gynecologic Oncology, Department of Obstetrics and Gynecology, Columbia University College of Physicians and Surgeons, New York, NY, USA

Columbia University Medical Center, New York, NY, USA

Jamie Capasso, D.O. Department of Internal Medicine, Irvine Medical Center, University of California, Orange, CA, USA

Elizabeth L. Dickson, M.D. Division of Gynecologic Oncology, Department of Obstetrics, Gynecology and Women's Health, University of Minnesota Medical Center, Fairview, Minneapolis, MN, USA

Ramez N. Eskander, M.D. Division of Gynecologic Oncology, Department of Obstetrics and Gynecology, Irvine Medical Center, University of California, Orange, CA, USA

Sara M. Jordan, M.D. Gynecologic Oncologist, Southwest Gynecologic Oncology Associates, Inc., Albuquerque, NM, USA

Lauren Krill, M.D., M.S. Division of Gynecologic Oncology, Department of Obstetrics and Gynecology, Irvine Medical Center, University of California, Orange, CA, USA

Quan Li, Pharm.D. Department of Pharmacy, The James Cancer Hospital, The Ohio State University, Columbus, OH, USA

Solomon Liao, M.D., A.A.H.P.M. Department of Internal Medicine, Irvine Medical Center, University of California, Orange, CA, USA

Susan G.R. McDuff, M.D., Ph.D. Department of Radiation Medicine and Applied Sciences, University of California San Diego Health System, La Jolla, CA, USA

Michael T. McHale, M.D. Department of Reproductive Medicine, UC San Diego Moores Cancer Center, La Jolla, CA, USA

Sally A. Mullany, M.D. Division of Gynecologic Oncology, Department of Obstetrics, Gynecology and Women's Health, University of Minnesota Medical Center, Fairview, Minneapolis, MN, USA

Rosene D. Pirrello, B.Pharm., R.Ph. Department of Pharmacy Services, UC Irvine Health Department of Pharmacy Services, Irvine Medical Center, University of California, Orange, CA, USA

Leslie M. Randall, M.D. Department of Gynecologic Oncology, Irvine Medical Center, University of California, Orange, CA, USA

Ana I. Tergas, M.D., M.P.H. Division of Gynecologic Oncology, Department of Obstetrics and Gynecology, Columbia University College of Physicians and Surgeons, New York, NY, USA

Krishnansu S. Tewari, M.D., F.A.C.O.G., F.A.C.S. The Division of Gynecologic Oncology, The Gynecologic Oncology Group at UC Irvine, Irvine Medical Center, University of California, Orange, CA, USA

Kristy K. Ward, M.D., M.A.S. Department of Reproductive Medicine, UC San Diego Moores Cancer Center, La Jolla, CA, USA

Jack L. Watkins, Pharm.D., B.C.O.P. Department of Clinical Effectiveness, University of Texas MD Anderson Cancer Center, Houston, TX, USA

Rebecca Liddicoat Yamarik, M.D., M.P.H. Providence Trinity Care Hospice, Torrance, CA, USA

Catheryn M. Yashar, M.D. Department of Radiation Medicine and Applied Sciences, University of California San Diego Health System, La Jolla, CA, USA

Section 1
Disease Sites

Chapter 1
Epithelial Ovarian Cancer, Low Malignant Potential, and Sex Cord Stromal Tumors of the Ovary

Ramez N. Eskander and Robert E. Bristow

Epidemiology

- Ovarian cancer remains the most lethal gynecologic malignancy, and is the fifth leading cause of cancer death in women in the USA.
- In 2014 there will be an estimated 21,980 cases with 14,270 deaths [1].
- No effective screening strategies exist, and therefore the majority of patients (approximately 75 %) present with advanced stage disease requiring surgical resection and adjuvant chemotherapy.
- An individual's lifetime risk of developing ovarian cancer is 1.8 % (approximately 1 in 70).
- The risk of malignancy, in the context of an adnexal mass, is significantly greater in postmenopausal women, when compared to premenopausal patients.

R.N. Eskander, M.D. (✉) • R.E. Bristow, M.D., M.B.A.
Division of Gynecologic Oncology, Department of Obstetrics and Gynecology, Irvine Medical Center, University of California, 101 The City Drive, Orange, CA 92868, USA
e-mail: eskander@uci.edu; rbristow@uci.edu

R.N. Eskander and R.E. Bristow (eds.), *Gynecologic Oncology: A Pocketbook*, DOI 10.1007/978-1-4939-1976-5_1,

Table 1.1. Risk factors associated with development of epithelial ovarian cancer [2].

Risk factor
Nulliparity
Early menarche
Late menopause
Increasing age
White race
Family history
Personal history of breast cancer
Hormone replacement therapy[a]
Fertility drugs[a]
Talc[a]

[a]Controversial

- Incidence increases with age, with peak incidence in women aged 56–60 years [1]. Risk of adnexal mass being malignant rises to 1 in 3 in women older than 40 years of age.
- Several risk factors associated with the development of ovarian cancer have been identified (Table 1.1).

Early Detection and Screening for Ovarian Cancer

- Screening and diagnostic methods explored in ovarian cancer include pelvic examination, transvaginal ultrasound (TVUS), cancer antigen 125 (CA 125), as well as multi-marker panels and bioinformatics.
- Sensitivity and specificity of pelvic exam alone poor.
- CA 125 with limited sensitivity (only ½ of early ovarian cancers produce sufficient CA 125 to produce a positive test).
- Noncancerous lesions also result in false positive CA 125.
- Two large prospective randomized trials completed in the USA and UK studied screening in average risk patients with a combination of CA 125 and TVUS [3].

PLCO Cancer Screening Trial

- 78,216 women aged 55–74 years randomized to 6 annual rounds of screening with CA 125 and TVUS for 4 years (n=39,105) or a group with usual care (n=39,111).
  - Participants followed for maximum of 13 years.
  - Primary outcome: ovarian cancer mortality.
  - At conclusion of study number of deaths similar in each group.
    - 3.1/10,000 in screening and 2.6/10,000 in control group (RR 1.18; 95 % CI 0.82–1.71).
    - No reduction in ovarian cancer mortality.
  - Absence of stage shift in screening group may indicate poor sensitivity of the screening protocol in this population.

UK Collaborative Trial of Ovarian Cancer Screening

- Examined the efficacy of multimodal screening including annual CA 125 with risk of ovarian cancer algorithm (ROCA) and TVUS as a second line test versus screening with TVUS alone.
  - ROCA measures the change in CA 125 over time rather than single cutoff value.
  - At the 2013 ASCO annual meeting the results of the UK FOCSS phase 2 study were presented [4].
- UK FOCSS 2 modified screening by employing Q4 month assessments with online system notifying physicians when additional/testing referral was required.
- A total of 4,531 women were enrolled.
- Patients with >10 % lifetime risk of ovarian cancer + age >35.
- Sensitivity ranged from 75 to 100 % and specificity 96.1 % with PPV of 13 %.

Despite Promising Results, Several Limitations

- Heterogeneous population with risk based on family history, BRCA mutation, and/or Lynch syndrome.
- Average age at entry was 44, which is younger than average age of onset of ovarian cancer, even in BRCA patients.
- Study algorithm intense and not likely generalizable.

- Currently, no organization recommends screening average-risk women for ovarian cancer.
- In 2012 USPSTF recommended against screening for ovarian cancer (D recommendation) given lack of reduction in ovarian cancer related mortality in completed studies.

Genetics and Hereditary Ovarian Cancer

- Hereditary breast and ovarian cancer (HBOC) was initially a clinical diagnosis based on family history of multiple relatives with early onset breast cancer and/or ovarian cancer at any age.
- Germ line BRCA1 and BRCA2 mutations account for approximately 15 % of invasive ovarian carcinomas.
- Conversely, BRCA1 and BRCA2 mutations are *not* associated with borderline ovarian neoplasms.
- BRCA1 and BRCA2 mutations lead to a 15–50 % lifetime risk of ovarian cancer.
- A number of additional genes (~10 in total) have been shown to cause hereditary ovarian cancer, and to account for up to 29 % of hereditary ovarian cancer cases.
  - Most common alternate mutations include RAD51C, TP53, CHEK2, BRIP1 [5].
  - Research into panel testing and next-generation sequencing ongoing.
- Nearly 1/3 of women with hereditary ovarian cancer have no relatives with cancer.
- 35 % of women with hereditary ovarian cancer are older than 60 years at diagnosis.

- Per the SGO clinical practice statement (2014)—all women diagnosed with ovarian, Fallopian tube, or primary peritoneal cancer should be offered genetic counseling with consideration of genetic testing regardless of age or family history.
- BRCA1

Location	Chromosome 17q21
Function and mutation	BRCA functions in homologous recombination and DAN repair. 80 % of mutations are loss of function nonsense or frameshift alterations
Incidence	Accounts for 45 % of site specific breast cancer and is mutated in 90 % of HBOC cases
Risk	Confers approximately 50 % chance of ovarian cancer and 85 % chance of breast cancer by age 70 39–46 % chance of ovarian cancer in patients with proven mutation Associated with other cancers including: pancreas, prostate, uterine, esophageal, stomach, and colon
Prevention	5 years of OCP use leads to 50 % reduction in risk of ovarian cancer Risk reducing surgery (BSO vs. TAH/BSO) recommended at completion of childbearing or by age 35 If decline surgery, screening with Q6 month TVUS and CA 125 should be performed

- BRCA2

Location	Chromosome 13q12
Function and mutation	BRCA functions in homologous recombination and DAN repair. 80 % of mutations are loss of function nonsense or frameshift alterations
Risk	Confers approximately 40–85 % lifetime risk of breast cancer Lower, but markedly increased risk of ovarian cancer, of 10–20 % in proven mutation carriers
Prevention	5 years of OCP use leads to 50 % reduction in risk of ovarian cancer Risk reducing surgery (BSO vs. TAH/BSO) recommended at completion of childbearing or by age 35 If decline surgery, screening with Q6 month TVUS and CA 125 should be performed

- *Lynch syndrome (HNPCC)* has also been linked to the development of ovarian cancer.
  - In families with history of early onset endometrial or colon cancer (<50 years), physicians should beware of Lynch syndrome.
  - Results from mutations in DNA mismatch repair genes: MLH1, MLH3, MSH2, MSH6, PMS2 [6, 7].
    - Lifetime risk of colon cancer 30–54 %.
    - Lifetime risk of endometrial cancer 42–69 %.
    - Lifetime risk of ovarian cancer 9–12 %.
  - Over 50 % of women with lynch syndrome will present with endometrial cancer as their first malignancy.
- Lynch syndrome.

Location	MSH2—chromosome 2p16 MLH1—chromosome 3p21 (above are the two most common Lynch associated mutations)
Function and mutation	Mutation results in mismatch repair defects—microsatellite repeats that result in genetic instability and uncontrolled proliferation, invasion, or metastases
Risk	Confers approximately 9–12 % lifetime risk of ovarian cancer At risk for additional malignancies including: endometrial, colon, upper urologic, GI, pancreas, and liver Lifetime risk of any Lynch associated cancer approaches 75 %
Prevention	Screening recommendations include: • Colonoscopy at age 25 (or 10 years prior to earliest age of dx of colon cancer) annually • For MSH6 mutations screening begins at age 30 due to late onset with this mutation • Consider annual EMB as well as TVUS and CA125 for evaluation of endometrial and ovarian cancer beginning at age 30–35 years • Annual UA and skin exam • Consider upper endoscopy

Presenting Signs and Symptoms

- Despite initial descriptions of ovarian cancer as a silent disease, recent investigation has shown that patients commonly report pelvic, abdominal, and menstrual symptoms prior to diagnosis [8].
  - Goff et al. developed an ovarian cancer symptom index that included [9]:
    - Abdominal pain.
    - Pelvic pain.
    - Urinary frequency and/or urgency.
    - Increased abdominal size/bloating.
    - Decreased appetite/early satiety.
  - The index had a sensitivity of 56.7 % for early ovarian cancer and 79.5 % for advanced stage ovarian cancer.
- Despite the above, over 75 % of patients will be diagnosed with advanced stage disease at presentation.

Pathologic Considerations

- Epithelial ovarian cancers represent 80–90 % of ovarian cancers, while germ cell tumors represent 3–5 %, and sex cord stromal tumors an additional 5–6 %.
- Approximately 75–80 % of epithelial ovarian cancers are serous histology.
- Tumors metastatic to the ovary (including endometrial, cervical, breast, GI (Krukenberg), and lymphoma) account for the remaining 5 % of ovarian malignancies.

Epithelial Ovarian Cancer

- High grade serous (75–80 %).
- Endometrioid (10 %).
- Clear cell (10 %).
- Mucinous (3 %).
- Low grade serous (<5 %).

- Transitional cell/Brenner (<1 %).
- High grade serous and low grade serous carcinomas are now considered different neoplasms with independent pathogenesis.

High Grade Serous Carcinoma

- Most common type of ovarian neoplasm and rarely confined to the ovary (<10 %) at the time of diagnosis.
- Can range in size from microscopic to >25 cm.
- Typically cystic and multilocular.
- Microscopic examination traditionally shows papillary, glandular, microcystic, and solid patterns.
- Psammoma bodies may be present but traditionally to a lesser degree than with low grade serous lesions.
- Marked cytologic atypia and prominent mitoses are common.
- Diffusely express p53 and p16.
- Can additionally express WT-1, estrogen, and Pax-8.

Low Grade Serous Carcinoma

- Uncommon and accounts for less than 5 % of ovarian cancers [10].
- Commonly diagnosed in advanced stage with poor long term prognosis.
- Commonly found in association with borderline component.
- Microscopically characterized by destructive stromal invasion.
- Lower mitotic activity and less nuclear atypia than high grade lesions.
- Molecular studies show common mutations in KRAS and BRAF.

Mucinous Carcinoma

- Nearly all present with early stage disease (Stage I).
- Tend to be large (>20 cm) at the time of presentation/resection.

- Bilateral in 5–10 % of cases (bilaterally may indicate GI metastases to ovary).
- Microscopically cells resemble those of endocervix, intestine, or gastric pylorus.
- Commonly express GI markers including CDX2 and CK20.
- Over 75 % have a KRAS mutation.

Endometrioid Carcinoma

- Commonly identified at an early stage with significantly better prognosis.
- Typically low grade, but chemosensitive.
- Associated with endometrial cancer 15–20 % of the time.
- Grossly solid and/or cystic and may arise in background of endometriosis.
- Microscopically resembles low grade endometrioid adenocarcinoma of the uterus.
- Typically express vimentin, ER, PR, and CA 125.
- The most common somatic mutations are found in beta-catenin and PTEN (analogous to endometrial adenocarcinoma).
- Bilateral in up to 15 % of cases.

Clear Cell Carcinoma

- Similar to endometrioid histology, clear cell commonly presents at an early stage with good prognosis.
- But, if presents in advanced stage, worse prognosis and outcome compared to serous or endometrioid carcinoma (not as chemo-responsive to platinum).
- Often associated with and arising from endometriosis.
- Traditionally large and cystic on gross inspection.
- Sheets of cells with clear cytoplasm characterize the solid pattern.
- Lack expression of ER and WT-1.
- Associated with mutation in ARID1A.

TABLE 1.2. Characteristics associated with serous and mucinous LMP.

Serous LMP	Mucinous LMP
Comprise 65 % of LMP	
Mean age at presentation: 35–40 years	
Ovary confined and slow growing	
10 % with areas of microinvasion	10–20 % with microinvasion
35 % with peritoneal implants	Harbor KRAS mutations
Low Ki67 and weak p53 expression	Positive CK7, CDX2, and CK20 expression
10-year survival 95–100 %	

Borderline or Low Malignant Potential (LMP) Neoplasms

- Can be serous or mucinous (Table 1.2).

Germ Cell Tumors

- Account for 3–5 % of ovarian cancers, with the majority (70 %) presenting as Stage I lesions (ovary confined disease).
- Most common age at presentation 10–30 years.
- These lesions are almost always unilateral aside from dysgerminoma, which is bilateral in up to 15 % of cases.
- Amongst malignant germ cell tumors: dysgerminoma, immature teratoma, yolk sac, and mixed account for 90 % of cases.

Tumor Markers

- hCG: embryonal, choriocarcinoma, mixed germ cell.
- AFP: yolk-sac/endodermal sinus, embryonal, mixed germ cell.
- LDH: dysgerminoma.
- Struma ovarii is a “monodermal” teratoma composed almost entirely of mature thyroid tissue.
  - Malignant change is rare but has been described.
- Non gestational choriocarcinoma is exceedingly rare, and has a propensity for early hematogenous spread.

Surgical Management of Ovarian Cancer

- The purpose of surgical exploration is diagnostic and therapeutic.
- Goal of resection is to define stage of disease and remove as much of the visible disease as possible, in order to achieve and R_0 state (microscopic residual disease).
- Staging traditionally defined by:
  - TAH + BSO.
  - Pelvic and para aortic LND.
  - Omentectomy.
  - Peritoneal biopsies (pelvic side wall, bladder serosa, cul-de-sac, pericolic gutters, and diaphragm).
  - Harvesting of ascites or procurement of cytology.
  - Biopsy of any suspicious lesions.
- In patients with more advanced disease, staging is replaced by attempts at aggressive surgical cytoreduction, which may require:
  - Small/large bowel resection (+/– ostomy), full thickness diaphragm resection or peritonectomy, splenectomy, peritoneal stripping, or collaborative efforts with additional teams to remove portions of the liver, pancreas, affected kidney/adrenal gland, etc.
- The FIGO staging system for ovarian cancer was revised in January 2014 and is shown below, with changes italicized:

Stage I: Tumor confined to ovaries			
Old		New	
IA	Tumor limited to one ovary, capsule intact, no tumor on surface, negative washings/ascites	IA	Tumor limited to one ovary, capsule intact, no tumor on surface, negative washings/ascites
IB	Tumor involves both ovaries otherwise like 1A	IB	Tumor involves both ovaries otherwise like 1A
IC	Tumor involves one or both ovaries with any of the following: capsule rupture, tumor on surface, positive washings/ascites	IC	Tumor limited to one or both ovaries
		ICI	Surgical spill
		IC2	Capsule rupture before surgery or tumor on ovarian surface
		IC3	Malignant cells in the ascites or peritoneal washings

Stage II: Tumor involves one or both ovaries with pelvic extension (below the pelvic brim) or primary peritoneal cancer			
Old		New	
IIA	Extension and/or implant on uterus and/or Fallopian tubes	IIA	Extension and/or implant on uterus and/or Fallopian tubes
IIB	Extension to other pelvic intraperitoneal tissues	IIB	Extension to other pelvic intraperitoneal tissues
IIC	11A or 11B with positive washings/ascites	Old stage IIC has been eliminated	

Stage III: Tumor involves one or both ovaries with cytologically or histologically confirmed spread to the peritoneum outside the pelvis and/or metastasis to the retroperitoneal lymph nodes			
Old		New	
IIIA	Microscopic metastasis beyond the pelvis	IIIA	(Positive retroperitoneal lymph nodes and/or microscopic metastasis beyond the pelvis)
		IIIAI	Positive retroperitoneal lymph nodes only IIIAI(i) Metastasis ≤10 mm IIIAI(ii) Metastasis ≥10 mm
		IIIA2	Microscopic, extrapelvic (above the brim) peritoneal involvement ± positive retroperitoneal lymph nodes
IIIB	Macroscopic, extrapelvic, peritoneal metastasis ≤2 cm in greatest dimension	IIIB	Macroscopic, extrapelvic, peritoneal metastasis ≤2 cm ± positive retroperitoneal lymph nodes. Includes extension to capsule of liver/spleen
IIIC	Macroscopic, extrapelvic, peritoneal metastasis ≥2 cm in greatest dimension and/or regional lymph node metastasis	IIIC	Macroscopic, extrapelvic, peritoneal metastasis ≥2 cm ± positive retroperitoneal lymph nodes. Includes extension to capsule of liver/spleen

Stage IV: Distant metastases excluding peritoneal metastases			
Old		New	
IV	Distant metastasis excluding peritoneal metastasis. Includes hepatic parenchymal metastasis	IVA	Pleural effusion with positive cytology
		1VB	Hepatic and/or *splenic parenchymal* metastasis, metastasis to extra-abdominal organs (including inguinal lymph nodes and lymph nodes outside of the abdominal cavity)

Other major recommendations are as follows:

- Histologic type including grading should be designated at staging.
- Primary site (ovary, Fallopian tube, or peritoneum) should be designated where possible.
- Tumors that may otherwise qualify for Stage I but involved with dense adhesions justify upgrading to Stage II if tumor cells are histologically proven to be present in the adhesions.

Paradigm of Surgical Cytoreduction and the Role of Neoadjuvant Chemotherapy

- Concept of cytoreductive surgery for ovarian cancer first introduced in 1934 (Meigs).
- This was followed by Griffiths who published a landmark study that demonstrated an inverse relationship between residual tumor and patient survival [11, 12].
- Residual disease after cytoreductive surgery is defined as the largest diameter of remaining tumor and is one of the most important prognosticators of outcome [13, 14].
  - Despite the above, a universal consensus on the definition of residual disease following surgery is lacking.
  - The Gynecologic Oncology Group (GOG) defines optimal residual disease as tumor ≤1 cm in the largest diameter at completion of surgery [15, 16].

TABLE 1.3. Importance of cytoreductive surgery [15, 18, 25].

Study	Type	Included studies	Findings
Hoskins et al. [15]	Ancillary data study of GOG 97 + GOG 52	*GOG 97*: Cisplatin 50 mg/m^2 + Cyclophosphamide 500 mg/m^2 every 3 weeks × 8 cycles versus Cisplatin 100 mg/m^2 + Cyclophosphamide 1,000 mg/m^2 every 3 weeks × 8 cycles *GOG 52*: Cisplatin 75 mg/m^2 every 3 weeks × 6 cycles versus Cisplatin 75 mg/m^2 + Paclitaxel 135 mg/m^2 every 3 weeks × 6 cycles	Complete resection to NGR disease (5-year survival 60 %) Optimal but visible disease (5-year survival 35 %) Suboptimal residual disease (5-year survival 20 %)
Chang et al. [18]	Meta analysis	18 Studies included and analyzed	Each 10 % increase in complete gross resection resulted in a 28 % improvement in the median survival time

GOG gynecologic oncology group, *NGR* no gross residual; optimal = 0.1 cm to ≤2 cm; suboptimal = 2 cm

Adapted from: Hodeib M, Eskander RN, Bristow RE. New Paradigms in the surgical and adjuvant treatment of ovarian cancer. Minerva Ginecol April 2014;66:179–92) Reprinted by permission of Edizioni Minerva Medica from April;66(2):179–92

- Contemporary data suggest that the most favorable survival outcomes are associated with complete cytoreduction to no gross residual disease [17–24] (Table 1.3) [25].
- Achieving optimal cytoreduction depends heavily on the skill, education/training, experience, and personal philosophy of the operating surgeon.
- Despite the impact of cytoreduction on oncologic outcome, maximal cytoreduction rates (no visible residual disease) vary significantly in the literature, ranging from 50 to 85 %.
- Unfortunately, major surgical procedures are associated with morbidity and mortality.

- In 2010, a retrospective review evaluating the incidence of major complications after the performance of extensive upper abdominal surgical procedures during primary cytoreduction for advanced stage ovarian cancer:
  - Grade 3–5 complications occurred in 31 (22 %) patients, including 2 mortalities (1.4 %).

Role of Neoadjuvant Chemotherapy

- In a subset of patients with advanced stage ovarian cancer, primary surgical cytoreduction is not feasible due to:
  - Tumor biology/disease distribution (unresectable intrathoracic metastases, multifocal liver parenchymal disease).
  - Medical comorbidities.
  - Lack of access to appropriate surgical specialist.
- In these setting, neoadjuvant chemotherapy is commonly administered.
- Additionally, given the potential morbidity associated with surgical cytoreduction, as well as the variability in achieving microscopic residual disease, an interest in the administration of neoadjuvant chemotherapy has emerged over the last decade.
- To date, 2 prospective phase 3, randomized clinical trials have been performed in Europe comparing neoadjuvant chemotherapy to up-front surgery in patients with advanced stage ovarian cancer (Table 1.4) [25].
- Neither trail showed primary cytoreduction to be superior to neoadjuvant chemotherapy with respect to oncologic outcome.
- Vergote et al. [26]—The hazard ratio for death in the group assigned to neoadjuvant chemotherapy followed by interval debulking, as compared with the group assigned to primary debulking surgery followed by chemotherapy, was 0.98 (90 % CI, 0.84 to 1.13; P=0.01 for non inferiority), and the hazard ratio for progressive disease was 1.01 (90 % CI, 0.89–1.15).

TABLE 1.4. Phase 3 clinical trials investigating neoadjuvant chemotherapy [25–27].

Study	Design	PFS	OS	Surgical outcome	Adverse events
Vergote et al. [26]	PS versus NACT, Stage III or IV disease, extra-pelvic metastasis >2 cm, regional lymph node mets, CA125:CEA ratio >25	12 m in both arms	PS = 29 m NACT = 30 m	PS arm → optimal residual disease = 41.6 %; complete cytoreduction = 18.4 % NACT arm → optimal residual disease = 80.6 %	PS arm: death 2.5 % NACT arm: death 0.7 % PS arm: hemorrhage 7.4 % NACT arm: Hemorrhage 4.1 %
CHORUS [27]	NACT versus PS; Stage III or IV disease, serum CA125:CEA ratio >25, anticipated use of carboplatin chemotherapy, performance status sufficient to allow treatment	PS = 10.3 m NACT = 11.7 m	PS = 22.8 m NACT = 24.5 m	NACT was non-inferior to PS → NACT associated with improved optimal cytoreduction rates + decreased morbidity	PS arm: death 5.6 % NACT arm: 0.5 %

NACT neoadjuvant chemotherapy, *PS* primary surgery, *PFS* progression free survival, *OS* overall survival, *mets* metastases
Adapted from: Hodeib M, Eskander RN, Bristow RE. New Paradigms in the surgical and adjuvant treatment of ovarian cancer. Minerva Ginecol April 2014;66:179–92) Reprinted by permission of Edizioni Minerva Medica from April;66(2):179–92

Limitations

- A cohort of patients were excluded post randomization (Argentina cohort 48/718 enrolled patients).
- Biased interpretation of perioperative mortality.
- A variety of chemotherapy regimens were allowed.
- Significant heterogeneity in surgical outcomes.

- *MRC CHORUS* (2013 ASCO annual meeting) randomized phase 3 trial, comparing neoadjuvant chemotherapy (NACT) to primary surgery (PS) for newly diagnosed advanced ovarian cancer (Abstract 5,500) was discussed [27].
  - When exploring outcomes, no significant difference in progression free survival or overall survival was identified.
  - Furthermore, the authors reported a 5.6 % 28-day mortality rate in the primary surgery arm, compared to 0.5 % in the neoadjuvant arm.

Limitations

- Low microscopic residual disease rate in the primary surgery arm.
- Identical median surgical times in both arms (120 min), calling into question the surgical effort with up-front surgery.
- 20 % of subjects had a PS of 2–3, representing an unfavorable population.

- Currently, we await the results of Japanese Clinical Oncology Group (JCOG) protocol 0602, once again evaluating the question of up-front surgery versus neoadjuvant chemotherapy.

Evolution of Adjuvant Chemotherapy in the Treatment of Epithelial Ovarian Cancer

Early Stage High-Risk Cancer

- Benefit of chemotherapy in the management of patients with early stage, high-risk disease, has been studied in three large clinical trials (Table 1.5) [28].

TABLE 1.5. Randomized clinical trials evaluating adjuvant treatment of early stage EOC [28–32].

Study	Trial design	Status
First-line adjuvant therapy		
ICON 1 [29]	477 patients randomized: adjuvant chemotherapy versus observation after surgery	HR 0.66 favoring adjuvant chemotherapy (surgical staging not required)
ACTION [30]	448 patients randomized: Ia and Ib grade II–III, all grades of Ic–IIa and all clear cell carcinomas—adjuvant chemotherapy versus observation	Recurrence-free interval HR 0.63 favoring adjuvant chemotherapy arm. No difference in overall survival (only 1/3 of group optimally staged)
GOG 157 [31]	457 patients with Stage Ia and Ib grade 3, Ic all grades, clear cell, and completely resected stage II, randomized to 3 versus 6 cycles of CT	No difference in HR for recurrence or death (29 % inadequately staged)
GOG 175 [32]	542 patients with Ia/Ib grade 3, clear cell, all Ic and Stage II EOC randomized to CT+maintenance T versus CT followed by observation	No difference in recurrence or 5 year survival

CT carboplatin/paclitaxel, *T* paclitaxel, *GOG* Gynecologic Oncology Group, *ICON* International Collaborative Ovarian Neoplasm, *ACTION* Adjuvant Chemotherapy Trial in Ovarian Neoplasia, *HR* hazard ratio
Reprinted with permission from Cambridge University Press. Eskander RN, Di Saia PJ. Chemotherapy of ovarian cancer. In: Deligdisch L, Kase NG, Cohen CJ, editors. Altchek's Diagnosis and Management of Ovarian Disorders, 3rd Edition. New York: Cambridge University Press; 2013; pp. 415–424

- These patients are defined as having Stage Ia and Ib grade II–III tumors, all grades of Ic–IIa and all clear cell carcinomas.
  - International Collaborative Ovarian Neoplasm Trial 1 (ICON1) [29].
  - The Adjuvant Chemotherapy Trial in Ovarian Neoplasia (ACTION) [30].
    - Surgical staging was not required in the ICON1 trial, and a proportion of these women likely had occult disease making them Stage III.

- In the ACTION trial, only 1/3 of the total group was optimally staged.
- Within the optimally staged population, no benefit was seen in those treated with adjuvant chemotherapy.
- Notably, 57 % of patients in the combined studies were treated with single agent carboplatin in the adjuvant setting, with a remaining 27 % treated with cisplatin.

– The trials initiated by the *Gynecologic Oncology Group (GOG) included protocol 157* [31] which examined 3 versus 6 cycles of adjuvant chemotherapy in patients with early stage disease.

- 29 % of patients had incomplete or inadequately documented surgical staging.
- The recurrence rate after 6 cycles was 24 % lower (HR 0.761; 95 % CI 0.51–1.13, P=0.18).
- The overall death rate was similar for the two regimens (HR: 1.02; 95 % CI: 0.662–1.57).

– Most recently, the *GOG completed protocol 175*, which compared the recurrence-free interval (RFI) and safety profile in patients with completely resected high-risk early-stage ovarian cancer treated with intravenous carboplatin and paclitaxel with or without maintenance low-dose paclitaxel for 24 weeks [32].

- The 5 year recurrence risk was 20 % in the maintenance paclitaxel arm, versus 23 % in the observation arm (HR 0.807; 95 % CI: 0.565–1.15).
- The probability of surviving 5 years was 85.4 and 86.2 %, respectively.
- The rates of neurologic, dermatologic, and infectious toxicities were significantly more common in the maintenance arm.

Advanced Stage Epithelial Ovarian Cancer

- Patients presenting with advanced stage ovarian cancer are managed with maximal surgical resection followed by adjuvant platinum and taxane based chemotherapy.

- Prior to the discovery and introduction of cisplatin patients were treated with the alkylating agents melphalan, thiotepa, cyclophosphamide, or chlorambucil as single agents.
- Our understanding of the therapeutic benefits of regimens containing cisplatin and paclitaxel originated following the results of *Gynecologic Oncology Group (GOG) protocol 111* [33]
  - Three hundred and eighty-six women with Stage III sub-optimally debulked or Stage IV disease were randomly assigned to receive 6 cycles of cisplatin (75 mg/m^2) plus paclitaxel (135 mg/m^2 over 24 h) or cisplatin (75 mg/m^2) plus cyclophosphamide (750 mg/m^2).
  - The paclitaxel-containing regimen showed a statistically significant improvement in overall response, clinical complete response (CR), PFS and OS (PFS 18 vs. 13 months, OS 38 vs. 24 months, respectively).
- *OV-10*, a European–Canadian trial, studied 680 patients treated with cisplatin (75 mg/m^2) and paclitaxel (175 mg/m^2 over 3 h) or cisplatin (75 mg/m^2) plus cyclophosphamide (750 mg/m^2) [34].
  - The paclitaxel containing arm showed an improvement in overall response, clinical CR, PFS (16 months vs. 12 months) and OS (36 months vs. 26 months).
- Following completion of GOG 111, the GOG opened protocol 158 [35].
  - This was a non-inferiority trial comparing carboplatin (AUC 7.5) and paclitaxel (175 mg/m^2 over 3 h) to cisplatin (75 mg/m^2) and paclitaxel (135 mg/m^2 over 24 h).
  - Median PFS (20.7 vs. 19.4 months for carboplatin and cisplatin, respectively) and OS (57.4 vs. 48.7 months, respectively) were not significantly different between study groups.
  - The combination of carboplatin and paclitaxel was less toxic, easier to administer and not inferior to the previous standard of cisplatin and paclitaxel.

- In patients who were optimally cytoreduced (residual disease at completion of surgery <1.0 cm) the median survival was nearly 5 years in the carboplatin containing arm.

- The combination of carboplatin and paclitaxel was then studied with gemcitabine, topotecan or liposomal doxorubicin in sequential doublets or triplets in *GOG 182/ICON5* [36].
  - This international trial recruited >4,000 women with advanced stage epithelial ovarian cancer.
  - There was no improvement in either PFS or OS associated with any experimental regimen.
  - Compared with standard paclitaxel and carboplatin, addition of a third cytotoxic agent provided no benefit in PFS or OS after optimal or suboptimal cytoreduction.

Intraperitoneal Chemotherapy

- In addition to intravenous (IV) therapy, the GOG also investigated intraperitoneal (IP) treatment options.
- Following completion of 2 randomized phase III intergroup trials comparing IV to IV+IP therapy that showed positive results, the *GOG opened protocol 172*, which compared IV paclitaxel (135 mg/m^2) over 24 h with IV cisplatin (75 mg/m^2) on day 2, versus IV paclitaxel (135 mg/m^2) over 24 h, followed by IP cisplatin (100 mg/m^2) on day 2 and IP paclitaxel (60 mg/m^2) on day 8 (Table 1.6) [25, 37–39].

  All patients had optimally resected disease with residual tumor limited to less than or equal to 1 cm in size.
  - Median survival for the IV only and IV+IP arms were 49.5 and 66.9 months, respectively.
  - The RR of death was 0.71 in the IP group (P=0.0076).
  - Tolerability for IP chemo was a concern as grade 3 and 4 hematologic, metabolic, and gastrointestinal toxicities were significantly more common in the IP arm. Only 42 % of patients allocated to the IP arm completed 6 cycles of chemotherapy.

Table 1.6. Studies investigating intraperitoneal chemotherapy [25, 37–39].

Study	N	Design	PFS	OS	Grade 3, and 4 adverse events
Markman et al. [37]	462	IV AP q 3 weeks × 6 cycles or IV carboplatin every 28 days for two courses, then IV paclitaxel and IP cisplatin	IP arm = 28 m IV arm = 22 m RR 0.78, P=0.01	IP arm = 63 m IV arm = 52 m RR 0.81, P=0.05	IP arm = Leukopenia 77 %, thrombocytopenia 49 %, GI event = 37 %, Neurologic event 12 %
Alberts et al. [38]	546	IP cisplatin + IV cyclophosphamide versus IV cisplatin + IV cyclophosphamide in FIGO Stage III patients	NR	IP arm = 49 m, 95 % CI, 42–56 m IV arm = 41 m, 95 % CI 34–47 m	IP arm = Leucopenia 40 %, thrombocytopenia 8 %, GI event 18 %
Armstrong et al. [39]	415	IV AP versus IV paclitaxel + IP cisplatin × 6 cycles every 3 weeks residual tumor limited to ≤1 cm	IV arm = 18.3 m IP arm = 23.8 m 95 % CI = 0.80 [0.64–1.0], P=0.05	IV arm = 49.5 m IP arm = 66.9 m 95 % CI = 0.75 [0.58–0.97] P=0.03	IP arm = Leukopenia 76 %, GI event = 46 %, metabolic event = 27 %, neurologic event = 19 %

AP cisplatin/paclitaxel, *IV* intravenous, *IP* intraperitoneal, *OS* overall survival, *PFS* progression free survival, *m* months, *NR* not recorded

Adapted from: Hodeib M, Eskander RN, Bristow RE. New Paradigms in the surgical and adjuvant treatment of ovarian cancer. Minerva Ginecol April 2014;66:179–92) Reprinted by permission of Edizioni Minerva Medica from April;66(2):179–92

- The results of the above study, in combination with previous positive studies exploring IP chemotherapy, resulted in a National Cancer Institute (NCI) clinical announcement recommending that women with optimally cytoreduced Stage III ovarian cancer be considered for IV+IP therapy.
- In an effort to improve compliance and tolerability of IP therapy, several investigators proposed alternate treatment dosing regimens.
- Barlin et al. investigated oncologic outcomes associated with a modified outpatient IP regimen in 102 patients with optimally cytoreduced epithelial ovarian cancer [40].
  - The modified regimen consisted of IV paclitaxel (135 mg/m^2) over 3 h on day 1 compared with a 24 h infusion, IP cisplatin (75 mg/m^2) on day 2 decreased from 100 mg/m^2 and IP paclitaxel (60 mg/m^2) on day 8 given every 21 days for 6 cycles.
  - The median PFS and OS were 29 and 67 months and 80 % of subjects were able to complete 4 or more cycles of IV plus IP therapy.
- Currently, the *GOG completed accrual on protocol 252*, the results of which will help better determine the role of intraperitoneal chemotherapy in patients who have had a complete cytoreductive surgery as well as the potential role of both dose dense paclitaxel and the antiangiogenic agent bevacizumab (discussed later in the chapter).

Hyperthermic Intraperitoneal Chemotherapy (HIPEC)

- The concept of HIPEC, although new in the treatment of ovarian cancer, has been around over 40 years.
- Initially investigated in patients with peritoneal carcinomatosis due to GI malignancies, peritoneal mesothelioma, and *pseudo-myxoma peritonei* [41–44].
- Currently, use of HIPEC at the time of surgical cytoreduction followed by conventional intravenous chemotherapy is being studied.

- The use of HIPEC relies on several important principles:
  - Direct and preferential cytotoxic effect of hyperthermia on tumor cells.
  - Synergistic effects of hyperthermia when used with conventional cytotoxic agents without an associated increase in toxicity.
  - Increased drug penetration from 3 to 5 mm, secondary to hyperthermia [45–52].
  - Has also been hypothesized that the presence of extensive adhesions postoperatively results in both impaired drug distribution and significant pain and toxicity when traditional IP chemotherapy is given.
    - In theory, use of HIPEC at the time of primary surgery will help aid in uniform distribution and systemic peritoneal coverage, potentially enhancing the antitumor efficacy of the drugs used.
- The first phase 2 clinical trial exploring the use of HIPEC in patients with primary advanced ovarian cancer was completed in 2007 (Table 1.7) [25, 42].
  - Forty-seven patients were enrolled in this open, prospective, single-center nonrandomized study; 22 underwent primary and 25 secondary CRS plus immediate HIPEC (cisplatin 75 mg/m^2) followed by systemic chemotherapy.
  - Major complications (gastrointestinal fistula, intra-abdominal bleeding and thrombosis) occurred in 21.3 % of the patients and the in-hospital mortality rate was 4.2 % (2 patients with pulmonary embolism). The mean overall survival was 30.4 months, median survival was 24 months, and mean disease-free survival was 27.4 months [53].
- This was followed by a study investigating the morbidity and feasibility of CRS + HIPEC in patients with advanced stage primary EOC.
- Lim et al. treated 30 patients with residual tumor measuring <1 cm at the time of primary surgery, with intraoperative HIPEC (cisplatin 75 mg/m^2) at a temperature of 41.5 °C for 90 min [54].

TABLE 1.7. Cytoreductive surgery + HIPEC in the treatment of advanced ovarian cancer: phase 2 studies [25, 53–55] *HIPEC* hyperthermic intraperitoneal chemotherapy, *Temp* temperature, *OS* overall survival, *PFS* progression free survival, *EOC* epithelial ovarian cancer, *GI* gastrointestinal, *CV* cardiovascular, *NR* not recorded.

Study	N	Disease stage	Setting of treatment	HIPEC drug used and dose	Temp (°C)	Duration of treatment (min)	OS (mo)	PFS (mo)	Common grade 2–3 toxicities
Di Giorgio et al. [53]	47	3C–4 EOC	22 primary 25 recurrent	Cisplatin 75 mg/m^2	42–43	60	30.4 (mean)	27.4 (mean)	Pleural effusions (8.5 %), infectious (8.5 %), GI (10.6 %), bleeding (6.4 %)
Lim et al. [54]	30	3–4 EOC	30 primary (14 underwent neoadjuvant treatment)	Cisplatin 75 mg/m^2	41.5	90	NR	NR	Hematologic (86.7 %), GI (30 %), infectious (16.7 %) Pulmonary (23.3 %), CV (13.3 %)
Deraco et al. [55]	26	3–4 EOC	26 primary	Cisplatin 40 mg/L perfusate + doxorubicin 15 mg/L perfusate	42.5	90	Not reached 5-years OS 60.7 %	30 (median) 5-years PFS 15.2 %	Hematologic (4 %), GI (4 %), pulmonary (14.3 %), infectious (14.3 %)

Adapted from: Hodeib M, Eskander RN, Bristow RE. New Paradigms in the surgical and adjuvant treatment of ovarian cancer. Minerva Ginecol April 2014;66:179–92) Reprinted by permission of Edizioni Minerva Medica from April;66(2):179–92

- More recently, a multi-institutional phase 2 study was completed evaluating the impact of CRS + HIPEC on PFS and OS in 26 women with Stage III–IV EOC [55].
  - After a median follow-up of 25 months, 5-year overall survival was 60.7 % and 5-year progression-free survival 15.2 % (median 30 months).
- To date, no randomized phase 3 clinical trials have been completed evaluating the impact of HIPEC on survival in patients with advanced stage ovarian, Fallopian tube, or primary peritoneal carcinoma.

Antiangiogenesis Therapy in Ovarian Cancer

- Studies have shown that angiogenesis is essential for tumor invasion and metastasis, and is required for tumor growth beyond 1–2 mm [56, 57].
  - This process requires the recruitment of vasculature, circulating endothelial cells, and pro-angiogenic mediators.
- Preclinical animal models indicated that inhibition of angiogenesis resulted in tumor growth inhibition.
- Ultimately, bevacizumab, a humanized monoclonal antibody directed against VEGF, was synthesized, and used in early proof of concept studies.
- Bevacizumab neutralizes VEGF-A and blocks its signal transduction through both VEGFR-1 and VEGFR-2, as demonstrated by the inhibition of VEGF-induced cell proliferation, survival permeability, nitric oxide production, migration, and tissue factor production.
- Four discrete targets in the angiogenic cascade have been identified (Fig. 1.1) [58].
- Vascular endothelial growth factor (VEGF).
- Angiopoietin (Ang).
- Fibroblast growth factor (FGF).
- Platelet derived growth factor (PDGF).

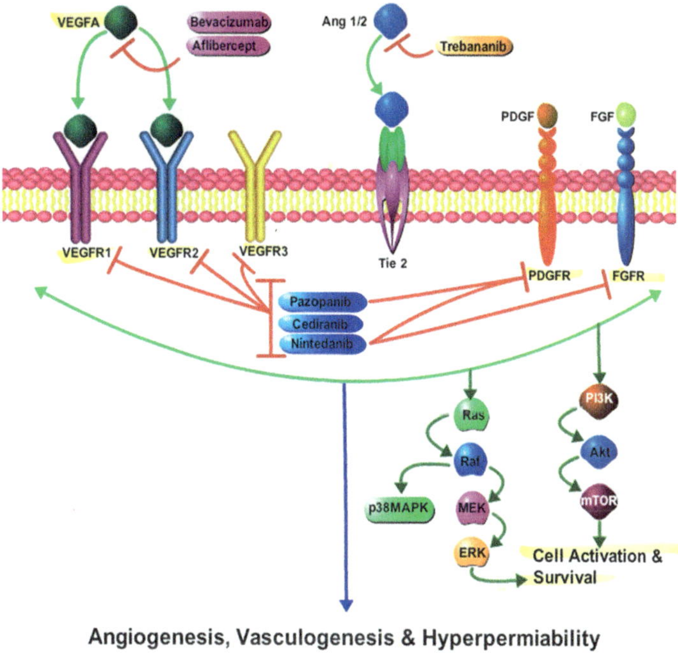

FIG. 1.1. Angiogenic pathway and targeted inhibitors [58]. The angiogenic cascade and antiangiogenic strategies in ovarian carcinoma. Both VEGF and non-VEGF dependent pathways are noted. Figure designed by RN Eskander and KS Tewari and created by RN Eskander and used with permission from RN Eskander and KS Tewari. RN Eskander, KS Tewari. Incorporation of anti-angiogenesis therapy in the management of ovarian carcinoma—Mechanistics, review of phase III randomized clinical trials, and regulatory implications. Gynecol Oncol 2013; 13(2): 496–505. Gynecologic Oncology by Society of Gynecologic Oncologists. Reproduced with permission of Academic Press.

- There are now eight positive phase 3 randomized clinical trials in OC involving five unique antiangiogenesis agents (five agents and their targets detailed in Fig. 1.1) [59–65].
- Table 1.8 details the pivotal phase 3 trials completed to date examining antiangiogenic agents in the treatment of advanced stage ovarian cancer [58].

TABLE 1.8. Phase 3 randomized trials of antiangiogenesis therapy in ovarian carcinoma [58–65].

Trial	N	Eligibility	Arms	Grade 3-4 AEs[a]	1° Endpoint	2° Endpoint
GOG 218 [59]	1873	Incompletely and completely[b] resected Stage III or any Stage IV; GOG PS 0-2	IV Carboplatin (AUC 5) + IV Paclitaxel (175 mg/m²) + placebo followed by maintenance placebo Q3 weeks IV Carboplatin (AUC 5) + IV Paclitaxel (175 mg/m²) + IV Bevacizumab (15 mg/kg) + Placebo maintenance Q3 weeks IV Carboplatin (AUC 5) + IV Paclitaxel (175 mg/m²) + IV Bevacizumab (15 mg/kg) + IV Bevacizumab (15 mg/kg) maintenance Q3 weeks	HTN; (22.9 %) GI events (2.6 %); Proteinuria (1.6 %); VTE (6.7 %)	Median PFS 10.3 versus 11.2 versus 14.1 months HR 0.717[c] (0.625–0.824); $P<0.001$	Median OS 39.3 versus 38.7 versus 39.7 months HR 0.915[c] (0.727–1.15); $P=0.45$
ICON 7 [60]	1528	Stage I–IIA (clear cell, grade 3); Stage IIB–IV; ECOG PS 0-2	IV Carboplatin (AUC 5) + IV Paclitaxel (175 mg/m²) Q3 weeks IV Carboplatin (AUC 5) + IV Paclitaxel (175 mg/m²) + IV Bevacizumab (7.5 mg/kg) + IV Bevacizumab (7.5 mg/kg) maintenance Q3 weeks	Bleeding (1 %); HTN (6 %) VTE (4 %); GIP (1 %) Neutropenia (17 %)	Median PFS 17.3 versus 19.0 months HR 0.81 (0.70–0.94); $P=0.0041$	Median OS 58.6 versus 58 months HR 0.99 (0.85–1.14) $P=0.85$
OCEANS [61]	484	Platinum sensitive recurrent ovarian cancer[d]; ECOG PS 0-1	IV Carboplatin (AUC 4) + IV Gemcitabine (1,000 mg/m²) + placebo Q3 weeks IV Carboplatin (AUC 4) + IV Gemcitabine (1,000 mg/m²) + IV Bevacizumab (15 mg/kg) Q3 weeks	HTN (17.4 %); proteinuria (8.5 %) Bleeding (5.7 %);F/A; (1.6 %); VTE (4 %)	Median PFS 8.4 versus 12.4 months HR 0.484) 0.388–0.605); $P<0.0001$	OS data immature ORR 78.5 % versus 57.4 %; $P<0.0001$ DOS 10.4 versus 7.4 months HR 0.534 (0.408–0.698)

AURELIA [62]	361	Platinum resistant recurrence[e]; ≤ 2 prior chemotherapy regimens; no e/o rectosigmoid involvement; ECOG PS 0-2	IV Paclitaxel (80 mg/m²) days 1, 8, 15, 22 Q 4 weeks or IV Topotecan (4 mg/m²) days 1, 8, 15 Q4 weeks or IV PLD (40 mg/m²) Q4 weeks Chemotherapy as above plus IV Bevacizumab (15 mg/kg) Q3 weeks	HTN (20.1 %); proteinuria (12.8 %); F/A (2.2 %); GIP (1.7 %) VTE (3.4 %)	Median PFS 3.4 versus 6.7 months HR 0.48 (0.36–0.60); *P* < 0.001	Median OS 13.3 versus 16.6 months HR 0.85 (0.66–1.08); *P* = 0.174
ICON 6 [65]	456	Platinum sensitive recurrence[d]; ECOG PS 0-1	Chemotherapy (choice of Platinum + Paclitaxel; Platinum + Gemcitabine; Carboplatin alone Q3 weeks) + PO Placebo + Continued PO Placebo Chemotherapy as above + PO Cedirinib 20 mg daily and maintenance PO placebo Chemotherapy as above + PO Cedirinib 20 mg daily + maintenance PO Cedirinib 20 mg	HTN (7 %); diarrhea (5 %); fatigue (20 %); voice change (21 %); bleeding (25 %)	Median PFS[f] 9.4 versus 12.5 months HR 0.57 (0.45–0.74); *P* = 0.024	Median OS[g] 17.6 versus 20.3 months HR 0.70 (0.51–0.99); *P* = 0.042

(continued)

Table 1.8. (continued)

Trial	N	Eligibility	Arms	Grade 3-4 AEs[a]	1° Endpoint	2° Endpoint
TRINOVA-1 [63]	919	Recurrent ovarian cancer (PFI < 12 months); ≤3 prior anticancer regimens; GOG PS 0-1	IV Paclitaxel days 1, 8, 15 Q4 weeks + IV Placebo weekly IV Paclitaxel days 1, 8, 15 Q4 weeks + IV Trebananib (15 mg/kg) weekly	Edema (5 %), ascites (20 %), pleural effusion (13 %)	Median PFS 5.4 versus 7.2 months HR 0.66 (0.57–0.77); $P<0.001$	ORR 29.8 % versus 38.4 % ($P=0.0071$) Median OS (interim analysis) 17.3 versus 19.0 months HR 0.86 (0.69–1.08); $P=0.19$
AGO-OVAR12/ LUME-Ovar 1 [64]	1366	Advanced stage (FIGO 2B-4) epithelial ovarian cancer; ECOG PS 0-2	Nintenanib 200 mg PO BID + Paclitaxel (175 mg/m^2) + Carboplatin (AUC 5 or 6) Q3 weeks + Nintenanib 200 mg PO BID for up to 120 weeks Placebo PO BID + Paclitaxel (175 mg/m^2) + Carboplatin (AUC 5 or 6) Q3 weeks + Placebo PO BID for up to 120 weeks	Neutropenia (44 %); Anemia (14 %); Thrombocytopenia (18 %); diarrhea (20 %); elevated ALT (15 %); elevated AST (7 %); HTN and fatigue (4 %)	Median PFS 17.3 versus 16.6 months HR 0.84 (0.72–0.98); $P=0.0239$ (RECIST and CA 125)	Not yet mature

N number, *AE* adverse events, *PFS* progression free survival, *OS* overall survival, *QOL* quality of life, *HTN* hypertension, *GIP* gastrointestinal perforation, *VTE* venous thromboembolism, *F/A* fistula/abscess, *ECOG* eastern Cooperative Oncology Group, *PS* performance status, *ORR* objective response rate, *DOR* duration of response, *e/o* evidence of, *PLD* pegylated liposomal doxorubicin, *PFI* progression free interval

Adapted from: RN Eskander, KS Tewari. Incorporation of anti-angiogenesis therapy in the management of ovarian carcinoma—Mechanistics, review of phase III randomized clinical trials, and regulatory implications. Gynecol Oncol 2013; 13(2): 496–505. Gynecologic Oncology by Society of Gynecologic Oncologists Reproduced with permission of ACADEMIC PRESS

[a]Investigational arms

[b]After protocol modification patients with optimally resected Stage III disease were eligible

[c]Comparison between the control arm and bevacizumab throughout arm

[c]Progression free interval at least 6 months

[e]Progression free interval less than or equal to 6 months

[f]Maintenance versus chemotherapy only arm

[g]Control versus bevacizumab throughout arms

- Despite the above, there is no FDA approved indication for use of antiangiogenic agents in gynecologic malignancies (although this is expected to change with GOG 240 and cervical carcinoma as detailed in the cervical cancer chapter).
- Table 1.9 outlines the FDA and European Medicines Agency approved indications for antiangiogenic therapy. It also outlines NCCN ovarian cancer recommendations regarding bevacizumab [58].

PARP Inhibition and Synthetic Lethality in Ovarian Cancer

- Germ line BRCA1 and BRCA2 mutations have long been recognized as conferring the greatest risk for both breast and ovarian cancer (as discussed previously).
- These genes are essential for cellular development, with pivotal roles in genomic stability.
- Absence of either BRCA1 or BRCA2 results in chromosomal rearrangements, and is lethal in embryonic development [66].
- Functional BRCA genes are required for error-free homologous recombination (HR).
  - While HR is not the only mechanism available for DNA damage repair, the alternative processes, nonhomologous end joining (NHEJ) and single-strand annealing (SSA), are error prone and frequently result in gross chromosomal rearrangements (GCR) [67, 68].
- As many as 24 % of patients with advanced stage ovarian cancer exhibit homologous recombination deficiency.
- The concept of synthetic lethality (Fig. 1.2) [69].
  - PARP-1 deficiency results in a failure to repair SS DNA breaks, which when left unrepaired, translate into DSDNA breaks (DSB) [70, 71].

TABLE 1.9. Approved indications for antiangiogenic agents under investigation [58].

Antiangiogenesis agent	US FDA	NCCN ovary	European Medicines Agency (EMA)
Bevacizumab (Avastin) [Genentech/ Roche]	Metastatic CRC; Metastatic RCC; Recurrent Glioblastoma; Metastatic NSCLC	Category 3 (frontline) Category 2B (recurrent, combined with C/G)	Advanced and recurrent OC; Metastatic CRC; Metastatic RCC; Metastatic NSCLC: Metastatic BC
Pazopanib (Votrient) [GlaxoSmithKline]	Advanced soft tissue sarcoma; Advanced RCC	–	Advanced soft tissue sarcoma; Advanced RCC
Cediranib (Recentin) [AstraZeneca]	–	–	–
Trebananib (AMG 386) [Amgen]	–	–	–
Nintedanib (Vargatef) [Boehringer Ingleheim]	–	–	–
VEGF-trap[a] (Aflibercept) [Regeneron]	Wet age-related macular degeneration	–	Metastatic CRC resistant or progressed after oxaliplatin containing regimen

CRC colorectal cancer, *RCC* renal cell carcinoma, *NSCLC* non-small-cell lung cancer, *OC* ovarian cancer, *BC* breast cancer, *C/G* carboplatin + gemcitabine, *NCCN* National Comprehensive Cancer Network

Adapted from: RN Eskander, KS Tewari. Incorporation of anti-angiogenesis therapy in the management of ovarian carcinoma—Mechanistics, review of phase III randomized clinical trials, and regulatory implications. Gynecol Oncol 2013; 13(2). 496-505. Gynecologic Oncology by Society of Gynecologic Oncologists. Reproduced with permission of Academic Press

[a]No phase 3 RCT

- Under normal conditions, these lesions would be repaired using high fidelity, BRCA dependent, HR mechanisms.
  - However, in BRCA deficient cells, these DSB are repaired using mutagenic nonhomologous repair processes, such as NHEJ and SSA, resulting in chromosomal instability, cell cycle arrest, and apoptosis.

- In a series of landmark publications, the clinical utility of PARP inhibition in BRCA deficient cell lines was descried [72–74].
- A series of phase 2 clinical trials subsequently confirmed the therapeutic efficacy of PARP inhibition in the recurrent disease setting [75–79] (Table 1.10) [69].
- As the efficacy and safety of PARP inhibition in patients with serous ovarian cancer and germ line BRCA mutation was confirmed in phase II studies, several prospective phase III trials were designed and are open for enrollment (Fig. 1.3, Table 1.11) [69].
- In June 2014 the ODAC (FDA oncology drug advisory committee) voted against accelerated approval of olaparib in the treatment of ovarian cancer patients with BRCA1/2 germ line mutations.
  - The primary criticisms included the subset analysis of the primary data set, risk of toxicity on treatment including secondary malignancy, and lack of an OS advantage.
  - The panel recommended that SOLO 2 be completed and the results interpreted before drug approval.

Treatment of Borderline Ovarian Tumors

- The recommended management of clinically apparent early-stage borderline ovarian tumors, in women who have completed childbearing, includes bilateral salpingo-oophorectomy with hysterectomy and surgical staging.
- For young patients with apparent early-stage disease who desire fertility preservation, unilateral oophorectomy or ovarian cystectomy with a staging procedure is an acceptable alternative.
  - Risk of recurrence as high as 30 % with cystectomy.
- For advanced-stage and recurrent disease, cytoreductive surgery is recommended.
- Adjuvant chemotherapy is reserved for selected cases only (e.g., unresectable disease, invasive metastatic implants, rapid growth rate with progressive symptomatology).

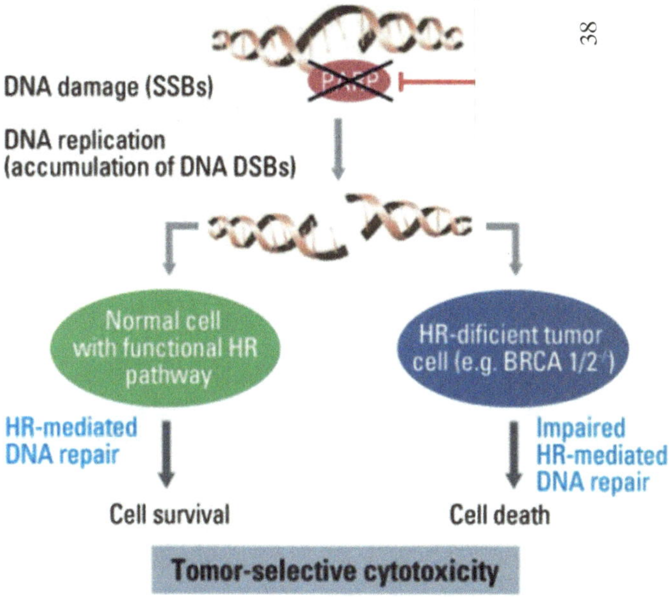

FIG. 1.2. PARP-1 deficiency results in a failure to repair single-stranded DNA breaks, which when left unrepaired, translate into double-stranded DNA breaks (DSB) at the replication fork [69]. Adapted from Eskander RN, Tewari KS. PARP inhibition and synthetic lethality in ovarian cancer. Expert Rev Clin Pharmacol. 2014. July 2: 1–10 [Epub ahead of print] 7(5); 2014; In press. Expert review of clinical pharmacology by Future Drugs Ltd. Reproduced with permission of Future Drugs Ltd in the format Republish in a book via Copyright Clearance Center.

- For patients with disease apparently confined to the ovaries, adjuvant chemotherapy is not recommended.
- Barnhill et al. reported a Gynecologic Oncology Group (GOG) prospective study in which 146 patients with Stage I serous borderline ovarian tumors were observed without adjuvant therapy [80].
  - With a median follow-up of 42.2 months, no patient developed recurrent disease.

TABLE 1.10. Phase 2 studies of PARP inhibitors in patients with ovarian cancer [69, 75–79].

Study	N	Drug dose and schedule	Objective response rate (ORR)	PFS	Grade 3/4 AEs
Gelmon et al. [77]	65	Olaparib 400 mg orally BID	41 % in BRCAm 24 % in BRCAwt	Not reported	Fatigue, nausea, emesis, and decreased appetite
Audeh et al. [75]	56	Olaparib 400 mg orally BID ($n=33$) Olaparib 100 mg orally BID ($n=24$)	33 % in 400 mg arm 13 % in the 100 mg arm	Not reported	Nausea, fatigue, and anemia[a]
Kaye et al. [78]	97	Olaparib 200 mg orally BID versus Olaparib 400 mg orally BID versus PLD 50 mg/m^2 every 28 days	25 % in 200 mg arm 31 % in the 400 mg arm 18 % in the PLD arm	6.5 months 8.8 months 7.1 months[b]	Nausea, fatigue, emesis, anemia[c]
Ledermann et al. [79]	265	Olaparib 400 mg orally BID versus placebo	12 % olaparib arm 4 % placebo	8.8 months versus 4.8 months (HR 0.35; $P<0.001$)	Nausea, fatigue, emesis, anemia
Coleman et al. [76]	52	Veliparib 400 mg orally BID	Total confirmed responders: 26 %	PFS 8.1 months OS 19 months	Nausea, emesis, neutropenia, thrombocytopenia

AEs adverse events, *PFS* progression free survival, *OS* overall survival, *BID* twice daily, *BRCAm* BRCA1 or BRCA2 mutation carrier, *BRCAwt* BRCA wild type, *PLD* pegylated liposomal doxorubicin

Adapted from Eskander RN, Tewari KS. PARP inhibition and synthetic lethality in ovarian cancer. Expert Rev Clin Pharmacol. 2014. July 2: 1–10 [Epub ahead of print] 7(5); 2014: In press. Expert review of clinical pharmacology by Future Drugs Ltd. Reproduced with permission of Future Drugs Ltd in the format Republish in a book via Copyright Clearance Center

[a]Only reported in the 400 mg arm

[b]Nonsignificant HR 0.88 with respect to survival

[c]Only in the olaparib arm

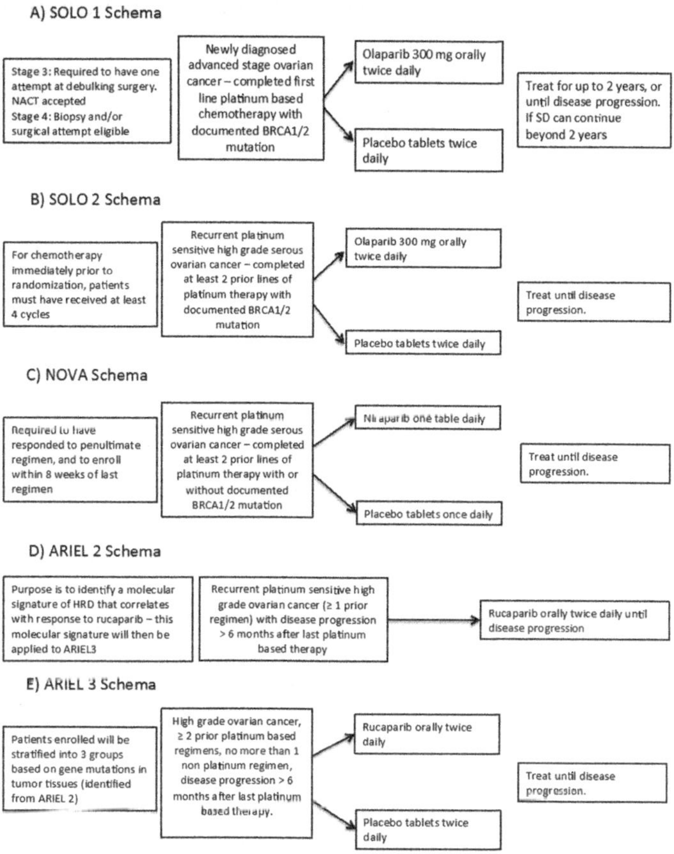

FIG. 1.3. Schema of phase 3 trials exploring PARP inhibition in patients with ovarian cancer [69]. Adapted from Eskander RN, Tewari KS. PARP inhibition and synthetic lethality in ovarian cancer. Expert Rev Clin Pharmacol. 2014. July 2: 1–10 [Epub ahead of print] 7(5); 2014: In press. Expert review of clinical pharmacology by Future Drugs Ltd. Reproduced with permission of Future Drugs Ltd in the format Republish in a book via Copyright Clearance Center.

TABLE 1.11. Phase 3 trials examining PARP inhibitors in the treatment of ovarian cancer [69].

Trial	Disease setting	Agent
SOLO 1 NCT01844986	Following a complete or partial response to first-line platinum-based chemotherapy	Olaparib
SOLO 2 NCT01874353	Platinum sensitive recurrent ovarian cancer	Olaparib
NOVA NCT01847274	Platinum sensitive recurrent ovarian cancer	Niraparib
ARIEL 3	To be defined	Rucaparib

Adapted from Eskander RN, Tewari KS. PARP inhibition and synthetic lethality in ovarian cancer. Expert Rev Clin Pharmacol. 2014. July 2: 1–10 [Epub ahead of print] 7(5); 2014: In press. Expert review of clinical pharmacology by Future Drugs Ltd. Reproduced with permission of Future Drugs Ltd in the format Republish in a book via Copyright Clearance Center

- To underscore this point, a large meta-analysis demonstrated a disease-free survival rate of 98.2 % and a disease-specific survival rate of 99.5 % for women with Stage I disease [81].
- Four prospective randomized trials conducted in Norway showed that for Stage I and II disease, the addition of adjuvant therapy did not improve survival and added toxicity, with overall survival rates of 99 and 94 % for no adjuvant therapy, and adjuvant therapy, respectively [82].
- Objective responses to platinum-based chemotherapy among patients with advanced-stage borderline ovarian tumors have been reported at the time of second look surgery.
  - Gershenson et al. reported complete responses to chemotherapy at second-look laparotomy in 8 of 20 patients with macroscopic residual disease after initial cytoreductive surgery and in 5 of 12 patients with microscopic residual disease after initial surgery [83].
  - Barakat and colleagues reported that 2 of 7 patients with macroscopic residual borderline ovarian tumors and 7 of 8 patients with microscopic disease had pathologic complete remissions at second-look laparotomy after platinum-based chemotherapy, with only one death due to progressive disease [84].

- Importantly, there was no difference in survival between patients who received chemotherapy and those who did not.
- Sutton et al. reported the GOG data using a subset of 32 women with advanced-stage borderline ovarian tumors that were optimally cytoreduced [85].
  - The patients were randomized to treatment with cisplatin and cyclophosphamide with or without adriamycin.
  - Fifteen of 32 patients underwent second-look surgery, and 9 showed evidence of persistent disease. However, at a median follow-up of 31.7 months, 31 of 32 patients were alive. Only one patient died and it was unrelated to the ovarian disease process.
- Due to the low percentage of actively dividing cells that are present in borderline ovarian tumors, these are thought to be relatively resistant to standard cytotoxic agents.
- Furthermore, adjuvant chemotherapy in patients with ovarian serous borderline tumors with invasive peritoneal implants showed no improvement in time to recurrence or overall survival.
- As noted earlier, even patients with advanced-stage disease can be expected to have excellent overall survival rates.

Treatment of Ovarian Germ Cell Tumors

- Malignant ovarian germ cell tumors are rare and aggressive, but very curable at all presenting stages of disease.
- They account for only 1–2 % of all ovarian cancers, and affect women of reproductive age, with nearly 70 % of ovarian germ cell tumors occurring in the first 2 decades of life.
- The recommended management of young patients with suspected malignant germ cell tumors of the ovary includes:
  - Intact removal of the tumor.
  - Sparing of the Fallopian tube if not adherent to the tumor.
  - Procurement of cytologic washings or harvesting of ascites fluid.

- Examination and palpation of the omentum with removal of suspicious areas.
- Examination and palpation of the iliac and aortocaval nodes with biopsy of abnormal areas.

- Following surgical cytoreduction, patients are managed with postoperative systemic chemotherapy, with 90–95 % cure rates, except in cases of Stage IA, grade I immature teratoma, and Stage IA dysgerminoma, where observation alone is acceptable.
- Our understanding regarding effective chemotherapy for the treatment of ovarian germ cell cancers paralleled advancements in adjuvant therapy for the more common testicular tumors.
- The combination regimen consisting of vincristine, actinomycin-D, and cyclophosphamide (VAC) was the first regimen to reproducibly cure patients with ovarian germ cell tumors.
- Gershenson et al. studied 80 patients with malignant nondysgerminomatous germ cell tumors of the ovary who were treated with the combination of vincristine, actinomycin-D, and cyclophosphamide (VAC) at The University of Texas M.D. Anderson Hospital and Tumor Institute [86].
  - Sixty-six patients received VAC as primary postoperative therapy with 46 patients (70 %) achieving a sustained remission.
- This regimen was then modified to include vinblastine, bleomycin, and cisplatin (VBP).
  - In a GOG trial, 97 patients with germ cell tumors were treated with 3–4 courses of vinblastine, bleomycin, and cisplatin (VBP) [87].
  - Of 35 patients with tumors other than dysgerminoma who had clinically measurable disease, 15 (43 %; CI, 26–61 %) had complete responses.
  - Forty of fifty-six second-look laparotomies (71 %; CI, 58–83 %) revealed no tumor or mature glial tissue.

The survival rate was 71 % (CI, 62–89 %) with a 51 % disease-free rate (CI, 41–62 %) at 2 years.

- Ultimately, a switch from VBP to combination bleomycin, etoposide, and cisplatin (BEP), resulted from experience with testicular tumors, where the etoposide containing regimen was shown to have a larger therapeutic index (particularly neurologic and GI toxicities).
- In a trial randomizing 261 men with disseminated germ-cell tumors to VBP versus BEP, 74 % of those receiving the regimen including vinblastine and 83 % of those receiving the regimen including etoposide became disease-free with or without subsequent surgery [88].
  - Among 157 patients with high tumor volume, 61 % became disease-free on the regimen that included vinblastine, as compared with 77 % on the regimen that included etoposide ($P<0.05$).
  - Survival among the patients who received etoposide was higher ($P=0.048$).
  - In addition, the etoposide regimen caused substantially fewer paresthesias ($P=0.02$), abdominal cramps ($P=0.0008$), and myalgias ($P=0.00002$).
- Despite the exquisite radiosensitivity of dysgerminomatous germ cell tumors, adjuvant chemotherapy in the form of BEP is preferred given the possible sterilizing effects of radiation in this predominantly young patient population.
- After adjuvant chemotherapy, Gershenson et al. reported resumption of normal menstrual activity in all 28 enrolled patients treated with the VAC regimen.
- Importantly, the likelihood of chemotherapy-induced amenorrhea is based on the specific chemotherapy administered as well as the patient's age.
  - The younger the patient at the time of exposure, the larger the oocyte reserve, facilitating recruitment and reestablishment of normal ovulation after completion of chemotherapy.

Treatment of Sex-Cord-Stromal Tumors

- Given the rare occurrence of these malignancies, information regarding adjuvant chemotherapy for patients with advanced stage or recurrent sex-cord-stromal tumors is limited.
- No prospective trials have been conducted and it is difficult to draw conclusions regarding optimal therapy due to limitations of retrospective trials, including the small patient numbers, and varying treatment regimens.
- Nonetheless, several regimens have been explored:
  - Combination adriamycin–cisplatin (AP).
  - Cyclophosphamide–adriamycin–cisplatin (CAP).
  - Cisplatin–vinblastine–bleomycin (PVB).
  - Bleomycin–etoposide–cisplatin (BEP).
- Response rates to the above regimens range from 37 to 100 % in patients with advanced stage or recurrent disease [89].
- More recently, combination carboplatin and paclitaxel has been used. GOG protocol 187 is currently open, investigating the potential benefits of single agent paclitaxel in patients with persistent or recurrent disease after up front therapy.
  - If paclitaxel appears to have an impact in this patient population, its use in primary treatment may be considered further.

References

1. Siegel R, Ma J, Zou Z, Jemal A. Cancer statistics, 2014. CA Cancer J Clin. 2014;64:9–29.
2. Schorge JO, Modesitt SC, Coleman RL, Cohn DE, Kauff ND, Duska LR, Herzog TJ. SGO white paper on ovarian cancer: etiology, screening and surveillance. Gynecol Oncol. 2010; 119:7–17.
3. Smith RA, Manassaram-Baptiste D, Brooks D, Cokkinides V, Doroshenk M, Saslow D, Wender RC, Brawley OW. Cancer screening in the United States, 2014: a review of current American Cancer Society guidelines and current issues in cancer screening. CA Cancer J Clin. 2014;64:30–51.

4. Eskander RN, Tewari KS. American Society of Clinical Oncology 2013: summary of scientific advancements in gynecologic cancer. Int J Gynecol Cancer. 2014;24:13–8.
5. Walsh T, Casadei S, Lee MK, Pennil CC, Nord AS, Thornton AM, Roeb W, Agnew KJ, Stray SM, Wickramanayake A, Norquist B, Pennington KP, Garcia RL, King MC, Swisher EM. Mutations in 12 genes for inherited ovarian, fallopian tube, and peritoneal carcinoma identified by massively parallel sequencing. Proc Natl Acad Sci U S A. 2011;108:18032–7.
6. Aarnio M, Sankila R, Pukkala E, Salovaara R, Aaltonen LA, de la Chapelle A, Peltomaki P, Mecklin JP, Jarvinen HJ. Cancer risk in mutation carriers of DNA-mismatch-repair genes. Int J Cancer. 1999;81:214–8.
7. Dunlop MG, Farrington SM, Carothers AD, Wyllie AH, Sharp L, Burn J, Liu B, Kinzler KW, Vogelstein B. Cancer risk associated with germline DNA mismatch repair gene mutations. Hum Mol Genet. 1997;6:105–10.
8. Clarke-Pearson DL. Clinical practice. Screening for ovarian cancer. N Engl J Med. 2009;361:170–7.
9. Goff BA, Mandel LS, Drescher CW, Urban N, Gough S, Schurman KM, Patras J, Mahony BS, Andersen MR. Development of an ovarian cancer symptom index: possibilities for earlier detection. Cancer. 2007;109:221–7.
10. Gershenson DM, Sun CC, Lu KH, Coleman RL, Sood AK, Malpica A, Deavers MT, Silva EG, Bodurka DC. Clinical behavior of stage II-IV low-grade serous carcinoma of the ovary. Obstet Gynecol. 2006;108:361–8.
11. Meigs J. Tumors of the female pelvic organs. New York: Macmillan; 1934.
12. Griffiths CT. Surgical resection of tumor bulk in the primary treatment of ovarian carcinoma. Natl Cancer Inst Monogr. 1975;42:101–4.
13. Fader AN, Rose PG. Role of surgery in ovarian carcinoma. J Clin Oncol. 2007;25:2873–83.
14. Bristow RE, Tomacruz RS, Armstrong DK, Trimble EL, Montz FJ. Survival effect of maximal cytoreductive surgery for advanced ovarian carcinoma during the platinum era: a meta-analysis. J Clin Oncol. 2002;20:1248–59.
15. Hoskins WJ, McGuire WP, Brady MF, Homesley HD, Creasman WT, Berman M, Ball H, Berek JS. The effect of diameter of largest residual disease on survival after primary cytoreductive surgery in patients with suboptimal residual epithelial ovarian carcinoma. Am J Obstet Gynecol. 1994;170:974–9.

16. Omura GA, Bundy BN, Berek JS, Curry S, Delgado G, Mortel R. Randomized trial of cyclophosphamide plus cisplatin with or without doxorubicin in ovarian carcinoma: a Gynecologic Oncology Group Study. J Clin Oncol. 1989;7:457–65.
17. Aletti GD, Dowdy SC, Gostout BS, Jones MB, Stanhope CR, Wilson TO, Podratz KC, Cliby WA. Aggressive surgical effort and improved survival in advanced-stage ovarian cancer. Obstet Gynecol. 2006;107:77–85.
18. Chang S-J, Bristow RE. Evolution of surgical treatment paradigms for advanced-stage ovarian cancer: redefining 'optimal' residual disease. Gynecol Oncol. 2012;125:483–92.
19. Chi DS, Eisenhauer EL, Lang J, Huh J, Haddad L, Abu-Rustum NR, Sonoda Y, Levine DA, Hensley M, Barakat RR. What is the optimal goal of primary cytoreductive surgery for bulky stage IIIC epithelial ovarian carcinoma (EOC)? Gynecol Oncol. 2006;103:559–64.
20. du Bois A, Reuss A, Pujade-Lauraine E, Harter P, Ray-Coquard I, Pfisterer J. Role of surgical outcome as prognostic factor in advanced epithelial ovarian cancer: a combined exploratory analysis of 3 prospectively randomized phase 3 multicenter trials: by the Arbeitsgemeinschaft Gynaekologische Onkologie Studiengruppe Ovarialkarzinom (AGO-OVAR) and the Groupe d'Investigateurs Nationaux Pour les Etudes des Cancers de l'Ovaire (GINECO). Cancer. 2009;115:1234–44.
21. Eisenkop SM, Spirtos NM, Friedman RL, Lin W-CM, Pisani AL, Perticucci S. Relative influences of tumor volume before surgery and the cytoreductive outcome on survival for patients with advanced ovarian cancer: a prospective study. Gynecol Oncol. 2003;90:390–6.
22. Wimberger P, Wehling M, Lehmann N, Kimmig R, Schmalfeldt B, Burges A, Harter P, Pfisterer J, du Bois A. Influence of residual tumor on outcome in ovarian cancer patients with FIGO stage IV disease: an exploratory analysis of the AGO-OVAR (Arbeitsgemeinschaft Gynaekologische Onkologie Ovarian Cancer Study Group). Ann Surg Oncol. 2010;17:1642–8.
23. Winter WE, Maxwell GL, Tian C, Carlson JW, Ozols RF, Rose PG, Markman M, Armstrong DK, Muggia F, McGuire WP. Prognostic factors for stage III epithelial ovarian cancer: a Gynecologic Oncology Group Study. J Clin Oncol. 2007;25:3621–7.
24. Winter WE, Maxwell GL, Tian C, Sundborg MJ, Rose GS, Rose PG, Rubin SC, Muggia F, McGuire WP. Tumor residual after surgical cytoreduction in prediction of clinical outcome in stage

IV epithelial ovarian cancer: a Gynecologic Oncology Group Study. J Clin Oncol. 2008;26:83–9.

25. Hodeib M, Eskander RN, Bristow RE. New paradigms in the surgical and adjuvant treatment of ovarian cancer. Minerva Ginecol. 2014;66:179–92.
26. Vergote I, Tropé CG, Amant F, Kristensen GB, Ehlen T, Johnson N, Verheijen RH, van der Burg ME, Lacave AJ, Panici PB. Neoadjuvant chemotherapy or primary surgery in stage IIIC or IV ovarian cancer. N Engl J Med. 2010;363:943–53.
27. Sean Kehoe JH, Nankivell M, Jayson GC, Kitchener HC, Lopes T. Chemotherapy or upfront surgery for newly diagnosed advanced ovarian cancer: results from the MRC CHORUS trial. J Clin Oncol 2013;31
28. Eskander RN, Di Saia PJ. Chemotherapy of ovarian cancer. In: Deligdisch L, Kase NG, Cohen CJ, editors. Altchek's diagnosis and management of ovarian disorders. 3rd ed. New York: Cambridge University Press; 2013. p. 415–24.
29. Colombo N, Guthrie D, Chiari S, Parmar M, Qian W, Swart AM, Torri V, Williams C, Lissoni A, Bonazzi C, Collaborators ICONI. International Collaborative Ovarian Neoplasm trial 1: a randomized trial of adjuvant chemotherapy in women with early-stage ovarian cancer. J Natl Cancer Inst. 2003;95:125–32.
30. Trimbos JB, Parmar M, Vergote I, Guthrie D, Bolis G, Colombo N, Vermorken JB, Torri V, Mangioni C, Pecorelli S, Lissoni A, Swart AM, 1 ICON, Neoplasm EOfRaToCC-ACuO. International Collaborative Ovarian Neoplasm trial 1 and adjuvant chemotherapy in ovarian neoplasm trial: two parallel randomized phase III trials of adjuvant chemotherapy in patients with early-stage ovarian carcinoma. J Natl Cancer Inst. 2003;95:105–12.
31. Bell J, Brady MF, Young RC, Lage J, Walker JL, Look KY, Rose GS, Spirtos NM, Group GO. Randomized phase III trial of three versus six cycles of adjuvant carboplatin and paclitaxel in early stage epithelial ovarian carcinoma: a Gynecologic Oncology Group study. Gynecol Oncol. 2006;102:432–9.
32. Mannel RS, Brady MF, Kohn EC, Hanjani P, Hiura M, Lee R, Degeest K, Cohn DE, Monk BJ, Michael H. A randomized phase III trial of IV carboplatin and paclitaxel × 3 courses followed by observation versus weekly maintenance low-dose paclitaxel in patients with early-stage ovarian carcinoma: A Gynecologic Oncology Group Study. Gynecol Oncol. 2011;122(1):89–94.
33. McGuire W, Hoskins W, Brady M, Kucera P, Partridge E, Look K, Clarke-Pearson D, Davidson M. Cyclophosphamide

and cisplatin compared with paclitaxel and cisplatin in patients with stage III and stage IV ovarian cancer. N Engl J Med. 1996;334:1–6.

34. Piccart MJ, Bertelsen K, James K, Cassidy J, Mangioni C, Simonsen E, Stuart G, Kaye S, Vergote I, Blom R, Grimshaw R, Atkinson RJ, Swenerton KD, Trope C, Nardi M, Kaern J, Tumolo S, Timmers P, Roy JA, Lhoas F, Lindvall B, Bacon M, Birt A, Andersen JE, Zee B, Paul J, Baron B, Pecorelli S. Randomized intergroup trial of cisplatin-paclitaxel versus cisplatin-cyclophosphamide in women with advanced epithelial ovarian cancer: three-year results. J Natl Cancer Inst. 2000;92:699–708.
35. Ozols R, Bundy B, Greer B, Fowler J, Clarke-Pearson D, Burger R, Mannel R, DeGeest K, Hartenbach E, Baergen R, Group GO. Phase III trial of carboplatin and paclitaxel compared with cisplatin and paclitaxel in patients with optimally resected stage III ovarian cancer: a Gynecologic Oncology Group study. J Clin Oncol. 2003;21:3194–200.
36. Bookman MA, Brady MF, McGuire WP, Harper PG, Alberts DS, Friedlander M, Colombo N, Fowler JM, Argenta PA, De Geest K, Mutch DG, Burger RA, Swart AM, Trimble EL, Accario-Winslow C, Roth LM. Evaluation of new platinum-based treatment regimens in advanced-stage ovarian cancer: a Phase III Trial of the Gynecologic Cancer Intergroup. J Clin Oncol. 2009;27:1419–25.
37. Markman M, Bundy BN, Alberts DS, Fowler JM, Clark-Pearson DL, Carson LF, Wadler S, Sickel J. Phase III trial of standard-dose intravenous cisplatin plus paclitaxel versus moderately high-dose carboplatin followed by intravenous paclitaxel and intraperitoneal cisplatin in small-volume stage III ovarian carcinoma: an intergroup study of the Gynecologic Oncology Group, Southwestern Oncology Group, and Eastern Cooperative Oncology Group. J Clin Oncol. 2001;19:1001–7.
38. Alberts DS, Liu PY, Hannigan EV, O'Toole R, Williams SD, Young JA, Franklin EW, Clarke-Pearson DL, Malviya VK, DuBeshter B. Intraperitoneal cisplatin plus intravenous cyclophosphamide versus intravenous cisplatin plus intravenous cyclophosphamide for stage III ovarian cancer. N Engl J Med. 1996;335:1950–5.
39. Armstrong DK, Bundy B, Wenzel L, Huang HQ, Baergen R, Lele S, Copeland LJ, Walker JL, Burger RA. Intraperitoneal cisplatin and paclitaxel in ovarian cancer. N Engl J Med. 2006;354:34–43.

40. Barlin JN, Dao F, Zgheib NB, Ferguson SE, Sabbatini PJ, Hensley ML, Bell-McGuinn KM, Konner J, Tew WP, Aghajanian C, Chi DS. Progression-free and overall survival of a modified outpatient regimen of primary intravenous/intraperitoneal paclitaxel and intraperitoneal cisplatin in ovarian, fallopian tube, and primary peritoneal cancer. Gynecol Oncol. 2012;125(3):621–4.
41. Verwaal VJ, van Ruth S, de Bree E, van Sloothen GW, van Tinteren H, Boot H, Zoetmulder FAN. Randomized trial of cytoreduction and hyperthermic intraperitoneal chemotherapy versus systemic chemotherapy and palliative surgery in patients with peritoneal carcinomatosis of colorectal cancer. J Clin Oncol. 2003;21:3737–43.
42. Spratt JS, Adcock RA, Muskovin M, Sherrill W, McKeown J. Clinical delivery system for intraperitoneal hyperthermic chemotherapy. Cancer Res. 1980;40:256–60.
43. Fujimoto S, Takahashi M, Mutou T, Kobayashi K, Toyosawa T, Isawa E, Sumida M, Ohkubo H. Improved mortality rate of gastric carcinoma patients with peritoneal carcinomatosis treated with intraperitoneal hyperthermic chemoperfusion combined with surgery. Cancer. 1997;79:884–91.
44. Fujimoto S, Takahashi M, Mutou T, Kobayashi K, Toyosawa T. Successful intraperitoneal hyperthermic chemoperfusion for the prevention of postoperative peritoneal recurrence in patients with advanced gastric carcinoma. Cancer. 1999;85:529–34.
45. Vernon C. Hyperthermia in cancer growth regulation. Biotherapy. 1992;4:307–15.
46. Shiu MH, Fortner JG. Intraperitoneal hyperthermic treatment of implanted peritoneal cancer in rats. Cancer Res. 1980;40:4081–4.
47. Robins HI. Role of whole-body hyperthermia in the treatment of neoplastic disease: its current status and future prospects. Cancer Res. 1984;44:4878s–83.
48. Ohno S, Siddik ZH, Kido Y, Zwelling LA, Bull JM. Thermal enhancement of drug uptake and DNA adducts as a possible mechanism for the effect of sequencing hyperthermia on cisplatin-induced cytotoxicity in L1210 cells. Cancer Chemother Pharmacol. 1994;34:302–6.
49. Nicoletto MO, Padrini R, Galeotti F, Ferrazzi E, Cartei G, Riddi F, Palumbo M, De Paoli M, Corsini A. Pharmacokinetics of intraperitoneal hyperthermic perfusion with mitoxantrone in ovarian cancer. Cancer Chemother Pharmacol. 2000;45:457–62.
50. Larkin JM. A clinical investigation of total-body hyperthermia as cancer therapy. Cancer Res. 1979;39:2252–4.

51. Kowal CD, Bertino JR. Possible benefits of hyperthermia to chemotherapy. Cancer Res. 1979;39:2285–9.
52. Johnson RJ, Subjeck JR, Moreau DZ, Kowal H, Yakar D. Radiation and hyperthermia. Bull N Y Acad Med. 1979;55:1193–204.
53. Di Giorgio A, Naticchioni E, Biacchi D, Sibio S, Accarpio F, Rocco M, Tarquini S, Di Seri M, Ciardi A, Montruccoli D, Sammartino P. Cytoreductive surgery (peritonectomy procedures) combined with hyperthermic intraperitoneal chemotherapy (HIPEC) in the treatment of diffuse peritoneal carcinomatosis from ovarian cancer. Cancer. 2008;113:315–25.
54. Lim MC, Kang S, Choi J, Song YJ, Park S, Seo S-S, Park S-Y. Hyperthermic intraperitoneal chemotherapy after extensive cytoreductive surgery in patients with primary advanced epithelial ovarian cancer: interim analysis of a phase II study. Ann Surg Oncol. 2009;16:993–991000.
55. Deraco M, Kusamura S, Virzi S, Puccio F, Macri A, Famulari C, Solazzo M, Bonomi S, Iusco DR, Baratti D. Cytoreductive surgery and hyperthermic intraperitoneal chemotherapy as upfront therapy for advanced epithelial ovarian cancer: multi-institutional phase-II trial. Gynecol Oncol. 2011;122:215–20.
56. Eskander RN, Randall LM. Bevacizumab in the treatment of ovarian cancer. Biologics. 2011;5:1–5.
57. Folkman J. Tumor angiogenesis: therapeutic implications. N Engl J Med. 1971;285:1182–6.
58. Eskander RN, Tewari KS. Incorporation of anti-angiogenesis therapy in the management of advanced ovarian carcinoma—mechanistics, review of phase III randomized clinical trials, and regulatory implications. Gynecol Oncol. 2014;132:496–505.
59. Burger RA, Brady MF, Bookman MA, Fleming GF, Monk BJ, Huang H, Mannel RS, Homesley HD, Fowler J, Greer BE, Boente M, Birrer MJ, Liang SX. Incorporation of bevacizumab in the primary treatment of ovarian cancer. N Engl J Med. 2011;365:2473–83.
60. Perren TJ, Swart AM, Pfisterer J, Ledermann JA, Pujade-Lauraine E, Kristensen G, Carey MS, Beale P, Cervantes A, Kurzeder C, du Bois A, Sehouli J, Kimmig R, Stahle A, Collinson F, Essapen S, Gourley C, Lortholary A, Selle F, Mirza MR, Leminen A, Plante M, Stark D, Qian W, Parmar MK, Oza AM. A phase 3 trial of bevacizumab in ovarian cancer. N Engl J Med. 2011;365:2484–96.
61. Aghajanian C, Blank SV, Goff BA, Judson PL, Teneriello MG, Husain A, Sovak MA, Yi J, Nycum LR. OCEANS: a randomized, double-blind, placebo-controlled phase III trial of chemotherapy

with or without bevacizumab in patients with platinum-sensitive recurrent epithelial ovarian, primary peritoneal, or fallopian tube cancer. J Clin Oncol. 2012;30:2039–45.

62. Pujade-Lauraine E, Wagner U, Aavall-Lundqvist E, Gebski V, Heywood M, Vasey P, Volgger B, Vergote I, Pignata S, Ferrero A, Sehouli J, Lortholary A, Kristensen G, Jackisch C, Joly F, Brown C, Le Fur N, du Bois A. Pegylated liposomal Doxorubicin and Carboplatin compared with Paclitaxel and Carboplatin for patients with platinum-sensitive ovarian cancer in late relapse. J Clin Oncol. 2010;28:3323–9.
63. Monk BJ, Poveda A, Vergote I, Raspagliesi F, Fujiwara K, Bae DS, Oaknin A, Navale L, Warner DJ, Oza AM. A phase III, randomized, double-blind trial of weekly paclitaxel plus the angiopoietin 1 and 2 inhibitor, trebananib, or placebo in women with recurrent ovarian cancer: TRINOVA-1. Ann Oncol. 2013;24:799–808.
64. Andreas du Bois GK, Ray-Coquard I, Reuss A, Pignata S, Colombo N, Denison U, Vergote I, del Campo JM, Ottevanger P, Merger M, Harter P. AGO-OVAR 12: a randomized placebo-controlled GCIG/engot-intergroup phase III trial of standard frontline chemotherapy +/– nintedanib for advanced ovarian cancer. Late Breaking Abstract. Int J Gyn Cancer. 2013; 23(Suppl 1): LBA 1.
65. Ledermann JA, Hackshaw A, Kaye S, Jayson G, Gabra H, McNeish I, Earl H, Perren T, Gore M, Persic M, Adams M, James L, Temple G, Merger M, Rustin G. Randomized phase II placebo-controlled trial of maintenance therapy using the oral triple angiokinase inhibitor BIBF 1120 after chemotherapy for relapsed ovarian cancer. J Clin Oncol. 2011;29:3798–804.
66. Pothuri B. BRCA1- and BRCA2-related mutations: therapeutic implications in ovarian cancer. Ann Oncol. 2013;24(24 Suppl 8): viii22–7.
67. Venkitaraman AR. Cancer susceptibility and the functions of BRCA1 and BRCA2. Cell. 2002;108:171–82.
68. Khanna KK, Jackson SP. DNA double-strand breaks: signaling, repair and the cancer connection. Nat Genet. 2001;27:247–54.
69. Eskander RN, Tewari KS. PARP inhibition and synthetic lethality in ovarian cancer. Expert Rev Clin Pharmacol. 2014;7(5): 613–22.
70. Hoeijmakers JH. Genome maintenance mechanisms for preventing cancer. Nature. 2001;411:366–74.
71. Dantzer F, de La Rubia G, Menissier-De Murcia J, Hostomsky Z, de Murcia G, Schreiber V. Base excision repair is impaired in mammalian cells lacking Poly(ADP-ribose) polymerase-1. Biochemistry. 2000;39:7559–69.

72. McCabe N, Lord CJ, Tutt AN, Martin NM, Smith GC, Ashworth A. BRCA2-deficient CAPAN-1 cells are extremely sensitive to the inhibition of poly (ADP-ribose) polymerase: an issue of potency. Cancer Biol Ther. 2005;4:934–6.
73. Farmer H, McCabe N, Lord CJ, Tutt AN, Johnson DA, Richardson TB, Santarosa M, Dillon KJ, Hickson I, Knights C, Martin NM, Jackson SP, Smith GC, Ashworth A. Targeting the DNA repair defect in BRCA mutant cells as a therapeutic strategy. Nature. 2005;434:917–21.
74. Bryant HE, Schultz N, Thomas HD, Parker KM, Flower D, Lopez E, Kyle S, Meuth M, Curtin NJ, Helleday T. Specific killing of BRCA2-deficient tumours with inhibitors of poly(ADP-ribose) polymerase. Nature. 2005;434:913–7.
75. Audeh MW, Carmichael J, Penson RT, Friedlander M, Powell B, Bell-McGuinn KM, Scott C, Weitzel JN, Oaknin A, Loman N, Lu K, Schmutzler RK, Matulonis U, Wickens M, Tutt A. Oral poly(ADP-ribose) polymerase inhibitor olaparib in patients with BRCA1 or BRCA2 mutations and recurrent ovarian cancer: a proof-of-concept trial. Lancet. 2010;376:245–51.
76. Coleman RL, Sill M, Aghajanian C, Gray HJ, Tewari KS, Rubin SC, Rutherford TJ, Chan JK, Chen HX, Swisher EM A phase II evaluation of the potent, highly selective PARP inhibitor veliparib in the treatment of persistent or recurrent epithelial ovarian, fallopian tube, or primary peritoneal cancer in patients who carry a germline BRCA1 or BRCA2 mutation – a Gynecologic Oncology Group study. Presented at: SGO 45th Annual Meeting on Women's Cancer, Tampa, FL; 2014. Abstract 136.
77. Gelmon KA, Tischkowitz M, Mackay H, Swenerton K, Robidoux A, Tonkin K, Hirte H, Huntsman D, Clemons M, Gilks B, Yerushalmi R, Macpherson E, Carmichael J, Oza A. Olaparib in patients with recurrent high-grade serous or poorly differentiated ovarian carcinoma or triple-negative breast cancer: a phase 2, multicentre, open-label, non-randomised study. Lancet Oncol. 2011;12:852–61.
78. Kaye SB, Lubinski J, Matulonis U, Ang JE, Gourley C, Karlan BY, Amnon A, Bell-McGuinn KM, Chen LM, Friedlander M, Safra T, Vergote I, Wickens M, Lowe ES, Carmichael J, Kaufman B. Phase II, open-label, randomized, multicenter study comparing the efficacy and safety of olaparib, a poly (ADP-ribose) polymerase inhibitor, and pegylated liposomal doxorubicin in patients with BRCA1 or BRCA2 mutations and recurrent ovarian cancer. J Clin Oncol. 2012;30:372–9.

79. Ledermann J, Harter P, Gourley C, Friedlander M, Vergote I, Rustin G, Scott C, Meier W, Shapira-Frommer R, Safra T, Matei D, Macpherson E, Watkins C, Carmichael J, Matulonis U. Olaparib maintenance therapy in platinum-sensitive relapsed ovarian cancer. N Engl J Med. 2012;366:1382–92.
80. Barnhill DR, Kurman RJ, Brady MF, Omura GA, Yordan E, Given FT, Kucera PR, Roman LD. Preliminary analysis of the behavior of stage I ovarian serous tumors of low malignant potential: a Gynecologic Oncology Group study. J Clin Oncol. 1995;13:2752–6.
81. Seidman JD, Kurman RJ. Ovarian serous borderline tumors: a critical review of the literature with emphasis on prognostic indicators. Hum Pathol. 2000;31:539–57.
82. Tropé C, Kaern J, Vergote IB, Kristensen G, Abeler V. Are borderline tumors of the ovary overtreated both surgically and systemically? A review of four prospective randomized trials including 253 patients with borderline tumors. Gynecol Oncol. 1993;51:236–43.
83. Gershenson DM, Silva EG. Serous ovarian tumors of low malignant potential with peritoneal implants. Cancer. 1990;65:578–85.
84. Barakat RR, Benjamin I, Lewis JL, Saigo PE, Curtin JP, Hoskins WJ. Platinum-based chemotherapy for advanced-stage serous ovarian carcinoma of low malignant potential. Gynecol Oncol. 1995;59:390–3.
85. Sutton GP, Bundy BN, Omura GA, Yordan EL, Beecham JB, Bonfiglio T. Stage III ovarian tumors of low malignant potential treated with cisplatin combination therapy (a Gynecologic Oncology Group study). Gynecol Oncol. 1991;41:230–3.
86. Gershenson DM, Copeland LJ, Kavanagh JJ, Cangir A, Del Junco G, Saul PB, Stringer CA, Freedman RS, Edwards CL, Wharton JT. Treatment of malignant nondysgerminomatous germ cell tumors of the ovary with vincristine, dactinomycin, and cyclophosphamide. Cancer. 1985;56:2756–61.
87. Williams SD, Blessing JA, Moore DH, Homesley HD, Adcock L. Cisplatin, vinblastine, and bleomycin in advanced and recurrent ovarian germ-cell tumors. A trial of the Gynecologic Oncology Group. Ann Intern Med. 1989;111:22–7.
88. Williams SD, Birch R, Einhorn LH, Irwin L, Greco FA, Loehrer PJ. Treatment of disseminated germ-cell tumors with cisplatin, bleomycin, and either vinblastine or etoposide. N Engl J Med. 1987;316:1435–40.
89. Colombo N, Parma G, Zanagnolo V, Insinga A. Management of ovarian stromal cell tumors. J Clin Oncol. 2007;25:2944–51.

Chapter 2
Cervical Cancer

Sara M. Jordan and Krishnansu S. Tewari

Anatomy

- Cervix (Latin for "neck") = neck of the uterus.
  - Average 2–4 cm in length and the point where the cervix joins the uterus is called the isthmus.
  - The intravaginal portion of the cervix is called the exocervix and is covered with stratified squamous epithelium identical to the lining of the vagina.
  - The stroma of the cervix consists of stratified muscle and connective tissue.
  - Blood supply to the cervix:
    - Via the broad ligament and parametrium which support the cervix laterally.

S.M. Jordan, M.D. (✉)
Southwest Gynecologic Oncology Associates, Inc.,
201 Cedar Street SE, Suite 304, Albuquerque, NM 87106, USA
e-mail: sara.jordan@uci.edu

K.S. Tewari, M.D., F.A.C.O.G., F.A.C.S.
The Division of Gynecologic Oncology, The Gynecologic Oncology Group at UC Irvine, Irvine Medical Center, University of California, 101 The City Drive, Orange, CA 92868, USA
e-mail: ktewari@uci.edu

R.N. Eskander and R.E. Bristow (eds.), *Gynecologic Oncology: A Pocketbook*, DOI 10.1007/978-1-4939-1976-5_2,

Epidemiology

- Worldwide cervical cancer remains the second most common cancer of women with a mortality rate of 52 % [1].
  - 86 % of cervical cancers are diagnosed in the developing world [1].
  - Global incidence and mortality depend on presence of screening and vaccination programs. These interventions have led to a 75 % decrease in incidence and mortality of cervical cancer in the past 50 years in developed countries [2].
- There will be 12,360 new cases of cervical cancer and 4,020 cervical cancer related deaths in the USA in 2014 [3].
- In the USA, cervical cancer is the third most common gynecologic malignancy (after uterine and ovarian cancer) and the 12th most common cancer of women.
  - The mortality from cervical cancer in the USA has declined from 15/100,000 in 1945 to 3.4/100,000 in 1991.
- Cervical cancer is the only malignancy for which the causative agent is known.
- The etiologic agent resulting in cervical cancer has been identified as a sexually transmitted oncogenic virus, human papillomavirus (HPV).
  - HPV is a circular, double-stranded DNA virus when in its' infectious state. Viral DNA integration into host DNA leads to a malignant phenotype. Once integrated, HPV E6 codes for a protein that degrades p53 and HPV E7 codes for a protein that complexes with pRB releasing transcription factor E2F causing the cell to be immortal (Table 2.1). Low risk strains of HPV (types 6 and 11) cause genital warts whereas high risk strains (types 16, 18, 31, 45, and less commonly 33, 35, 39, 51, 54, 55, 56, 58, 59 66, and 68), if integrated into host DNA, cause cervical dysplasia and cervical carcinoma (Fig. 2.1) [4].

TABLE 2.1. HPV genome.

E1	E2	E4	E5	E6	E7	L1	L2
ATPase	Regulator of E6 and E7	Disrupts cytokeratin matrix for release of virions	Potentiation of membrane bound EGF receptors	Bind and inactivate p53	Bind pRB leading to E2F activity	Major capsid (conserved)	Minor capsid (variable)

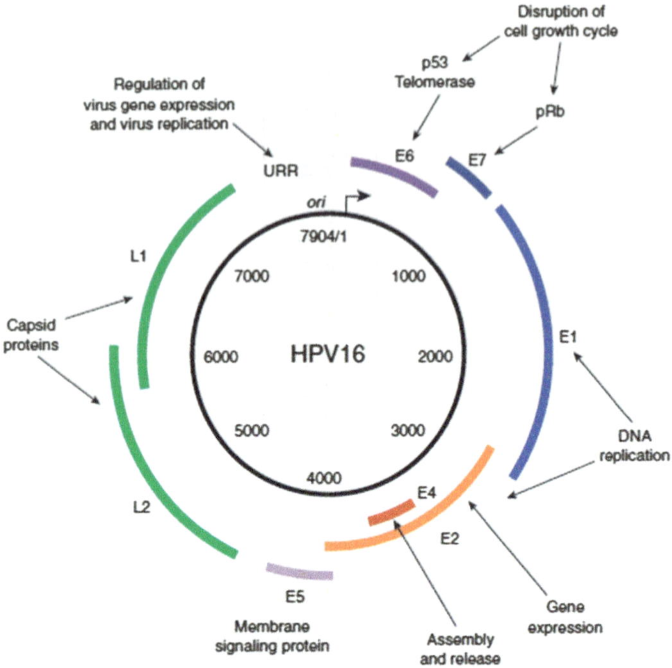

FIG. 2.1. Human papillomavirus genome [4]. Reprinted from Clinical Gynecologic Oncology, 7th Edition, Di Saia PJ, Creasman WT. Chapter 3 Invasive Cervical Cancer, Monk BJ, Tewari KS, Copyright 2007, with permission from Elsevier. Clinical gynecologic oncology by Di Saia PJ, Creasman WT. Reproduced with permission of Elsevier Mosby in the format reuse in a book/textbook via Copyright Clearance Center.

- HPV is detectable in over 95 % of squamous cell carcinomas and 30–40 % of adenocarcinomas.
- High-risk strains cause a mutation of cells in the squamocolumnar junction leading to cervical dysplasia and cancer.
- Incidence of progression without treatment:
  - CIN1 (16 %), CIN2 (30 %), CIN3 (70 %).
  - CIN3 → invasive disease: 0–20 years.

- Risk factors:
  - Lower socioeconomic status.
  - Multiple sexual partners, early age of first intercourse, promiscuous partners, co-infection with other sexually transmitted diseases.
  - Tobacco use.
  - Immunocompromised conditions (HIV or pharmacologic).
- The greatest risk for developing cervical cancer is infrequent or no prior screening.
  - In many South American, African, and Asian countries, cervical cancer is the leading cause of cancer related death in women.

Prevention

- Abstinence prevents HPV related cervical carcinomas, but the large majority of women are sexually active and therefore at risk for exposure to HPV infection.
- Two US Food and Drug Administration (FDA)-approved vaccines indicated to prevent cervical cancer (Table 2.2).
  - Quadravalent Vaccine: GARDASIL.
    - FDA approved in 2006.
    - In 2007 the Females United to Unilaterally Reduce Endo/Ectocervical Disease (FUTURE) II reported results from a randomized, double-blind trial of 12,167 women aged 15–26 years who received Gardasil or placebo. For 3-year follow-up, vaccine efficacy for preventing dysplasia or invasive disease was 98 % in the per-protocol population (44 % for the intention-to-treat population).
    - FUTURE I was a phase III, randomized, double-blind, placebo-controlled trial involving 5,455 women aged 16–24 years. Vaccine efficacy for preventing anogenital warts as well as dysplasia or invasive disease associated with HPV types 16 or 18 was 100 %.

TABLE 2.2. HPV directed vaccines.

	Gardasil	Cervarix
HPV types	6,11, 16, 18	16, 18
Dose schedule	0.5 mL IM 0, 2, 6 months	0.5 mL IM 0, 1–2, 6 months
Indications	Cervical cancer, CIN, AIS, Vulvar cancer, VIN, Vaginal cancer, VAIN, Anogenital warts	Cervical cancer, CIN, AIS
Population approved	Males and females aged 9–26 years	Females aged 9–25 years
Advisory Committee on Immunization Practices (ACIP) recommendations	Females aged 11 and 12 years with catch-up vaccination for females aged 13–26 years. Permissive for boys aged 9–26 years	
Technology used	Yeast	Insect cell substrate
Adjuvant	Amorphous hydroxyphosphate sulfate (Merck and Co., Inc)	Aluminum hydroxide + 3 = deacetylated monophosphoryl lipid A (MPL, Coixa/GSK)

  - In a double-blind, randomized trial of 3,817 women aged 24–45 years, GARDASIL efficacy against infection related to HPV-6, -11, -16, and -18 was 90.5 %.
  - Merck is currently comparing the efficacy of GARDASIL to a nanovalent HPV vaccine.

- Bivalent Vaccine: CERVARIX.

  - Phase II, randomized, double-blind, controlled trial known as Papilloma TRIal against Cancer In young Adults (PATRICIA) published in 2009. In this study, 18,644 women aged 15–25 years received placebo or were vaccinated with CERVARIX.
  - Vaccine efficacy against HPV-16 and -18 CIN II–IIII was 92.9 %.
  - Evidence of cross-protection efficacy.
  - There has not been a direct head-to-head efficacy trial between GARDASIL and CERVARIX.

Diagnosis

- *First* symptom of early cervical cancer: frequently thin, clear or blood-tinged vaginal discharge usually unrecognized by the patient.
- *Classic* symptom: intermittent, painless metrorrhagia or postcoital spotting, although this is not the most common symptom.
- With progression, bleeding becomes heavier, more frequent, and ultimately continuous. Usually if this bleeding occurs in a postmenopausal woman, it leads to earlier medical attention.
- Late stage disease involves spread into the parametria or the pelvic sidewalls and causes *flank or leg pain*, which is usually a sign of involvement of the ureters or sciatic nerve. Bladder or rectal invasion frequently leads to *hematuria*, *rectal bleeding*, and possibly vesicovaginal or rectovaginal *fistula*. Lymphedema may be a sign of late stage or recurrent disease due to venous blockage from extensive sidewall disease.
- Gross clinical appearance.
  - Most common: exophytic, large, friable polypoid lesion arising from the ectocervix (Fig. 2.2). These lesions may arise within the endocervcial canal creating a barrel-shaped lesion.
    - Lesions within the endocervical canal are more commonly adenocarcinomas, which arise in the endocervical mucous-producing gland cells. Because of the origin within the cervix, the lesion may be present for longer time before it is clinically evident.
  - Firm cervix with little visible ulceration or mass.
  - An ulcerative tumor that erodes through the cervix.

Screening

- Prevention, screening, and early treatment are imperative.
- Cervical dysplasia and cancer is slow to progress, able to be diagnosed early with current screening modalities, and almost always cured when diagnosed early.

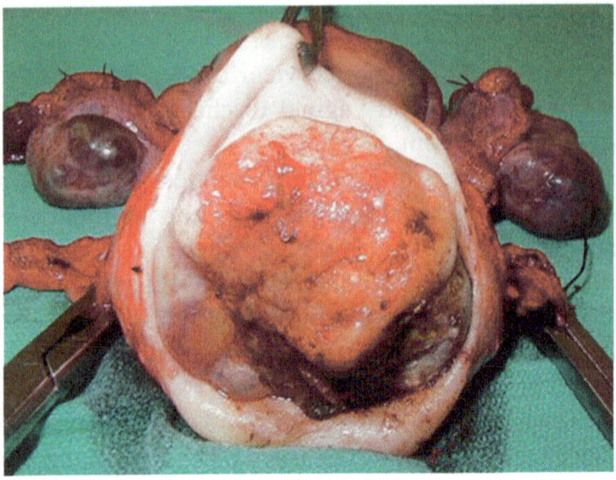

FIG. 2.2. Gross image of invasive cervical carcinoma (Image provided courtesy of Dr. Krishnansu S. Tewari).

- Late diagnosis most frequently results in incurable disease and death.
- Cytology, using the Papanicolaou (Pap) smear, and colposcopy are both valuable screening tools.
- Cervical cancer screening guidelines according to American Society for Colposcopy and Cervical Pathology (ASCCP) (Table 2.3).
- Abnormal pap smears may require further workup with colposcopy with possible need for biopsy.
- Colposcopy involves use of 5 % acetic acid applied to the cervix and inspection with a colposcope that magnifies the cervix and allows for visualization with color filters.
  - A satisfactory colposcopy requires that the entire squamocolumnar junction (SCJ) be visualized.
  - Concerning findings for which biopsy should be obtained:
    - Acetowhite changes.
    - Irregular contour.
    - Atypical vessels.
    - Coarse mosaicism or punctation.
    - Large multiquadrant lesions.

TABLE 2.3. ASCCP cervical cancer screening guidelines.

Population	Screening recommendation
<21 years	No screening
21–29 years	Cytology every 3 years without HPV testing
30–65 years	Cytology and HPV co-testing every 5 years
>65 years	No screening if negative adequate prior screening (as long as no prior history of CIN or cervical cancer)
After hysterectomy	No screening (as long as cervix removed and no prior history of CIN or cervical cancer)
After HPV vaccination	Same as unvaccinated women

TABLE 2.4. Rates of pelvic and para aortic lymph node metastases by stage [4].

Stage	Rate of pelvic lymph node metastases (%)	Rate of para aortic lymph node metastases (%)
I	15	6
II	29	17
III	47	30

Reprinted from Clinical Gynecologic Oncology, 7th Edition, Di Saia PJ, Creasman WT. Chapter 3 Invasive Cervical Cancer, Monk BJ, Tewari KS, Copyright 2007, with permission from Elsevier. Clinical gynecologic oncology by Di Saia PJ, Creasman WT. Reproduced with permission of Elsevier Mosby in the format reuse in a book/textbook via Copyright Clearance Center

- An endocervical curettage (ECC) should be done as long as the patient is not pregnant.
- Cervical dysplasia or early invasive cervical cancer (Stage IA1) can be treated with loop electrosurgical excision procedure (LEEP) or cold knife cone (CKC).
- ASCCP guidelines (www.asccp.org) should be used to triage abnormal cytology and histology.

Pathology (Refer to Table 2.4) [4]

- There are *four main routes of spread* of cervical carcinoma:
  - Direct spread into the vaginal mucosa.
  - Spread into the myometrium, particularly with lesions originating in the endocervix.

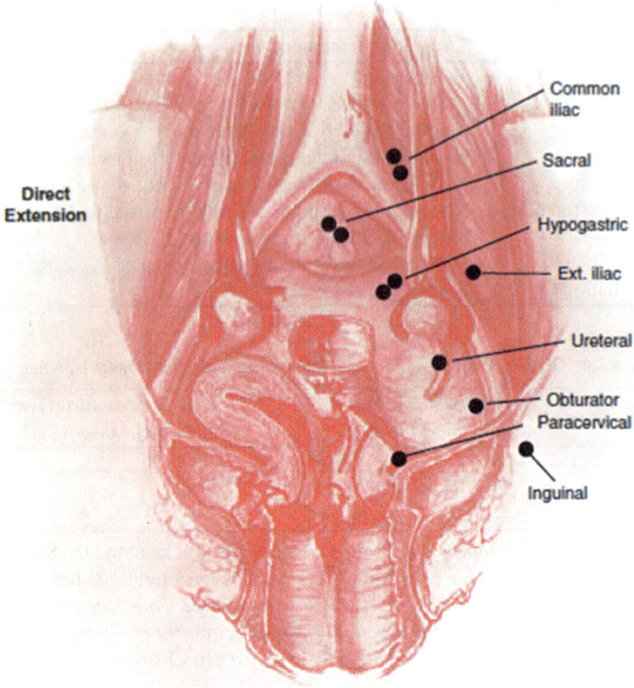

FIG. 2.3. Patterns of lymphatic spread in cervical carcinoma [4]. Reprinted from Clinical Gynecologic Oncology, 7th Edition, Di Saia PJ, Creasman WT. Chapter 3 Invasive Cervical Cancer, Monk BJ, Tewari KS, Copyright 2007, with permission from Elsevier. Clinical gynecologic oncology by Di Saia PJ, Creasman WT. Reproduced with permission of Elsevier Mosby in the format reuse in a book/textbook via Copyright Clearance Center.

- Spread into the paracervical and parametrial lymphatics and then further (primarily: obturator, hypogastric, external iliac, and sacral nodes and secondarily: common iliac, inguinal, and para-aortic nodes) (Fig. 2.3) [4].
- Direct extension into adjacent structures (parametria, bladder, bowel).

Table 2.5. Five-year survival according to stage and mode of treatment [5].

Stage	Surgery only (%)	Radiation only (%)	Surgery + radiation (%)
Ib1	94.5	80.1	83.6
Ib2	91.4	73.7	76.7
IIa	72.6	64.5	76.2
IIb	73.0	64.2	64.3

Reprinted with permission from International Federation of Gynecology and Obstetrics, in International Journal of Gynecology and Obstetrics. Benedet JL, Odicino F, Maisonneuve P, et al. in Carcinoma of the cervix uteri. International Journal Gynecology and Obstetrics. Oct 2003;83 Suppl 1:41–78

- Adenocarcinomas arise from the endocervical mucous-producing glands and, because they originate within the endocervical canal, it takes longer until these tumors are clinically evident. This growth pattern results in the classic barrel-shaped cervix.
- No difference in survival between cervical adenocarcinomas and squamous carcinomas after correction for stage (see Tables 2.5 and 2.6 [5]).
  - 1998 FIGO Annual Report of over 10,000 squamous cell carcinomas and 1,138 adenocarcinomas noted no difference in survival in Stage I cancers.

Staging

- Cervical cancer is clinically staged based on (Table 2.7):
- Exam.
- CKC or LEEP.
- Imaging—CXR, IVP, CT urogram, Barium enema.
- Cystoscopy.
- Proctosigmoidoscopy.

PET/CT Staging

- In 2005 the Centers for Medicare and Medicaid Services approved coverage for FDG-PET for staging newly diagnosed and locally advanced cervical cancers and screening for cervical cancer recurrence.

TABLE 2.6. Histologic types of cervical cancer.

Pathology	Prevalence
Nonglandular	
Squamous cell	65–85 %
Verrucous	Rare
Sarcomatoid	Rare
Glandular	
Endocervical	10–25 %
Endometrioid	Rare
Clear cell	Rare
Mucinous	Rare
Serous	Rare
Adenoid cystic	Rare
Villoglandular	Rare
Other, mixed epithelial tumors	
Adenosquamous	5 %
Glassy cell	Rare
Small cell	Rare
Nonepithelial tumors	Rare
Carcinosarcoma, leiomyosarcoma, endometrial stromal sarcoma, germ cell tumors, melanoma, lymphoma, neuroendocrine	

TABLE 2.7. Cervical cancer staging according to the International Federation of Gynecology and Obstetrics (FIGO) revised in 2009.

FIGO Stage	Description
0	Carcinoma in situ
Ia1	Invasion of stroma <3 mm in depth and ≤7 mm in width
Ia2	Invasion of stroma >3 mm and ≤5 mm in depth and ≤7 mm in width
Ib1	Clinical lesions greater than Stage Ia but no greater than 4 cm
Ib2	Clinical lesions confined to the cervix that are greater than 4 cm
IIa	Involvement of the upper 2/3 vagina
IIb	Involvement of the parametria without sidewall involvement
IIIa	Extension to lower 1/3 vagina
IIIb	Extension to pelvic sidewall or hydronephrosis or non-functional kidney
IVa	Extension to bladder or rectum
IVB	Distant metastasis or disease beyond the pelvis

- Sensitivity of PET in detecting pelvic nodal metastases in patients with untreated cervical cancer = 80 %, sensitivity of CT = 48 % [6].
- A 2007 meta-analysis of 41 studies concluded that PET/CT had the highest sensitivity (82 %) and specificity (95 %) for detection of positive nodes compared to CT (50 and 92 %) and MRI (56 and 91 %). PET positive nodes have been found to be a prognostic biomarker predicting treatment response, pelvic recurrence risk, and survival [6].

Genetics

- There is no known genetic basis for cervical cancer.

Indication for and Modes of Treatment (Surgery/Chemotherapy/Radiation Therapy)

- During the past several decades, staging definitions and treatment recommendations for cervical cancer have changed significantly (Table 2.8).
- First radical hysterectomy was performed by Dr. Joe V. Meigs at Harvard University in 1944.
- Morbidity: 1–5 %.
- There are five traditional classes of radical hysterectomy as described by Piver and Rutledge (Table 2.9).
- Understanding of the eight pelvic spaces is critical in the completion of a radical hysterectomy (Fig. 2.4) [4].
- Pelvic lymph node dissection boundaries:
  - Lateral—genitofemoral nerve.
  - Medial—superior vesical artery.
  - Distal—Deep circumflex iliac vein.
  - Proximal—2 cm above bifurcation of common iliac artery.
  - Inferior—Obturator nerve.
- In the hands of an experienced surgeon, complication rates are less than 5 % (Table 2.10).

TABLE 2.8. Treatment of cervical cancer by stage.

Stage	Standard treatment	Fertility preserving treatment
IA1, –LVSI	Extrafascial hysterectomy	Cervical cone biopsy
IA1, +LVSI	Extrafascial hysterectomy, +/– pelvic lymph node dissection	Cervical cone biopsy and laparoscopic pelvic lymph node dissection
IA2, occult IB1	Modified radical hysterectomy with pelvic lymph node dissection, +/– adjuvant therapy	Radical trachalectomy with pelvic lymph node dissection
IB1, IB2, IIA	Radical hysterectomy with pelvic lymph node dissection, +/– adjuvant therapy	Radical trachalectomy with pelvic lymph node dissection only if IB1 $\leq$2 cm, and *not* small cell histology
IB2–IVA	Chemoradiation with HDR brachytherapy +/– pretreatment laparoscopic pelvic lymph node dissection	Radical hysterectomy with lymph node dissection and adjuvant therapy only if IB2–IIA
Isolated central pelvic recurrence	If prior radiation then proceed with pelvic exenteration with urinary diversion	If no prior radiation then proceed with chemoradiation
IVB, persistent, or non-central recurrence	Cisplatin and paclitaxel and bevacizumab +/– palliative radiotherapy for bleeding or bone metastases	Cisplatin and paclitaxel and bevacizumab +/– palliative radiotherapy for bleeding or bone metastases

TABLE 2.9. Piver and Rutledge classification of radical hysterectomy.

Class	Description	Indication
I	Extrafascial hysterectomy	CIN, early stromal invasion
II	Removal of medial half of the cardinal and uterosacral ligaments, upper 1/3 vagina	
III	Removal of entire cardinal and uterosacral ligaments, upper 1/3 vagina	Stage Ib and IIa
IV	Removal of all the periureteral tissue, superior vesical artery, ¾ vagina	Anteriorly occurring central recurrences
V	Removal of portions of the distal ureter and bladder	Central recurrent cancer, or primary disease involving portions of the distal ureter or bladder

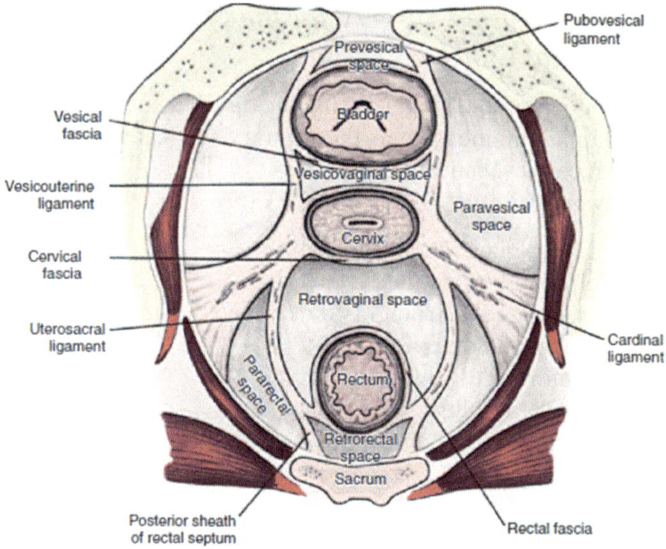

FIG. 2.4. Cross section of the pelvis to illustrate the 8 pelvic spaces [4]. Reprinted from Clinical Gynecologic Oncology, 7th Edition, Di Saia PJ, Creasman WT. Chapter 3 Invasive Cervical Cancer, Monk BJ, Tewari KS, Copyright 2007, with permission from Elsevier. Clinical gynecologic oncology by Di Saia PJ, Creasman WT. Reproduced with permission of Elsevier Mosby in the format reuse in a book/textbook via Copyright Clearance Center.

TABLE 2.10. Complications of radical hysterectomy.

Severe bladder atony	4 %
Lymphocyst requiring drainage	3 %
Ureterovaginal fistula	2 %
Thrombophlebitis	2 %
Ureterovaginal fistula	2 %
Vesicovaginal fistula	1 %
Bowel obstruction requiring surgery	1 %
Pulmonary embolus	1 %

Robotic-Assisted Surgery for the Management of Cervical Cancer

- Robotic-assisted surgery using the da Vinci surgical system is gaining momentum as the primary surgical approach to treat cervical cancer.
- Advantages:
  - 3D and magnified visualization.
  - Improved ergonomics.
  - Articulated instruments that mimic the human wrist.
  - Enhanced dexterity.
  - Tremor reduction.
  - Camera stability.
  - Steep learning curve.
- Disadvantages:
  - Increased operating time.
  - Increased cost.
  - Prolonged steep Trendelenberg.
  - Potential instrument malfunction.
- Evaluation of oncologic outcomes and cost–benefit analysis of the robotic approach is ongoing.

Ovarian Transposition

- The incidence of premature ovarian failure after pelvic radiation without ovarian transposition is high (nearly certain ovarian failure after 8 Gy single dose or 10 Gy fractionated dose).
- Ovarian transposition is an intraoperative procedure in which the infundibulopelvic ligament is mobilized and bilateral ovaries are sutured ("transposed") to the paracolic gutters. The new location of the ovaries is generally marked with staples in order to be visible on imaging and assist with postoperative radiation planning.
- Ovarian failure after transposition and pelvic radiation decreases but is still 28–50 %. If radiation is not required, risk of ovarian failure from transposition alone is 5 % [6].

Indications for Postoperative Adjuvant Therapy

- Recommendation for postoperative adjuvant pelvic radiation with or without radio sensitizing chemotherapy following radical hysterectomy is based on pathologic risk factors.
- High-intermediate risk factors (GOG 92):
  - Tumor diameter (>4 cm).
  - Depth of stromal invasion (>1/3).
  - Presence of lymphovascular space invasion.
- High-risk factors:
  - Positive margins.
  - Positive parametria.
  - Positive lymph nodes.
- A simple hysterectomy performed for a cervical cancer greater than Stage IA1 is considered a "cut through" hysterectomy and is not adequate therapy. Prognosis in this setting is poor and probability of curative radiotherapy is greatly decreased [6].

Clinical Trials Supporting Current Treatment Algorithms

Locally Advanced Cervical Cancer

- Five pivotal trials support the use of chemoradiation in locally advanced cervical cancer (Table 2.11) [7–11]:
- Radiation alone fails to control cervical cancer in 35–90 % of women with locally advanced disease [6].
- Concurrent radio sensitizing chemotherapy improves local control and often eradicates distant metastases.
- The rationale for radiosensitizing chemotherapy is based on the discovery that tumor radio sensitivity is enhanced through the formation of DNA–platinum adducts. Additionally, the addition of chemotherapy helps prevent the repair of sublethal damage in cancer tissue preferentially.

Table 2.11. Five pivotal trials supporting chemoradiation in locally advanced cervical cancer [7–11].

Trial	Eligibility	Arms	OS (months)	PFS (months)	Conclusion
GOG 109 [7]	IA2–IIA	• Adjuvant pelvic RT	71	63	Benefit of radio sensitizing cisplatin
		• Adjuvant pelvic RT + cisplatin 70 mg/m^2	81	80	
GOG 123 [8]	IB2	• Pre-op pelvic RT + cisplatin 40 mg/m^2/week	86	80	
		• Pre-op pelvic RT	72	64	
RTOG 9001 [9]	IB–IVA	• Pelvic RT + cisplatin 75 mg/m^2 + 5-FU 4 g/m^2/96 h (3 cycles)	73	67	Benefit of radiosensitizing cisplatin
		• Pelvic RT + extended field RT	58	40	
GOG 85 [10]	IIB–IVA	• Pelvic RT + cisplatin 50 mg/m^2 + 5-FU 4 g/m^2/96 h (2 cycles)	65	60	Cisplatin + 5-FU superior to hydroxyurea
		• Pelvic RT + hydroxyurea 3 g/m^2 (2×/week)	50	48	
GOG 120 [11]	IIB–IVA	• Pelvic RT + cisplatin 40 mg/m^2/week	60	60	Both cisplatin arms superior to hydroxyurea alone
		• Pelvic RT + cisplatin 50 mg/m^2 + 5-FU 4 g/m^2/96 h + hydroxyurea 2 g/m^2	58	60	
		• Pelvic RT + hydroxyurea 3 g/m^2 (2×/week)	34	45	

TABLE 2.12. Single agents evaluated in the treatment of advanced stage, persistent or recurrent cervical cancer categorized by trial outcome [12–23].

Positive signal[a]	Negative signal[b]
Thigpen et al. [12]: cisplatin	McGuire et al. [13]: carboplatin; iproplatin
Sutton et al. [14]: ifosfamide	Fracasso et al. [15]: oxaliplatin
Schilder et al. [16]: gemcitabine	Thigpen et al. [17]: Mitomycin-C
Bookman et al. [18]: topotecan	Look et al. [19]: irinotecan
Curtin et al. [20]: paclitaxel	Garcia [21]: docetaxel
McGuire et al. [22]: paclitaxel	
Muggia et al. [23]: vinorelbine	

[a]Agents included in subsequent combination trials given response rates
[b]Agents abandoned as single agent therapeutic options due to limited response and/or unacceptable toxicity

- The most common regimen is weekly cisplatin 40 mg/m^2 (maximum dose of 70 mg/week) given during radiation treatment.

Metastatic Cervical Cancer: Combination Cytotoxic Regimens

- In 1981 single agent cisplatin established as the chemotherapy backbone for the treatment of metastatic/advanced stage cervical cancer.
- Numerous single agent trials evaluating various agents subsequently conducted with mixed signals (Table 2.12) [12–23].
- Despite rigorous investigation, cisplatin remained the historical standard treatment.
- Ultimately, various combination regimens were studied to improve oncologic outcomes in this vulnerable population.
- Not curative, but progression free survival has improved with systemic chemotherapy (see Table 2.13) [24–28].
- Following publication of GOG 110 and GOG 149 it became evident that improvement in RR and PFS did not translate into improvements in OS.
- Thus, the importance of evaluating QOL on treatment emerged and subsequent trials tracked QOL, patient reported outcomes.

Combination regimens tested in phase III studies for the treatment advanced Stage (IVB), recurrent or persistent cervical cancer [24–28].

Trial	Regimen	RR (%)	OS (months)	PFS (months)
GOG 110 [24]	Cisplatin 50 mg/m²	17.8	8	3.2
	Cisplatin 50 mg/m² + DBD 180 mg/m²	21.1	7.3	3.3
	Cisplatin 50 mg/m² + Ifosfamide 5 g/m² + mesna	31.1	8.3	4.6
GOG 149 [25]	Cisplatin 50 mg/m² + Ifosfamide 5 g/m²	32	8.5	4.6
	Cisplatin 50 mg/m² + Ifosfamide 5 g/m² + Bleomycin 30 units	31.2	8.4	5.1
GOG 169 [26]	Cisplatin 50 mg/m²	19	8.8	2.8
	Cisplatin 50 mg/m² + Paclitaxel 135 mg/m²	36	9.7	4.8
GOG 179 [27]	Cisplatin 50 mg/m²	13	6.5	2.9
	Cisplatin 50 mg/m² + Topotecan 0.75 mg/m² d1–3	26	9.4	4.6
	MVAC	NA	NA	NA
GOG 204 [28]	Cisplatin 50 mg/m² + Paclitaxel 135 mg/m²	29.1	12.9	5.8
	Cisplatin 50 mg/m² + Topotecan 0.75 mg/m² d1–3	23.4	10.3	4.7
	Cisplatin 50 mg/m² + Gemcitabine 1,000 mg/m²	22.3	10.3	4.6
	Cisplatin 50 mg/m² + Vinorelbine 30 mg/m²	25.9	10	4.0

DBD dibromodulcitol, *RR* response rate, *OS* overall survival, *PFS* progression free survival, *d* day, *MVAC* methotrexate 30 mg/m² days 1, 15, and 22, vinblastine 3 mg/m² days 2, 15, and 22, doxorubicin 30 mg/m² day 2, and cisplatin 70 mg/m² day 2 given every 4 weeks, *NA* not applicable as study arm closed early

- *GOG 169* showed a near doubling of the RR with combination cisplatin + paclitaxel, without deterioration in QOL and this became the standard chemotherapeutic approach moving forward.
- *GOG 179* subsequently established cisplatin + topotecan as superior to cisplatin alone, and was the first trial in this disease setting to show an improvement in OS resulting in FDA approval of the regimen.

- OS advantage criticized, given what was described as a relative underperformance of the cisplatin control arm of GOG 179, in comparison to GOG 110 and GOG 169.
- This was attributed to increased use of radiosensitizing cisplatin, and "re-treatment" with platinum in patients enrolled and treated on GOG 179.
    - GOG 169: 31 % received prior radiosensitizing cisplatin.
    - GOG 179: 58 % received prior radiosensitizing cisplatin.

- *GOG 204* then developed and opened in May 2003 comparing four chemotherapy doublets.
    - 70 % received prior cisplatin containing chemoradiation.
    - Cisplatin + Paclitaxel regimen stood out with highest RR, and longest PFS and OS (despite lack of significance).
    - Response rate to combination cisplatin + paclitaxel attenuated in GOG 204 when compared to GOG 169, and once again attributed to increased prior cisplatin exposure in the patients enrolled on GOG 204 (i.e., these patients may have a degree of platinum resistance from prior platinum exposure).
- In an effort to mitigate nephrotoxicity and shorten chemotherapy infusion, JGOG conducted a non-inferiority phase 3 trial of cisplatin + paclitaxel versus carboplatin + paclitaxel.
    - Median OS and PFS nearly identical between study arms (HR 1.04; 95 % CI 0.8–1.35).
    - In a secondary analysis of 117 patients not receiving prior platinum therapy the cisplatin + paclitaxel regimen appeared superior to carboplatin + paclitaxel.
        - Median OS 23.2 versus 13 months (HR 1.57; 95 % CI 1.06–2.32).
- Unfortunately, despite the above, limited gains made in OS.

- Moore et al. attempted to help identify patients a priori who were unlikely to respond to cytotoxic therapy (*Moore criteria*).
  - Identified 5 factors independently prognostic of poor response: African-American, PS > 0, pelvic disease, prior radiosensitizer, and time interval from diagnosis to first recurrence <1 year.
  - Patients with 4–5 risk factors had a RR of only 13 %, and median PFS and OS of 2.8 and 5.5 months, respectively.

Exploration of Non-platinum Doublets

- With early closure of GOG 204, the cervical cancer committee was tasked with development of a replacement phase 3 protocol.
- *GOG 240* was designed as a 4 arm trial, with cisplatin + paclitaxel (with or without bevacizumab) being compared with topotecan + paclitaxel (with or without bevacizumab) [29] (Table 2.13) [24–28].
  - Four hundred and fifty-two patients accrued onto study. Notably the majority of patients on each backbone had a PS of 0, and 75 % of the entire cohort had previously received platinum (even between arms).
  - Topotecan + paclitaxel was not shown to be superior or inferior to cisplatin + paclitaxel (HR 1.20; 95 % CI 0.82–1.76).
  - Importantly, the investigators showed a significant improvement in OS in the bevacizumab containing arms relative to non-bevacizumab controls (17 months vs. 13.3 months, respectively; HR 0.71; 95 % CI 0.54–0.95; $p = 0.0035$).
  - Analogous improvements in PFS were identified (8.2 months bevacizumab containing arm and 5.9 months in control arm (HR 0.67; 95 % CI 0.54–0.82; $p = 0.0002$).
  - Exploratory sub-analysis indicated the beneficial effects of bevacizumab in patients with prior platinum

Table 2.14. GOG 240 Schema and regimens [29].

Trial	Eligibility	Arms	Conclusion
GOG 240	Metastatic, recurrent, or persistent SCC, AS, or adenocarcinoma	• Paclitaxel 135 mg/m^2 over 24 h or 175 mg/m^2 over 3 h • Cisplatin 50 mg/m^2 on day 1 or 2 • Paclitaxel 135 mg/m^2 over 24 h or 175 mg/m^2 over 3 h • Cisplatin 50 mg/m^2 on day 1 or 2 • Bevacizumab 15 mg/kg • Paclitaxel 175 mg/m^2 • Topotecan 0.75 mg/m^2 • Paclitaxel 175 mg/m^2 • Topotecan 0.75 mg/m^2 • Bevacizumab 15 mg/kg	Patients who received Bevacizumab had 3.7 month improvement in OS

exposure, recurrent or persistent disease, and squamous histology. Importantly, the benefits of bevacizumab persisted in patients with recurrent disease in a previously irradiated field, which was hypothesized to be relatively hypoxic.

  - These findings represent the first time a targeted anti-angiogenic agent has shown an improvement in OS in patients with gynecologic cancer.

- Current new standard of care is based on results from GOG 240 recommending cisplatin, paclitaxel, and bevacizumab (see Table 2.14.) [29].
- Toxicity of bevacizumab on GOG 240.
  - Within the bevacizumab-containing arms, there was an increase in grade ≥3 GI and GU fistula ($n = 5$), as well as grade ≥2 hypertension, grade ≥4 neutropenia and grade ≥3 thrombocytopenia. This did not translate into a significant deterioration in HRQOL (FACT-Cx TOI).
  - The most common adverse events included HTN and proteinuria. Rare but serious adverse events included thromboembolic disease and GI/GU fistulas.

Beyond Angiogenesis in Cervical Cancer

- To date, the largest study exploring non-bevacizumab anti-angiogenic agents in the treatment of cervical cancer was reported in August 2010.
  - Monk et al. studied pazopanib and lapatinib as single agents and in combination in patients with Stage IVB persistent/recurrent cervical carcinoma not amenable to curative therapy and at least one prior regimen in the metastatic setting [30]. The primary end point was progression-free survival (PFS), and secondary end points were overall survival (OS), response rate (RR), and safety.
    - One hundred and fifty-two were randomly assigned to the monotherapy arms: pazopanib ($n=74$) or lapatinib ($n=78$). Importantly, the futility boundary was crossed at the planned interim analysis for combination therapy compared with lapatinib therapy, and the combination arm was terminated.
    - Pazopanib improved PFS (HR 0.66; 90 % CI, 0.48–0.91; $p=0.013$) and OS (HR 0.67; 90 % CI, 0.46–0.99; $p=0.045$). Median OS was 50.7 weeks and 39.1 weeks and RRs were 9 and 5 % for pazopanib and lapatinib, respectively. The only grade 3 AE>10 % was diarrhea (11 % pazopanib and 13 % lapatinib). Grade 4 AEs were 9 % (lapatinib) and 12 % (pazopanib).
    - The results of this phase 2 study confirmed the activity of anti angiogenic agents in advanced and recurrent cervical cancer and demonstrated the benefit of pazopanib based on the prolonged PFS and favorable toxicity profile.
- Sunitinib, an analogous, oral multi-TKI, exerts its antiangiogenic effects via inhibition of VEGFR-1, -2, and -3, PDGF α and β, and related receptor tyrosine kinases [31].
  - A phase 2 clinical trial was developed investigating the efficacy and safety of sunitinib in patients with unresectable, locally advanced or metastatic cervical carcinoma [32].

- A total of 19 subjects were enrolled on this multicenter phase II study. Unfortunately, there were no documented objective responses on therapy, with significant morbidity (fistula rate of 26 %).
- Median time to progression was reported as 3.5 months. Given lack of signal, it was determined that sunitinib has insufficient activity as a single agent in cervical cancer to warrant further investigation.

Anti-vascular Strategies in the Treatment of Cervical Cancer

- Interest into the study of *vascular disrupting agents* (VDAs) emerged in an effort to circumvent acquired resistance to traditional antiangiogenic therapies.
- VDAs result in a rapid and selective shutdown of tumor vasculature via destruction of endothelial cells [33].
- One of the best-studied agents within this class is combretastatin A-4 phosphate (CA4P), a synthetic, phosphorylated prodrug of the natural product combretastatin A-4 (CA4) [34]. It functions by binding β–tubulin subunits, preventing microtubule formation resulting in cytoskeletal changes within endothelial cells [35]. The anti-vascular effects of CA4P have been demonstrated in both in vitro and in vivo models, and appear to be the result of endothelial damage, leading to increased vascular resistance, reduced tumor blood flow, and central tumor necrosis [34, 35].
- The most extensively studied VDA in the treatment of cervical cancer is the investigational anticancer drug 5,6-dimethylxanthenone-4-acetic acid (DMXAA) [36].

  - In a phase 1 trial exploring DMXAA in the treatment of several solid tumors, DMXAA (22 mg/kg by intravenous infusion over 20 min) resulted in a partial response in one patient with metastatic cervical squamous carcinoma. Given the clinical and preclinical data, six separate VDA have been synthesized and are in various stages of phase 1 and 2 clinical trials exploring their efficacy in patients with solid tumors [37].

Pelvic Exenteration for Centrally Recurrent Cancers

- Total pelvic exenteration can be offered to certain patients with central pelvic recurrence after prior pelvic radiation with or without prior radical hysterectomy.
- Contraindications:
  - Lymphatic metastases.
  - Extension of disease to the pelvic sidewalls.
  - Distant metastases.
- Patients must be carefully selected, as they must be highly motivated to manage multiple ostomies and potential postoperative complications.
- Total pelvic exenteration removes the bladder, uterus, vagina, and rectum and requires extensive reconstruction including urinary conduid (continent or non-continent), low rectal anastomosis or frequently end colostomy, and potential vaginoplasty with split thickness skin graft or myocutaneous flaps. The salvage rate is 60–70 % with a 2 % mortality from the procedure.

Neoadjuvant Chemotherapy

- In certain situations, neoadjuvant chemotherapy is beneficial prior to surgery for cervical cancer. The chemotherapy used is often based on the "Buenos Aires Protocol":
  - Cisplatin 50 mg/m^2 day 1.
  - Vincristine 1 mg/m^2 day 1.
  - Bleomycin 5 mg/m^2 days 1–3 (3 cycles at 10 day intervals).

Cervical Cancer in Pregnancy

- Stage for stage, pregnancy does not worsen survival. Diagnosis is however often delayed during pregnancy.
- Recent studies suggest that there is no decrease in survival with treatment delay during pregnancy.
- Cesarean delivery is often recommended for invasive lesions due to friability of the tumor although vaginal delivery does not worsen prognosis.

- Consideration may be given for neoadjuvant chemotherapy during pregnancy, followed by surgical resection at the time of delivery.
- Ultimately, a multidisciplinary approach involving gynecologic oncology, maternal fetal medicine and neonatology is recommended in the management of these uncommon cases.

References

1. WHO/ICO Information Center of HPV and Cervical Cancer (HPV Information Center). Human Papillomavirus and Related Cancers in the World. Summary Report 2010.
2. Quinn M, Babb P, Jones J, Allen E. Effect of screening on incidence of and mortality from cancer of cervix in England: evaluation based on routinely collected statistics. BMJ. 1999; 318(7188):904–8.
3. Siegel R, Naishadham D, Jemal A. Cancer statistics. CA Cancer J Clin. 2013;63(1):11–30.
4. DiSaia PJ, Creasman WT. Clinical Gynecologic Oncology. 7th Edition, Mosby Publishers, Philadelphia, PA; 2007
5. Benedet JL, Odicino F, Maisonneuve P, et al. Carcinoma of the cervix uteri. Int J Gynaecol Obstet. 2003;83 Suppl 1:41–78.
6. DiSaia PJ, Creasman WT. Clinical Gynecologic Oncology. 8th edition. JExpert Consult online and print. Saunders Elsevier Inc., Philadelphia, PA, 2012
7. Peters 3rd WA, Liu PY, Barrett 2nd RJ, et al. Concurrent chemotherapy and pelvic radiation therapy compared with pelvic radiation therapy alone as adjuvant therapy after radical surgery in high-risk early-stage cancer of the cervix. J Clin Oncol. 2000;18(8):1606–13.
8. Keys HM, Bundy BN, Stehman FB, et al. Cisplatin, radiation, and adjuvant hysterectomy compared with radiation and adjuvant hysterectomy for bulky stage IB cervical carcinoma. N Engl J Med. 1999;340(15):1154–61.
9. Morris M, Eifel PJ, Lu J, et al. Pelvic radiation with concurrent chemotherapy compared with pelvic and para-aortic radiation for high-risk cervical cancer. N Engl J Med. 1999;340(15): 1137–43.
10. Whitney CW, Sause W, Bundy BN, et al. Randomized comparison of fluorouracil plus cisplatin versus hydroxyurea as an adjunct to radiation therapy in stage IIB-IVA carcinoma of the

cervix with negative para-aortic lymph nodes: a Gynecologic Oncology Group and Southwest Oncology Group study. J Clin Oncol. 1999;17(5):1339–48.

11. Rose PG, Bundy BN, Watkins EB, et al. Concurrent cisplatin-based radiotherapy and chemotherapy for locally advanced cervical cancer. N Engl J Med. 1999;340(15):1144–53.
12. Thigpen T, Shingleton H, Homesley H, Lagasse L, Blessing J. Cis-platinum in treatment of advanced or recurrent squamous cell carcinoma of the cervix: a phase II study of the Gynecologic Oncology Group. Cancer. 1981;48(4):899–903.
13. McGuire 3rd WP, Arseneau J, Blessing JA, et al. A randomized comparative trial of carboplatin and iproplatin in advanced squamous carcinoma of the uterine cervix: a Gynecologic Oncology Group study. J Clin Oncol. 1989;7(10):1462–8.
14. Sutton GP, Blessing JA, Adcock L, Webster KD, DeEulis T. Phase II study of ifosfamide and mesna in patients with previously-treated carcinoma of the cervix. A Gynecologic Oncology Group study. Invest New Drugs. 1989;7(4):341–3.
15. Fracasso PM, Blessing JA, Wolf J, Rocereto TF, Berek JS, Waggoner S. Phase II evaluation of oxaliplatin in previously treated squamous cell carcinoma of the cervix: a gynecologic oncology group study. Gynecol Oncol. 2003;90(1):177–80.
16. Schilder RJ, Blessing JA, Morgan M, Mangan CE, Rader JS. Evaluation of gemcitabine in patients with squamous cell carcinoma of the cervix: a Phase II study of the gynecologic oncology group. Gynecol Oncol. 2000;76(2):204–7.
17. Thigpen T, Blessing JA, Gallup DG, Maiman M, Soper JT. Phase II trial of mitomycin-C in squamous cell carcinoma of the uterine cervix: a Gynecologic Oncology Group study. Gynecol Oncol. 1995;57(3):376–9.
18. Bookman MA, Blessing JA, Hanjani P, Herzog TJ, Andersen WA. Topotecan in squamous cell carcinoma of the cervix: a phase II study of the Gynecologic Oncology Group. Gynecol Oncol. 2000;77(3):446–9.
19. Look KY, Blessing JA, Levenback C, Kohler M, Chafe W, Roman LD. A phase II trial of CPT-11 in recurrent squamous carcinoma of the cervix: a gynecologic oncology group study. Gynecol Oncol. 1998;70(3):334–8.
20. Curtin JP, Blessing JA, Webster KD, et al. Paclitaxel, an active agent in nonsquamous carcinomas of the uterine cervix: a Gynecologic Oncology Group Study. J Clin Oncol. 2001;19(5):1275–8.

21. Garcia AA, Blessing JA, Vaccarello L, Roman LD. Phase II clinical trial of docetaxel in refractory squamous cell carcinoma of the cervix: a Gynecologic Oncology Group Study. Am J Clin Oncol. 2007;30(4):428–31.
22. McGuire WP, Blessing JA, Moore D, Lentz SS, Photopulos G. Paclitaxel has moderate activity in squamous cervix cancer. A Gynecologic Oncology Group study. J Clin Oncol. 1996;14(3):792–5.
23. Muggia FM, Blessing JA, Method M, et al. Evaluation of vinorelbine in persistent or recurrent squamous cell carcinoma of the cervix: a Gynecologic Oncology Group study. Gynecol Oncol. 2004;92(2):639–43.
24. Omura GA, Blessing JA, Vaccarello L, et al. Randomized trial of cisplatin versus cisplatin plus mitolactol versus cisplatin plus ifosfamide in advanced squamous carcinoma of the cervix: a Gynecologic Oncology Group study. J Clin Oncol. 1997;15(1):165–71.
25. Bloss JD, Blessing JA, Behrens BC, et al. Randomized trial of cisplatin and ifosfamide with or without bleomycin in squamous carcinoma of the cervix: a gynecologic oncology group study. J Clin Oncol. 2002;20(7):1832–7.
26. Moore DH, Blessing JA, McQuellon RP, et al. Phase III study of cisplatin with or without paclitaxel in stage IVB, recurrent, or persistent squamous cell carcinoma of the cervix: a gynecologic oncology group study. J Clin Oncol. 2004;22(15):3113–9.
27. Long 3rd HJ, Bundy BN, Grendys Jr EC, et al. Randomized phase III trial of cisplatin with or without topotecan in carcinoma of the uterine cervix: a Gynecologic Oncology Group Study. J Clin Oncol. 2005;23(21):4626–33.
28. Monk BJ, Sill MW, McMeekin DS, et al. Phase III trial of four cisplatin-containing doublet combinations in stage IVB, recurrent, or persistent cervical carcinoma: a Gynecologic Oncology Group study. J Clin Oncol. 2009;27(28):4649–55.
29. Tewari KS, Sill MW, Long 3rd HJ, et al. Improved survival with bevacizumab in advanced cervical cancer. N Engl J Med. 2014;370(8):734–43.
30. Monk BJ, Mas Lopez L, Zarba JJ, et al. Phase II, open-label study of pazopanib or lapatinib monotherapy compared with pazopanib plus lapatinib combination therapy in patients with advanced and recurrent cervical cancer. J Clin Oncol. 2010;28(22):3562–9.

31. Chow LQ, Eckhardt SG. Sunitinib: from rational design to clinical efficacy. J Clin Oncol. 2007;25(7):884–96.
32. Mackay HJ, Tinker A, Winquist E, et al. A phase II study of sunitinib in patients with locally advanced or metastatic cervical carcinoma: NCIC CTG Trial IND.184. Gynecol Oncol. 2010; 116(2):163–7.
33. Chaplin DJ, Pettit GR, Parkins CS, Hill SA. Antivascular approaches to solid tumour therapy: evaluation of tubulin binding agents. Br J Cancer Suppl. 1996;27:S86–8.
34. Bilenker JH, Flaherty KT, Rosen M, et al. Phase I trial of combretastatin a-4 phosphate with carboplatin. Clin Cancer Res. 2005;11(4):1527–33.
35. Salmon HW, Siemann DW. Effect of the second-generation vascular disrupting agent OXi4503 on tumor vascularity. Clin Cancer Res. 2006;12(13):4090–4.
36. Zhou S, Kestell P, Baguley BC, Paxton JW. 5,6-Dimethylxanthenone-4-acetic acid (DMXAA): a new biological response modifier for cancer therapy. Invest New Drugs. 2002;20(3): 281–95.
37. Lippert 3rd JW. Vascular disrupting agents. Bioorg Med Chem. 2007;15(2):605–15.

Chapter 3
Cancer of the Vulva and Vagina

Lauren Krill and Leslie M. Randall

Abbreviations

AJCC	American Joint Committee on Cancer
CCA	Clear cell adenocarcinoma
DVT	Deep vein thrombosis
EBRT	External beam radiation
5-FU	5-Fluorouracil
GM	Gracilis myocutaneous flap
GOG	Gynecologic Oncology Group
HPV	Human papillomavirus
FIGO	International Federation of Gynecology and Obstetrics
IFLND	Inguinofemoral lymphadenectomy
IMRT	Intensity-modulated radiotherapy
ISSVD	International Society for the Study of Vulvar Diseases
LDH	Lactate dehydrogenase
LSG	Lymphoscintigraphy
MRI	Magnetic resonance imaging
PE	Pulmonary embolism
PET	Positron emission tomography

L. Krill, M.D., M.S. (✉) • L.M. Randall, M.D.
Division of Gynecologic Oncology, Department of Obstetrics and Gynecology, Irvine Medical Center, University of California, 101 The City Drive, Orange, CA 92868, USA
e-mail: lsmithkr@uci.edu; lrandall@uci.edu

R.N. Eskander and R.E. Bristow (eds.), *Gynecologic Oncology: A Pocketbook*, DOI 10.1007/978-1-4939-1976-5_3,

RT	Radiation therapy
SCC	Squamous cell carcinomas
SEER	Surveillance Epidemiology End Report
SLN	Sentinel lymph node
SLNB	Sentinel lymph node biospy
SRS	Stereotactic radiosurgery
TNM	TNM classification of malignant tumors
USA	United States of America
VAIN	Vaginal intraepithelial neoplasia
VIN	Vulvar intraepithelial neoplasia
WHO	World Health Organization

Vulvar Cancer

Epidemiology

- Vulvar carcinoma accounts for approximately 4 % of gynecologic malignancies.
- In the USA during 2013, there will be 4,700 new diagnoses of vulvar cancer and approximately 990 related deaths [1].
- The most common histology is squamous cell carcinoma (SCC) followed by melanoma and adenocarcinoma (Fig. 3.1).
- Peak incidence is between 65 and 75 years of age and the median age at diagnosis is 68.
- Recent series suggest vulvar cancers etiologically related to human papillomavirus infection (HPV) infection present at a younger age than non-HPV related cancers [3].
- Risk factors for invasive vulvar cancer depend on two distinct etiologic pathways:
  - Keratinizing, well-differentiated carcinomas arise in the background of vulvar dystrophy, such as lichen sclerosus or squamous hyperplasia.
  - Non-keratinizing carcinomas develop from malignant transformation of dysplastic conditions related to HPV infection, smoking, or immunosuppresion.

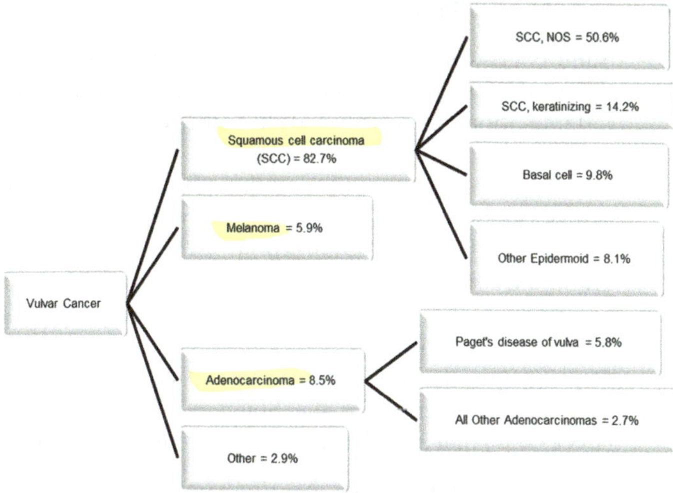

FIG. 3.1. Histolopathologic Types of Carcinoma of the Vulva: SEER Data 1988–2001 [2]. Data source: Kosary CL. Cancer of the Vulva. In: Ries LAG, Young JL, Keel GE, Eisner MP, Lin YD, Horner M-J (editors). SEER Survival Monograph: Cancer Survival Among Adults: U.S. SEER Program, 1988–2001, Patient and Tumor Characteristics. National Cancer Institute, SEER Program, NIH Pub. No. 07-6215, Bethesda, MD, 2007 [2].

 - Quadrivalent HPV vaccination is effective against HPV types 16, 18, 6, and 11 and the expectation is that immunization will decrease the incidence of vulvar cancers related to HPV in the future.

Diagnosis/Screening

- *Screening:* There is no screening test for vulvar cancer.
  - Patients with a history of cervical or vaginal cancer should be monitored closely with systematic inspection of the vulva with or without colposcopy.
  - Regular surveillance should also be standard practice for patients with lichen sclerosus or past history of vulvar intraepithelial neoplasia (VIN).

- Natural History/Preinvasive lesions.
  - Tumors grow slowly over several years, resulting from either prolonged mucosal HPV infection or chronic inflammation due to vulvar dystrophies or autoimmune processes.
  - VIN is often a precursor lesion that precedes malignant transformation to invasive SCC of the vulva and as such the World Health Organization (WHO) prefers to grade VIN the same as cervical intraepithelial lesions according to the degree of abnormality (e.g., VIN 1, VIN2, and VIN3).
  - Current terminology was modified in 2004 by the International Society for the Study of Vulvar Diseases (ISSVD) [4] that introduced three different subcategories:
    - VIN, usual type (warty, basaloid, or mixed).
    - VIN, differentiated is now used to describe what was previously referred to as VIN simplex type (not HPV related).
    - VIN, unclassified encompasses VIN that cannot be classified into either of the above groups including pagetoid type cells.
    - The VIN 1 category was eliminated (because the diagnosis is not reliably reproducible and the findings are associated with HPV effect or reactive changes, not a precancerous lesion).
  - Thus, the term VIN is reserved for histologically high-grade squamous cell lesions.
    - VIN 2 and VIN 3 were combined since they are difficult to differentiate and would both be treated as high-grade preinvasive dysplasia.
    - Instead, VIN is divided into two diagnostic categories (usual and differentiated type) that more accurately reflect the etiology (+/– HPV) and clinical characteristics of the SCC variants they are associated with (see details in Sect. 1.4).

- Clinical presentation.
  - Vulvar cancer may be asymptomatic but pruritis is the most common symptom.
  - Approximately 50 % present with a lump or ulcer on the vulva (or less commonly in the groin from metastases to lymph nodes).
  - Clinicians should have a low threshold to biopsy any suspicious vulvar abnormalities, because the appearance of malignant lesions is often similar to that of benign processes.
    - Frequently, this may result in delays in diagnosis from patients ignoring symptoms or physicians attempting topical therapy without definitive diagnosis.
- Pretreatment evaluation.
  - Pathologic diagnosis is obtained using wedge or Keyes biopsy.
  - Clinical assessment with thorough history and physical exam including palpation of groin lymph nodes and complete pelvic with Pap smear if cervix remains in situ and colposcopy of the entire cervix, vagina, and vulva.
  - Imaging with PET or MRI for the evaluation of lymph nodes and soft tissues as appropriate.
  - Imaging is more sensitive than physical exam for detecting inguinal lymph node involvement; however, inflammatory processes may lead to false positive findings.
  - Prior to initiating treatment, it is important to disclose the risks and benefits of treatment with particular attention to counseling on sexual function after treatment.
- Mode of spread.
  - The majority of vulvar cancers are confined to the vulva.
  - Initially local spread extends to contiguous skin and larger lesions can invade adjacent structures vagina, urethra, and rectum.

- Pattern of lymphatic spread is typically predictable and stepwise to ipsilateral superficial inguinal nodes followed by deep inguinal/femoral and pelvic nodes. Anatomic variations occur in a small percentage of women.
- Metastatic sites including pelvic nodes (external, hypogastirc, obturator, and common iliac) are considered distant site involvement.
- Hematogenous dissemination is rare except in malignant melanoma.

Staging

- The International Federation of Gynecology and Obstetrics (FIGO) employ a surgical staging scheme that incorporates major determinants of prognosis such as primary tumor size and laterality, lymph-node metastasis, and distant spread to other organs (see Table 3.1) [5].
- Depth of invasion is strictly measured from the epithelial-stromal junction of the most superficial dermal papillae to the deepest point of invasion.
- Complete staging requires resection of the primary tumor and complete inguinofemoral and pelvic lymphadenectomy to accurately determine nodal status if lesions are >1 mm in depth.
- However, excisional biopsy of sentinel lymph nodes is frequently used to assign stage and guide further treatment in an effort to avoid the morbidity associated with complete groin dissections (for detailed discussion see Sect. 1.5).
- Accurate surgical staging is critical. Detecting the presence or absence of lymph node involvement at initial diagnosis is not only prognostic, but can also impact therapeutic efficacy by permitting modifications to the treatment plan and improving the probability of cure.
  - The prognostic significance of the number and size of nodal metastases are reflected in the recent revisions made to the FIGO staging system.

TABLE 3.1. FIGO staging classification of vulvar cancer and 5-year overall survival.

Stage[a] (TNM)	Description	Treatment	5-Year survival (%)
I (T1)	Tumor confined to vulva or perineum		79–92
IA	Tumor confined to vulva or perineum; lesion ≤2 cm with stromal invasion ≤1 mm, no nodal metastasis	Radical local excision	
IB	Tumor confined to vulva or perineum; lesion >2 cm or stromal invasion >1 mm, with negative nodes	Radical local excision with ipsilateral or bilateral inguinofemoral lymphadenectomy (IFLND)[b]	
II (T2)	Tumor of any size with extension to adjacent perineal structures (lower 1/3 urethra, lower 1/3 vagina, anus) with negative nodes	Radical local excision with bilateral IFLND	58–78
III (T3)	Tumor of any size with or without extension to adjacent perineal structures with positive inguinofemoral lymph nodes		43–55
IIIA	(1) With 1 lymph node metastasis (≥5 mm) or (2) One to two lymph node metastasis(es) (<5 mm)	Radical local excision with ipsilateral or bilateral IFLND[b] Adjuvant pelvic and bilateral groin RT[c]	
IIIB	(1) With two or more lymph node metastases (≥5 mm) or (2) Three or more lymph node metastases (<5 mm)		
IIIC	With positive nodes with extracapsular spread		

(continued)

TABLE 3.1. (continued)

Stage[a] (TNM)	Description	Treatment	5-Year survival (%)
IVA (T4)	(1) Tumor invades upper urethra and/or vaginal mucosa, bladder mucosa, rectal mucosa, or fixed to pelvic bone fixed or (2) Ulcerated inguinofemoral lymph nodes	Radical local excision with bilateral IFLND, remove all enlarged groin and pelvic nodes Unresectable nodes should receive preoperative RT +/– chemotherapy	13–28
IVB	Spread to distant sites or pelvic lymph nodes	Supportive care +/– palliative chemotherapy or radiation	

[a]FIGO Stage and TNM classification, *T* primary tumor, *N* regional lymph nodes (N0-no palpable nodes; N1-Nodes palpable in either groin, not enlarged, mobile; N2-Palpable enlarged firm nodes in either or both groins; N3-fixed or ulcerated nodes), *M* distant metastases (M0-none; M1 palpable deep pelvic nodes; M1b-other distant metastases)

[b]Performance of bilateral IFLND depends on the location of the lesion, size, and unilateral Groin status

[c]Observation may be sufficient after surgery for one intracapsular micrometastasis (<5 mm) but reported series are too small to draw definitive conclusions and current studies are on-going

- Depth of invasion and lymphovascular space involvement are prognostic measures for the risk of nodal disease.

The incidence of groin lymph node metastases are: 10, 26, 64, and 89 % for Stages I–IV, respectively.

- Fifteen to 20 % of patients with positive groin nodes also have metastases to pelvic nodes; almost all patients with positive pelvic nodes will have clinically suspicious groin nodes and on pathology ≥3 positive groin nodes and invasion >4 mm [6, 7].
- Overall, the incidence of metastasis to pelvic lymph nodes is less than 10 % and pelvic lymphadenectomy is no longer performed routinely, as this did not translate into improved survival outcomes.

Pathology/Histology

- *Squamous cell carcinomas* (*SCC*) account for 80–90 % of vulvar malignancies.
  - Keratinizing subtype—represents more than 70 % of SCC; is not related to HPV and occurs in older women. These lesions tend to be unifocal, and a significant number are associated with atrophic lesions, such as lichen sclerosus. Precursor lesion is differentiated VIN (or VIN simplex type). Microscopically, it consists of invasive nests of malignant squamous epithelium and central keratin pearls.
  - Warty and basaloid carcinomas are associated with high-risk HPV types, predominantly HPV 16, 18, and 33. Precursor lesion is the classic or usual type of VIN. May be multifocal, occurs in younger women for whom the risk of progression to invasive carcinoma is approximately 6 % but the risk is higher in older women or immunosuppressed populations.

- *Verrucous Carcinoma* is a distinct variant of squamous carcinoma that occurs in postmenopausal women that present as large, fungating masses that may be misidentified as condyloma.
  - Commonly associated with HPV 6 or 11.
  - The histologic appearance of verrucous carcinoma includes large nests of squamous cells with abundant cytoplasm, small bland nuclei, mitoses are rare but squamous pearls are common. This may be differentiated from condyloma acuminata by the absences of fibrovascular cores (connective tissues within the proliferating papillary masses of the tumor) that are typical of condyloma acuminata. To establish the diagnosis biopsies must be sufficiently deep to obtain underlying stroma.
  - Lymph node metastasis is exceedingly rare, but deep local invasion and local tumor recurrences are common.
  - Treatment consists of radical local excision. Lymphadenectomy is of limited value except with clinically suspicions lymph nodes. Radiation therapy is contraindicated because it is ineffective and may lead to increased aggressive behavior within this tumor.
- *Basal Cell Carcinoma* constitutes <10 % of vulvar cancers.
  - Unlike other basal cell carcinomas of the skin ultraviolet light exposure plays no role in carcinogenesis, but histologically these lesions are identical.
  - Grossly, appears as flesh colored to pearly white nodules or plaques that are often ulcerated centrally.
  - They are usually local invasive and rarely metastasize, and wide local excision is the recommended treatment.
  - The prognosis is good despite a 20 % risk of local recurrence.
- *Bartholin's Gland Carcinomas* are rare representing less than 1 % of vulvar neoplasms
  - Cell types that give rise to Bartholin's gland carcinomas include adenomatous, squamous, adenosquamous, and adenoid cystic.

- Enlargement in the Bartholin gland in postmenopausal women is presumed to be a neoplasm until proved otherwise and biopsy of all suspicious lesions is recommended in women age 40 and older.
- Unfortunately, given the extensive vascular and lymphatic supply in this area, metastatic disease is common

- *Malignant Melanoma* of the vulva is uncommon, but is the second most common primary cancer of the vulva (5–10 %).

  - Melanomas are typically raised lesions, with irregular pigmentation and borders or ulcerations that probably arise from junctional or compound nevi. They usually occur on the labia majora or clitoris, but also on mucosal surfaces.
  - Histology is similar to melanomas of other skin areas but in difficult cases be confirmed in conjunction with immunohistochemisty staining for melanoma markers S-100 antigen and Melanoma specific (HMB) antibody.

    - There are several microstaging systems for vulvar melanoma that are summarized in Table 3.2.

  Clark's and Breslow systems are based on depth of invasion and tumor thickness, respectively. Chung modified Clark's level to account for morphologic differences in the vulva and vagina [11].
  - Prognosis depends primarily on tumor size, thickness and on the presence or absence of lymph node involvement which is captured in the American Joint Committee on Cancer (AJCC) TNM criteria [12] that further subdivide staging of cutaneous melanomas by tumor ulceration, mitotic rate, microscopic tumor burden in lymph nodes, and lactate dehydrogenase (LDH) levels in metastatic disease (see Table 3.3).
  - Radical local excision is standard for the primary lesion [13] and if limited to the vulva with negative lymph nodes the survival is good. Although nodal status has prognostic significance, regional lymphadenectomy has a more prognostic role than therapeutic and sentinel lymph node biopsy should be considered.

TABLE 3.2. Microstaging classification systems of melanoma of the vulva [8–10].

	Clark [8]	Chung [9]	Breslow [10]
I	Intraepithelial	Intraepithelial	<0.76 mm
II	Tumor extends into papillary dermis	Invasion ≤1 mm from granular layer	0.76–1.50 mm
III	Tumor filling dermal papillae	Invasion 1.1–2 mm from granular layer	1.51–2.25 mm
IV	Tumor extends into reticular dermis	Invasion >2 mm deeper than granular layer	2.26–3.0 mm
V	Tumor extends into subcutaneous fat	Into subcutaneous fat	>3.0 mm

TABLE 3.3. American Joint Committee on Cancer TNM staging for cutaneous melanoma [12].

Stage group	TNM clinical staging			Thickness (mm)	Ulceration	Mitotic rate
IA	T1a	N0	M0	<1.0	None	<1 mitoses/mm^2
IB	T1b	N0	M0	<1.0	Present	>1 mitoses/mm^2
	T2a	N0	M0	1.01–2.0	None	
IIA	T2b	N0	M0	1.01–2.0	Present	
	T3a	N0	M0	2.0–4.0	None	
IIB	T3b	N0	M0	2.0–4.0	Present	
	T4	N0	M0	>4.0	None	
IIC	T4	N0	M0	>4.0	Present	
III	Any T	N1-3[a]	M0			
IV	Any T	Any N	M1			

[a]Clinical staging includes microstaging of the primary melanoma after excision. Further classification of regional lymph nodes is included in final Pathologic Staging (for details please refer to the 7th Edition Final Version of 2009 AJCC Melanoma Staging and Classification originally published by the American Society of Clinical Oncology. J Clin Oncol Vol 27; 2009) [12]

- Five-year survival is lower than for cutaneous melanomas and vulvar SCC at 36 % [11].
- The prognosis is very poor with positive inguinal or pelvic nodes and most of these patients die as a result of their disease.
- In high risk patients or recurrent settings, the use of radiation, chemotherapy, biologic agents and immunotherapies are tailored to the individual patient.

- *Extramammary Paget's Disease of the Vulva* is rare.
  - Well demarcated patches of erythematous thickened areas and islands of white epithelium with foci of excoriation and induration are apparent on gross examination.
  - On histology these lesions contain diagnostic cells (Paget cells) with copious pale cytoplasm that infiltrate the epithelium and are interspersed among normal keratinocytes and often mixed inflammatory infiltrates of lymphocytes and plasma cells are noted in the underlying dermis. If the disease is limited to the epithelium, its clinical course is usually prolonged and indolent but approximately one-third of patients will develop recurrences after surgery.
  - Rarely the disease may have an invasive component or secondary infiltration of the vulvar skin with pagetoid cells that can result from an underlying primary adenocarcinoma of the apocrine glands.
  - The prevalence of these conditions reported in the literature varies widely and the risk of concomitant carcinomas at other sites has become fairly controversial.
  - The largest series reviewed 100 cases of Paget's disease of the vulva and the prevalence of invasive Paget's disease was 12 % and concurrent adenocarcinoma was identified in 4 % of patients [14].
  - Invasive Paget's disease in women can be associated with concomitant carcinoma at other sites (e.g., breast, colon, or genitourinary cancer); thus, the workup should include colonoscopy, cystoscopy, mammogram, and colposcopy.
  - Treatment includes wide local excision or simple vulvectomy with 2- to 3-cm borders of uninvolved tissue in most cases, however, if an underlying adenocarcinoma or invasive Paget's disease is identified radical excision and inguinal lymphadenectomy is required.

Treatment Algorithm

Therapy for Early Vulvar Cancer Stage I and II

The management of all invasive vulvar cancers involves careful consideration of the most appropriate surgical procedure for (1) excision of the primary tumor and (2) assessment of regional lymph nodes.

Primary Tumor

- Historically this involved en bloc radical vulvectomy and bilateral inguinofemoral lymphadenectomy using a butterfly-shaped incision (Fig. 3.2a) to remove vulva and groin lymph nodes with the intervening skin; results in high survival rates but unacceptable morbidity for many patients.
- Radical local excision (modified radical vulvectomy) is favored in contemporary practice and involves excision of the entire lesion with clinical margins of 1–2 cm laterally and dissection down to the perineal membrane (deep fascia of the urogenital diaphragm). Separate groin incisions (Fig. 3.2b) allow the intervening skin bridges between the vulva and unilateral or bilateral groin dissection to remain intact for improved healing.
- Survival appears to be equivalent in retrospective series between radical local incision and radical vulvectomy but using three separate incisions has significantly improved surgical morbidity and mortality [16, 17].

Treatment of Positive or Narrow Margins

- Shrinkage of tissue margins occurs in formalin-fixated specimens for histopathologic sectioning (microscopic 8 mm margins in fixed tissue specimens correspond to 1 cm clinical margins).
- Microscopic margins less than 8 mm are associated with significantly higher rates of local recurrence (48 %). None of the women in this study with negative surgical margins ≥8 mm experienced a local recurrence [18].

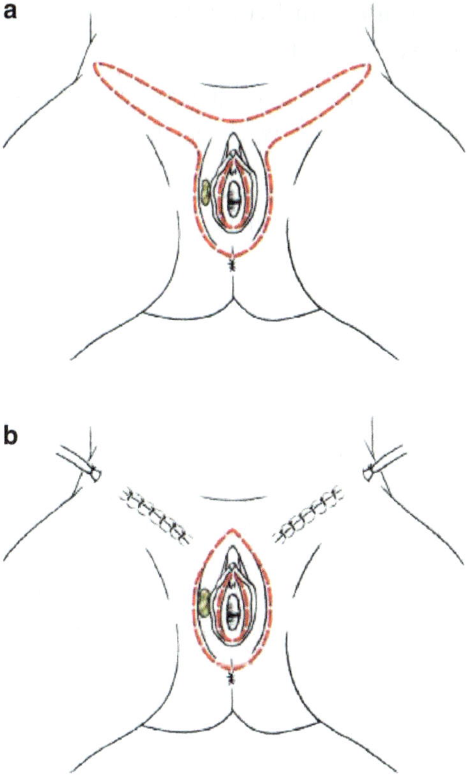

FIG. 3.2. Incisions for resection of vulvar cancer [15]. (**a**) Incision for en bloc radical vulvectomy with inguinal femoral lymphadenectomy. (**b**) Three separate incisions for the vulva or hemi-vulvectomy and both sides of the groin. Reprinted with kind permission from Springer Science and Business Media. From Horowitz IR. Female Genital System. In: Wood WC, Skandalakis JE, Staley CA, editors. Berlin: Springer; 2010 pp 637–78. [15].

- Re-excision is recommended to ensure complete resection of the primary lesion with adequate tumor-free margins.
- Postoperative radiation may be used if re-excision is not possible or if further surgery is declined by the patient.
- RT improves local control in high risk patients but local recurrences are frequently salvaged with additional surgery or radiation.

Management of Groin Lymph Nodes in Early Vulvar Cancer

- Appropriate treatment of the groin is the single most important factor in reducing mortality from vulvar cancer.
- The optimal approach is to determine the most appropriate operation for each individual patient—to maximize the likelihood of cure and minimize morbidity.
  - *Microinvasive or Stage IA* tumors have an extremely low incidence of lymphatic involvement (<1 %) therefore inguinofemoral lymphadenectomy (IFLND) may be omitted [19].
  - Patients with *Stage IB and Stage II* should undergo at least ipsilateral IFLND (with lateralized lesion >1 cm from midline) but the incidence of positive nodes in the contralateral groin is minimal and therefore unilateral dissection is acceptable.
  - Bilateral dissection is required for tumors that are <2 cm from midline or large (>4 cm), and for clinically suspicious lymph nodes.
  - If a positive unilateral lymph node is identified then dissection of the contralateral side is recommended as the risk of metastasis in this setting is as high as 18 %.
  - If all nodes are negative, no further treatment is necessary.
  - There is a high incidence of complications related to complete groin dissection and radiation but unexpected groin failures are universally fatal.

- Adjuvant pelvic and bilateral groin RT is recommended for patients with affected groin lymph nodes after IFLND with more than two micrometastases (<5 mm), one macrometastasis (>5 mm) or extracapsular spread given the evidence to date. However, there is significant morbidity associated with complete lymphadenectomy and RT.
- Radiation fields should include inguinal and femoral nodes as well as pelvic nodes distal to and including the bifurcation of the common iliac vessels using various methods.

- The recommended dose is dependent on the size and extent of nodal disease, approximate range is 50–60 Gy. Primary radiation of advanced gross vulvar disease requires 60–70 Gy for local control.
- Intensity-modulated radiotherapy (IMRT) may be used to reduce the dose to the femoral head and neck, pelvic bone, bladder, and rectum.

Alternative Methods for Approaching Lymph Nodes

Post-treatment complications related to the treatment of vulvar cancer have prompted investigators to study alternative methods to selectively identify patients who benefit from complete inguinofemoral lymphadenectomy versus those who may be spared unnecessary morbidity without compromising survival.

- *Primary Groin Radiation* (without groin dissection) after radical vulvectomy is less morbid acutely but is associated with significantly higher rates of groin recurrence and inferior survival compared to primary groin lymphadenectomy [20]. Investigators had hypothesized that prophylactic radiation of intact groins could be used to avoid lymph node dissection in low risk patients (to treat occult metastasis) but it is not recommended based on the results of *GOG 88* that closed prematurely due to the number of groin recurrences with RT compared to surgical dissection.
- *Superficial Lymphadenectomy* has been studied in an effort to reduce the extent of groin dissection.
- GOG 74.
- Prospective study of ipsilateral superficial lymphadenectomy and radical local excision for Stage I disease.
- The rate of recurrence diagnosed in the groin after negative superficial lymphadenectomy was 7 %. Significantly higher than historical controls in which groin relapse occurred in less than 1 % following en bloc radical vulvectomy and bilateral inguinofemoral lymphadenectomy.

- The number of patients who experienced recurrence in the operated groin may be attributed to anatomic variation in lymphatic drainage of the vulva and suggests the sentinel node is not always an ipsilateral superficial inguinal node and may actually be located in the deep femoral nodes or contralateral groin in 15 % of women.

Sentinel Lymph Node Biopsy

- The use of sentinel lymph node biopsy (SLNB) is based on the concept that the sentinel node is the first node to receive lymphatic drainage from the primary tumor and will be the first node to develop metastasis and can therefore be used to patients who do not need full regional lymphadenectomy.
- The practice of SLNB in early-stage vulvar cancer has increased in Europe and the U.S. following the publication of two landmark trials discussed below:
- GOG 173.
- Patients with primary tumor with >1 mm invasion and 2–6 cm in size underwent intraoperative lymphatic mapping and SLNB followed by unilateral or bilateral lymphadenectomy [21].
- Protocol: Intradermal injection of isosulfan blue (or 1 % methylene blue) is made at the leading edge of the primary tumor closest to the ipsilateral groin or on both sides for midline tumors; multiple peri-tumoral injections up to 2.5 ml on each side are permitted. Massage injection sites gently. The groin incision should be made a minimum of 5 min following injection, and if afferent lymphatic channel cannot be located in the groin a second injection of the primary site is permitted. Intraoperative radiolocalization can be performed after preoperative lymphoscintigraphy (LSG) with 0.5–1.0 ml of radiolabeled Tc99 microsulfur colloid, if done on the day of surgery, or the radionuclide is injected 1–6 h prior to the operation.
- Sentinel nodes were identified in 418 women out of 452 total subjects.
- Metastases were identified in 132 (31.6 %) node-positive women with 11 false-negative findings on SLNB.

- The sensitivity was 91.7 % which exceeded predetermined statistical target.
- The false-negative predictive value was 3.7 % overall and 2.5 % in tumors smaller than 4 cm and 7.4 % with larger tumors 4–6 cm in size.
- The combined method of detection using radio-colloid and blue dye improved the identification of sentinel lymph nodes.
- GROINSS V.
- Prospective observational study, patients underwent SLNB and resection of primary tumor for early-stage vulvar cancer (T1 or T2 <4 cm); inguinofemoral lymphadenectomy was performed only for patients with positive SLNB.
- Groin recurrences were observed in 3 % of patients with negative SLNB.
- Overall survival at 3 years was 97 % with substantially fewer postoperative complications.
- SLNB identifies patients with positive nodes who require full dissection and potentially additional treatment.
- Results in decreased perioperative morbidity including wound breakdown and lymphedema in node-negative patients who are unlikely to benefit from elective complete lymphadenectomy.
- Candidates for SLNB may benefit from preoperative LSG in order to determine if unilateral or bilateral dissection is appropriate.
- Ancillary study of GOG 173 confirmed bilateral IFLND is not always necessary and LSG is informative:
- *Laterally ambiguous* primary tumors (do not involve the midline but are less than 2 cm away) with exclusively ipsilateral drainage noted on LSG may safely undergo unilateral SLN.
- No SLN or positive groin nodes were identified in the contralateral side after full dissection in these patients [22].
- Furthermore, interesting variations in lymphatic patterns revealed more than one in five patients with *lateral* primary tumors will have bilateral drainage identified on LSG preoperatively; approximately one third of *midline* tumors demonstrated unilateral lymphatic drainage on LSG.

- Pathologic ultrastaging with serial step-sectioning (40–500 μm, interval varies by protocol) of SLN allows for detection of microscopic foci of tumor.
- The clinical relevance for the detection of isolated micrometastasis (<5 mm) is under investigation in vulvar cancer but given evidence to date, should be managed as metastatic disease; these patients are candidates for further therapy until the results of on-going observational studies on this topic, GOG270 and GROINSS VII, are available.
- The number and size of microscopic metastases has been correlated with the risk of recurrence and decrease disease-specific survival [23].
- There is small but definite risk for *false-negative results* with SLNB, especially with larger tumors, and after candid informed consent discussions regarding the risks, benefits and alternatives to SLNB some patients may elect to have full dissections despite the risk of treatment-related morbidity.
- Complete inguinofemoral lymphadenectomy technique:
- A linear skin incision is made parallel to the inguinal ligament 1 cm above the groin crease along the medial four-fifths of a line drawn between the anterior superior iliac spine and the pubic tubercle.
- Subcutaneous tissue is left and lymphoid tissue containing the superficial inguinal nodes are removed from along the saphenous vein inferior to the Camper's fascia and mobilized off the cribiform fascia that overlies the femoral vessels posteriorly. Preservation of the greater saphenous vein is common practice in order to minimize postoperative complications such as wound breakdown and chronic lymphedema without compromising oncologic outcomes [24, 25].
- The anatomic borders of the dissection form the femoral triangle, the inguinal ligament superiorly, the border of the Sartorius muscle laterally and adductor longus muscle medially.
- The deep inguinal or femoral nodes are located underneath the cribiform fascia medial to the femoral vein. The cribiform fascia can be opened along the Sartorius muscle at the time of superficial lymph node dissection; it is then

mobilized medially and the deep inguinal nodes are removed in continuity with the superficial nodes. Alternatively, the cribiform fascia may be preserved in order to reduce acute morbidity by opening the fascia medial to the femoral vein and removing only the adjacent nodes. The most proximal of the deep femoral nodes is commonly referred to as Cloquet's node.

Treatment for Advanced Vulvar Cancer

- *Stage III and IVA* primary tumors or bulky groin nodes may be treated with radical vulvectomy with bilateral groin dissection, chemoradiation, or pelvic exenteration.
  - Surgical excision of the primary tumor is preferred whenever feasible.
    - Resection of the primary lesion should result in clear surgical margins without sphincter damage resulting in fecal or urinary incontinence.
    - Notably, the distal 1 cm of the urethra may be removed without compromising urinary continence.
    - If primary surgery would require bowel or urinary stoma then primary chemoradiation should be considered to avoid exenteration.
    - Prior to surgery, cisplatin and 5 FU have been used effectively for neoadjuvant chemotherapy and for concomitant chemoradiation for the management of advanced lesions [26, 27].
  - Preoperative imaging is helpful in evaluating the status of the pelvic and groin lymph nodes prior to planning overall treatment.
    - Enlarged pelvic nodes on pretreatment imaging can be removed via extraperitoneal resection.
    - Clinically suspicious groin nodes should be surgically resected if possible (through separate incisions). However, complete lymphadenectomy with postoperative radiation may result in severe lymphedema

and therefore complete lymphadenectomy should be avoided if histologically positive nodes are confirmed on frozen section. Only enlarged groin and pelvic nodes should be removed followed by postoperative RT.

  - *GOG 37*: Pelvic and bilateral groin RT following radical vulvectomy and inguinal lymphadenectomy for node positive vulvar cancers significantly reduced local relapse rates and the number of cancer-related deaths compared to pelvic lymphadenectomy [28, 29].

- Alternatively, if vulvar tumors or fixed and ulcerated nodes are deemed unresectable, primary chemoradiation can be used to treat the primary tumor as well as groin and pelvic nodes.
- Postoperative resection of macroscopic residual disease may be performed in many cases after partial clinical response or a biopsy can be performed on the tumor bed to confirm complete clinical response.

  - *GOG 101:* patients with advanced nodal disease achieved high respectability rates following preoperative chemoradiation (cisplatin/5-FU) making unresectable nodes resectable (~95 %) with excellent control local control rates with complete pathologic response noted at time of surgery in the nodes and primary tumors of approximately 40 and 31 % of cases, respectively [27].
  - *GOG 205:* later showed combined RT and weekly cisplatin yielded high complete clinical response rates and complete pathologic responses in 64 and 50 % of patients (increased compared to 48 and 31 %, respectively, in GOG 101) with acceptable toxicity [30].

Vulvar Reconstruction

- Primary closure of vulvar defects without tension is usually possible with adequate planning and tissue mobilization. Healing by secondary intention or granulation is an alternative option to primary repair but the recovery phase is much longer.

- Closure of extensive dissections may be better accomplished in some cases using alternate tissue sources:
  - Skin Grafts
  - Split thickness or full thickness skin grafts can be harvested from the anteromedial thigh to cover defects in the vulva by relying on spontaneous connection between host and graft blood vessels.
  - Skin Flaps
  - There are many types of local and regional skin flaps. Local tissue advancement flaps derive their blood supply from the adjacent subcutaneous vascular networks. For example, Rhomboid Flaps—are transposition flaps developed by making V-shape incisions adjacent to the defect and dissecting subcutaneous tissue that can then be rotated over the defect and secured with absorbable sutures (Fig. 3.3).
  - Myocutaneous flaps—contain a segment of muscle that is supplied by a defined neurovascular bundle. Gracilis myocutaneous (GM) flaps are very common and versatile. They can be designed to cover virtually any defect of the vulva, perineum, vagina or groin. The short GM flap varies in size (length of 12–14 cm and width 5–7 cm) but is primarily used to cover unilateral vulvar or perineal defects not feasible by more conservative methods [11]. The long "classic" GM flap can be used for vaginal reconstruction (Fig. 3.4).

Postoperative Management

- Approximately 50–75 % will experience some type of early postoperative complications following radical vulvectomy and IFLND:
  - Wound dehiscence and infection.
  - Lymphocysts.
  - Osteitis pubis.

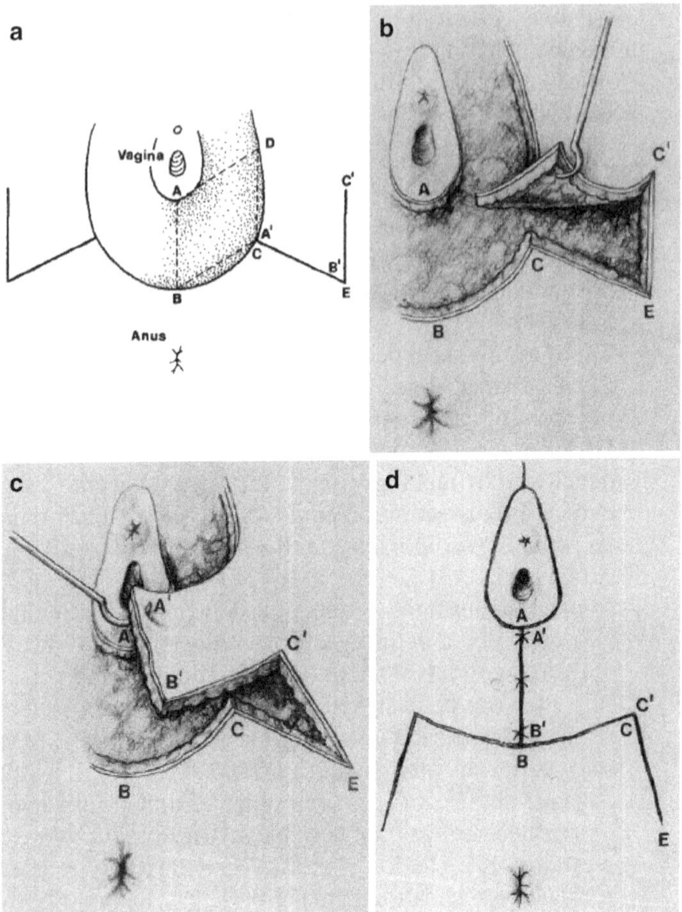

FIG. 3.3. Rhomboid flap closure for vulva [31, 32]. (**a**) Diagram of rhomboid flap design. (**b**) Flap raised. (**c**) Flap swung across to midline. (**d**) Flap in place. (**e**) Bilateral rhomboid flaps used to reconstruct the posterior vulvectomy defect and perineum. Appearance at the end of the procedure. Diagrams in Figs. 3.3a–3.3d reprinted with permission from Helm CW, Hatch KD, Partridge EE, Shingleton HM. The rhomboid transposition flap for repair of the perineal defect after radical vulvar surgery. Gynecol Oncol. 1993;50:164–7 [31]. Photo in Fig. 3.3e reprinted with permission from John HE, Jessop ZM, Di Candia M, et al. An algorithmic approach to perineal reconstruction—experience from two international centers. Ann Plast Surg. 2013;71:96–102 [32].

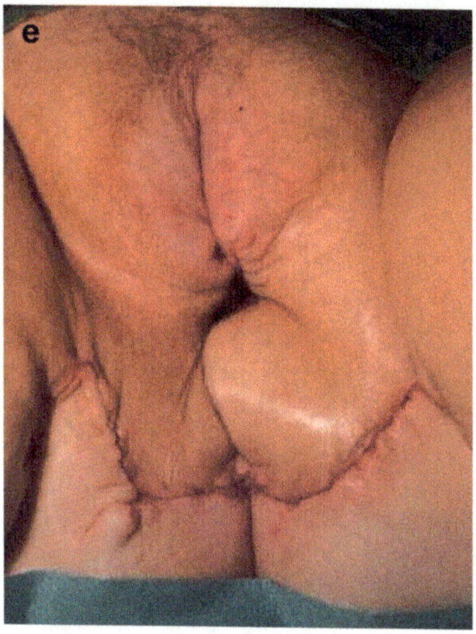

FIG. 3.3. (continued)

- Cellulitis and lymphangitis.
- Nerve injury/paresthesias.
- Lymphedema.
- Others including urinary tract infection, deep vein thrombosis (DVT), pulmonary embolism (PE), myocardial infarction, and hemorrhage.

• Preventative measures attempt to minimize immediate postoperative morbidity:

  - DVT and lymphedema prevention with thromboprophylaxis, compression stockings, and sequential pneumatic compression devices are particularly important because immobility in the immediate postoperative period; ambulation may be delayed at least 48 h depending of the surgical methods used. Delaying bowel function, restriction of body positioning and bed rest are intended to reduce contamination, stress, and tension on incisions but are also potentially problematic.
  - Closed suction drains and pressure dressing is used for groin incisions. Lymphocysts may form after IFLND in 7–40 % and may not be avoidable. Small asymptomatic

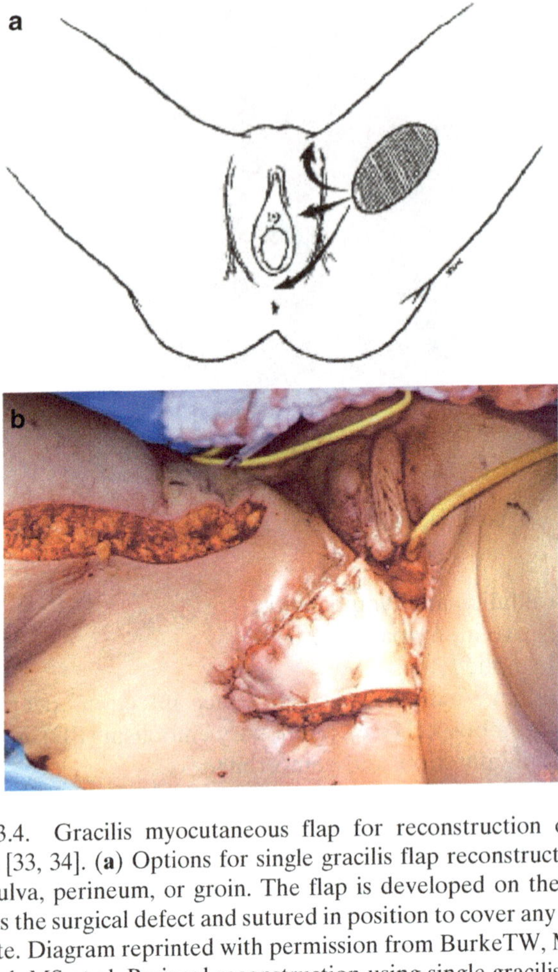

FIG. 3.4. Gracilis myocutaneous flap for reconstruction of the vulva [33, 34]. (**a**) Options for single gracilis flap reconstruction of the vulva, perineum, or groin. The flap is developed on the same side as the surgical defect and sutured in position to cover any external site. Diagram reprinted with permission from BurkeTW, Morris M, Roh MS et al. Perineal reconstruction using single gracilis myocutaneous flaps. Gynecol Oncol 1995;57:221–25 [33]. (**b**) Right sided gracilis myocutaneous flap tunneled after radical resection of post-radiation recurrence of vulvar carcinoma. Photo reprinted with permission from Fowler JM. Incorporating pelvic/vaginal reconstruction into radical pelvic surgery. Gynecol Oncol. 2009;115:154–61 [34].

lymphocysts may be observed. Incision and drainage can be used in this case of larger or symptomatic lymphocysts. Repeated aspiration increases the risk of infection and should be avoided, but injection of sclerosing agents may be indicated if lymphocysts persist.

- Wounds are routinely observed for infection or dehiscence and necrosis of skin flaps. Management is frequently outpatient with local care and healing by granulation. Debridement is rarely required.

Recurrent and Distant Metastatic Disease (IVB)

- Recurrences can be categorized into groups: local (vulva), groin, and distant.
- Local recurrences in the vulva can be surgically resected and achieve relative good outcomes (e.g., one study of patients with local recurrences reported survival of 51 % at 5 years) [35].
- Groin relapses are difficult to treat and even if detected early are associated with a high mortality rate.
- Distant metastases should be managed with systemic cytotoxic chemotherapy for palliation.

Post-treatment

- Surveillance following treatment should include physical exams, which is able to detect most recurrences, every 6 months for 2–3 years and then annually thereafter.
- Patient education regarding symptoms that require immediate evaluation should be clear—itching, pain, bleeding, visible changes, or palpable groin mass or swelling.

Complications from Treatment

- Overall incidence of significant long-term morbidity following treatment is 25 % and is correlated with the extent of therapy.

- Primary site complications after surgery—wound dehiscence is the most common.
- Groin complications: wound separation or infection, lymphedema, lymphocyst formation, and lymphangitis.
- There are limited effective treatment options for patients with debilitating lymphedema and the best progress in recent years has been seen in prevention, through removing fewer lymph nodes in less women.
- Irradiation leads to desquamation of vulvar skin to some degree in virtually all patients but regresses rapidly after completion of RT with acceptable cosmesis for most women.
- Premature ovarian failure may occur in young patients with RT and can also cause significant vaginal atrophy/dryness. There are no cancer related contraindications to hormone replacement therapy or vaginal estrogen.

Survival

- Median 5-year survival is 76 %, irrespective of histology.
- Survival rates by disease stage are listed in Table 3.1.
    - Histopathologic features of lymph node metastases including size, number and presence or absence of extracapsular spread have a significant impact on survival for patients with SCC of the vulva.
    - Patients with node-positive vulvar cancer showing only intracapsular positivity or metastasis less than 5 mm in diameter have a 5-year disease specific survival of almost 90 % that decreases to only 20 % in patients with larger or extracapsular metastases [36].

Preinvasive Disease of the Vulva (VIN) and Vaginal Intraepithelial Neoplasia (VAIN) Management

- The goal of therapy is to prevent the development of invasive cancer while preserving anatomy, normal tissue and function.

- Treatment of VIN or VAIN can be individualized to address location and extent of disease with the appropriate surgical or medical intervention.

VIN

- Surgical excision is the mainstay of therapy for high-grade lesions of the vulva. Options include wide local excision, simple vulvectomy, and CO_2 laser ablation.
  - Wide local excision is warranted if invasion cannot be excluded and is the preferred treatment of differentiated VIN because of the high malignant potential.
  - Laser ablation is beneficial in extensive multifocal lesions or if it is not feasible to obtain adequate margins with excision.
    - The CO_2 Laser using colposcopic guidance achieves precise control over the depth of desired destruction of 1–2 and 2–3 mm, for non-hair-bearing and hair-bearing areas, respectively. The intraepithelial lesion is effectively treated by vaporizing the epidermis, papillary dermis, and superficial reticular dermis, but the minimal residual thermal damage allows rapid healing with very little scarring. Postoperative pain management: oral narcotic analgesics, sitz baths, and topical 1 % lidocaine and 2 % silver sulfadiazine cream.
  - Vulvectomy is rarely indicated but may be used to manage extensive confluent lesions or patients who have failed all other therapies.
- Topical therapies: several drugs have been utilized to preserve vulvar anatomy but many are not FDA approved specifically for vulvar dysplasia.

Imiquimod

- Topical immune response modulator that affects local cytokine production and cell-mediated immunity that have indirect antitumor and antiviral effects.

- Dosing and administration: 0.25 g Imiquimod 5 % cream is applied topically only to the lesion 2–3 times per week before bedtime for 16 weeks, but the schedule can be modified based on side-effects and response. Sulfur precipitate 5 % in zinc oxide ointment can be applied the day after imiquimod to avoid super-infection [37].
- Adverse reactions are related mostly to inflammation at application site consisting of mild to moderate erythema, pruritis, erosion or painful ulceration.
- Several randomized controlled trials have shown that imiquimod is more effective than placebo for the treatment of VIN but it is still considered investigational for this purpose.

Topical 5-Fluorouracil (5-FU)

- 5-FU is a topical cream that causes chemical desquamation of VIN lesion and is very effective with response rates as high as 75 % but is not as well tolerated compared to other topical agents and is more commonly used for vaginal dysplasia (see below).
- Monitoring for intraepithelial or invasive squamous neoplasia every 6 months includes cervical and vaginal cytology (anal pap smears if involved) and careful inspection of the lower genital tract with colposcopy as needed. Smoking cessation and HIV testing should be encouraged.
- Approximately one-third of women will have recurrent VIN following treatment regardless of the modality.
- Long-term surveillance is recommended at 3 and 6 months following treatment then every 6 months for a total of 5 years and then annually thereafter.

VAIN

- Preinvasive squamous lesions of the vagina can also be treated by surgical excision, laser ablation, and topical therapy as well.

- Cure rates for all modalities are approximately 69–88 % [38].
- Exclusion of invasive disease is imperative prior to definitive therapy.
- If left untreated 30 % will progress to invasive cancer.
- Surgical management is the mainstay of treatment for VAIN.
  - Wide local excision (5 mm margins) or partial vaginectomy permits histologic diagnosis and exclusion of invasion. Specifically, surgery is indicated if there is any suspicion for invasion or involvement of the vaginal vault recesses after hysterectomy, in postmenopausal women or in those who have failed other therapies. Primary closure of the defect can usually be performed.
  - Laser vaporization-similar technique to that described for vulvar dysplasia as above. Generally well tolerated but side effect can include adhesions, synechiae, or stricture.
- Topical therapies for VAIN dosing, administration, and surveillance:
  - Topical treatment is simple and particularly useful for multifocal disease that does not involve the lower vagina, but complications can occur from chemical vulvovaginitis. The use of intermittent regimens and several preventive steps can be used to reduce these side effects.
  - 5-FU cream—Suppositories of 5 % 5-FU are placed in the top of the vagina at bedtime once per week for 10 weeks. Petroleum jelly should be applied liberally over the vulva, perineum, and anus to protect these areas. A tampon is then placed in the vagina to prevent leakage. The tampon is removed and the patient is advised to douche and bath the next morning to wash the cream out of the vagina.
  - Imiquimod—Recently, several investigators have reported reasonable side effect profiles and response rates in patients with VAIN using 0.25 mg of 5 % imiquimod cream intravaginally once weekly for 3 weeks [39]. Surveillance for resolution of any lesions

and irritation should be performed 8–12 weeks after completion of treatment.

- The most common adverse events of topical therapy are local irritation, burning or soreness, which are generally not severe enough to interrupt or discontinue therapy. As mentioned previously, petroleum jelly and zinc oxide cream can be used as prophylactic barrier to protect adjacent skin areas from ulceration during treatment and following treatment vaginal estrogen may reduce any residual discomfort.
- Historically, total vaginectomy and radiation have been used to treat VAIN but have fallen out of favor due the significant morbidity associated with these procedures.

Vaginal Cancer

Epidemiology

- Vaginal cancer is rare, representing only 1–2 % of female genital tract malignancies and is comprised of a heterogenous group of tumors.
- An estimated 2,890 new cases of vaginal cancer will be diagnosed in 2013 and approximately 840 related deaths will occur in the USA [1].
- The majority of primary vaginal cancers are SCC and the peak incidence occurs in the sixth and seventh decades of life.
  - Adenocarcinomas and other histologies are more common in younger patients.
- Primary lesions are classified as vaginal carcinomas only after the exclusion of cervical, urethral or vulvar origins. By convention, a neoplasm that involves both the cervix and the vagina is always considered to be a primary cervical cancer.
- The majority of vaginal neoplasms are metastases from other primary malignancies of the endometrium, cervix, or vulva. Less commonly, vaginal metastases can occur with non-gynecologic malignancies (kidney, breast, lung, etc).

- However, if the diagnosis occurs more than 5 years after a history of cervical carcinoma in situ or invasive cervical cancer (ICC) it is considered a new primary vaginal carcinoma.

Risk Factors for Invasive Vaginal Cancer

- Human papillomavirus infection (HPV): epidemiologic evidence suggests SCC of the vagina has strong relationship with HPV infection (nearly two-thirds are related to HPV16).
- History of ICC: Proposed mechanisms include the presence of occult residual disease, radiation induced tumorigenesis, or the development of new lesions from "field effect" related to shared exposure and/or susceptibility to carcinogenic stimuli in high-risk individuals.
- The natural history of preinvasive disease is difficult to characterize because VAIN is usually treated after it is diagnosed.
  - Despite treatment 3 % of VAIN 1 and 7 % of VAIN 2/3 progress to invasive cancer [40].
- Exposure to diethylstilbestrol (DES) in utero is a risk factor for clear cell adenocarcinoma of the vagina.

Diagnosis/Screening

Screening

- Routine screening programs have not been established. Pap smears are effective in detecting asymptomatic lesions. Abnormal results, especially with no gross cervical lesions, should prompt colposcopy of the vagina.
- Regular screening after hysterectomy for benign disease is not recommended. Although, it has been reported that 20–40 % of patients with primary vaginal cancer have had a prior hysterectomy for benign conditions [41].
- For history of DES exposure, annual Pap smear screening is indicated independent of sexual activity and HPV status and should begin at menarche or 14 years of age.

Clinical Presentation

- Painless vaginal discharge and postcoital or postmenopausal bleeding are common.
- Women with lesions involving compression or involvement of nearby organs may present with urinary complaints (e.g., dysuria, retention, or hematuria) or even gastrointestinal symptoms (e.g., tenesmus, constipation, melena) can occur.
- Pelvic pain may be associated with advanced disease.
- The remaining women are asymptomatic (approximately 5–10 %) and detected during routine physical examination or following abnormal Pap test.

Diagnosis

- Biopsy is needed to confirm diagnosis.

Pretreatment Evaluation

- Thorough history and physical with pelvic examination and visualization of the entire vagina that can be performed under anesthesia if needed.
- The gross morphology, dimensions, and location of the tumor including midline proximity and involved structures should be documented thoroughly during the clinical evaluation.
- Further diagnostic studies also include chest radiograph, possibly cystoscopy and proctosigmoidoscopy depending on tumor location, symptoms, and to confirm radiographic evidence of infiltration of other pelvic organs.
- Although, not used in staging computed tomography (CT), magnetic resonance imaging (MRI) or PET/CT can be used to assess lymph nodes and tumor volume for treatment planning.

Staging

- Staging is performed clinically rather than surgically based on the system established by the International Federation of Gynecology and Obstetrics (FIGO) [42] summarized in Table 3.4.

TABLE 3.4. FIGO staging classification of vaginal cancer and 5-year overall survival.

Stage	Description	Treatment	5-Year survival (%)
I	The carcinoma is confined to the vaginal wall	Surgical management[a] +/– adjuvant RT *or* primary RT with brachytherapy +/– EBRT	73–58
II	The carcinoma involves subvaginal tissue but does not extend to the pelvic sidewall	EBRT +/– brachytherapy +/– chemotherapy *or* surgical management[b] +/– adjuvant RT	58–78
III	The carcinoma extends to the pelvic sidewall[c]	EBRT +/– brachytherapy +/– chemotherapy	36–58
IV	The carcinoma extends beyond the true pelvis or involves the bladder or rectum; bullous edema not sufficient to be allotted to Stage IV		
IVA	Tumor invades bladder or rectal mucosa or there is direct extension beyond the true pelvis	EBRT +/– brachytherapy +/– chemotherapy *or* pelvic exenteration +/– RT +/– chemotherapy	18–21
IVB	Spread to distant organs	Supportive care +/– palliative chemotherapy or radiation	0–12

[a]Local excision with partial or total vaginectomy or Radical hysterectomy/vaginectomy +/– pelvic/inguinal node dissection (selection based on individual disease presentation)
[b]Radical hysterectomy/vaginectomy + parametrectomy +/– vulvectomy/inguinal node + pelvic lymphadenectomy, +/– para-aortic node dissection
[c]AJCC assigns involvement of the inguinal lymph nodes to Stage III

- Imaging can be used to evaluate lymph node status or distant metastasis.
- Sentinel lymph node biopsy is investigational and should be limited to research protocols.
- Vaginal cancer spreads by the following routes:
  - *Direct extension*. Advanced disease commonly involves local spread to adjacent pelvic soft tissues, bladder, rectum, and pelvic bones.

- *Lymphatic dissemination.* The pattern is dependent on a complex network of efferent lymphatics in the vagina and varies based on primary tumor location within the vagina.
  - Lymphatic metastasis from lesions in the upper third of the vagina spread to pelvic and para-aortic lymph nodes.
  - Tumors in the distal third of the vagina first spread to inguinofemoral and then pelvic nodes (reported rates are between 30 and 35 %).
- *Hematogenous spread* to distant organs is typically seen in advanced stages of the disease (e.g., lung, liver, or bone).

Pathology

- *Squamous Cell Carcinomas* represent 80–90 % of primary vaginal carcinomas and the histology resembles SCC of the cervix.
- *Adenocarcinoma* (clear cell, endometrioid, mucinous, and serous).
  - Accounts for approximately 10 % of primary vaginal cancers and peak incidence in the second decade of life.
  - Clear cell adenocarcinoma (CCA) may arise from areas of adenosis (97 %) which is commonly associated with exposure to diethylstilbestrol in utero.
  - Histology is identical to CCA of the ovary and endometrium, abundant clear cytoplasm due to large quantities of glycogen and hobnail cells with bulbous nuclei line the glandular lumina.
  - Prognosis of CCA is good and the overall survival is 78 %.
  - However, primary non-clear cell adenocarcinoma has worse prognosis, with high rates of distant metastasis (39 %) and lower 5-year overall survival rate of 34 % compared to 58 % in SCC [43].

- *Melanoma* constitutes 3 % of vaginal cancers and less than1% of malignant melanomas in women, highly aggressive tumors usually pigmented lesions in the distal vagina. Survival, like other melanomas, is related to depth of invasion and Clark's classification and staging per AJCC system. Overall 5 year survival is approximately 10 %.
- *Embryonal Rhabdomyosarcoma* (Sarcoma botryoides) is the most common malignant neoplasm of the vagina in infants. The gross appearance is confluent polypoid mass resembling a bunch of grapes and histologically consists of primitive spindle rhabdomyoblasts and myxomatous stroma.
- Other rare epithelial tumors include adenosquamous, adenoid cystic, neuroendocrine tumors and verrucous carcinomas.

Treatment: Overview of Indication for and Modes of Treatment

- Invasive vaginal cancers can be treated with *surgery and/ or radiation (RT)*.
- These methods are highly effective and even curative in early stage tumors, but there is no standard treatment with proven efficacy for metastatic disease.
- Chemotherapy for advanced vaginal cancer is not curative, and there are no standard drug regimens.
- Prospective clinical trial data is not available due to the low incidence of primary vaginal cancers and current treatment guidelines are mostly based on retrospective studies.
- Furthermore, head to head efficacy studies are not feasible to compare different modalities.
- Treatment planning decisions are influenced by many factors: clinical stage, tumor size and location, proximity to other important anatomic structures and psychosexual considerations (e.g., maintenance of a functional vagina).

Surgery

- Several surgical series have reported comparable or superior survival outcomes to primary RT in appropriately selected patients [44–47]. However, inherent selection bias may result from more unfavorable cases being managed by RT instead of aggressive surgery.
- An analysis of the National Cancer Data Base ($n=4{,}885$) demonstrated a statistically significant difference in 5-year survival between surgery and RT:
  - Stage I: surgery = 90 % versus RT alone = 63 %; both surgery and RT = 79 %.
  - Stage II: survival was also higher with surgery = 70 % compared to RT = 57 % [48].
- For Stage I disease surgery is preferred if negative surgical margins can be achieved with wide local excision or total vaginectomy with vaginal reconstruction for small superficial (<2 cm size or ≤0.5 cm thick) lesions but radical hysterectomy, partial vaginectomy and pelvic lymphadenectomy are required for larger and deeply invasive tumors (>0.5 cm thickness) [40].
- If narrow margins are noted after surgical resection adjuvant radiation is recommended.
- Carcinoma involving the distal third of the vagina necessitates dissection of groin nodes.
- Gross adenopathy should be excised and then irradiated.
- For Stage II–IV disease radical surgery may be the treatment of choice (radical hysterectomy/vaginectomy or pelvic exenteration with diverting surgeries) in very select patients (e.g., small volume central disease or rectovaginal or vesicovaginal fistula is present) alone or combined with irradiation.
- Pretreatment surgical staging and ovarian transposition is a reasonable approach in young patients who require radiation therapy.
- Neoadjuvant chemotherapy followed by radical surgery has been advocated by some as an alternative to primary RT or primary surgery in advanced disease [49].

Radiation

- Radiotherapy has historically been the treatment of choice for the majority of patients with vaginal cancer and can be delivered by external beam radiation (EBRT) or brachytherapy.
- Proper treatment planning should be tailored to the extent of disease, account for the depth of invasion, and aim to minimize acute and long term radiation sequelae.
- Several studies have reported combined modality therapy is better than EBRT or brachytherapy alone [50, 51].
  - EBRT delivers 4500–5000 Gy to the true pelvis using anteroposterior parallel-opposed fields extending to the level of L5-S1 superiorly, distally to approximately 3–4 cm below the caudad extent of disease, and 1–2 cm lateral to the pelvic brim, anterior to pubic symphysis and posterior to the junction of S2-3 [52].
  - In addition to EBRT, brachytherapy is important for locoregional control and methods for interstitial and intracavitary brachytherapy must be individualized.
  - However, brachytherapy alone is an accepted choice of treatment for favorable stage I tumors [41].
- For adequate local control the minimum dose of 75Gy is used to treat the primary tumor, if feasible, given normal tissue tolerances and the proximity of the bladder, urethra, and rectum to the vagina.
- In bulky Stage II–IVA disease, additional parametrial boost with midline shielding can be used to deliver up to 60 Gy to the pelvic sidewall. Similarly, boost to areas of positive nodes (pelvic or inguinal lymph nodes) should be given.
- RT to the inguinofemoral region should be considered electively if the primary tumor involves the middle to lower third of the vagina.
- Intensity modulated radiation therapy (IMRT) may lead to higher tumor control with less local normal tissue effects.
- RT is commonly administered along with concurrent cisplatin chemosensitization. Other agents that have been

used alone or in combination with RT, including 5-fluorouracil (5-FU) and mitomycin C.

  - The efficacy of cisplatin chemosensitization has not been rigorously evaluated in randomized controlled trials in vaginal cancer specifically.
  - It is common practice because of the proven benefit in disorders with analogous pathophysiology like cervical cancer [41].
  - Subsequent examination of Surveillance, Epidemiology End Report (SEER) data on primary vaginal cancers has confirmed an apparent survival advantage that coincided with the advent of this practice since 2000 [53].

- Palliative RT and supportive care is the preferred therapy for Stage IVB.

Recurrent Disease

- The risk of pelvic recurrence in Stage I and II vaginal cancers are 10–20 % and 30–40 %, respectively.
- Stage III–IVA even with high doses of RT pelvic control rates are relatively low; 50–70 % have persistent disease or locoregional recurrence and 25–40 % have failures at distant sites [54].
- The long-term prognosis is very poor for patients with distant recurrences or recurrences in previously radiated fields.
- RT options for patients with recurrent disease are limited due to toxicity and require extreme caution, but may be utilized in patients unable or unwilling to have surgery.
  - Stereotactic radiosurgery (SRS), also known as CyberKnife, may be considered in this setting.
- Pelvic exenteration may be an effective treatment for previously irradiated but isolated central pelvic recurrences or persistent disease.
- Surgery with intraoperative RT has also been reported in small series.

- Chemotherapy is limited typically to salvage treatment and is relatively ineffective.
  - *GOG 26:* There is a single phase II GOG study in recurrent vaginal SCC of cisplatin 50 mg/m^2 IV q 3 weeks. Most patients showed no response, one complete response (in patient with no prior therapy), and the remaining 5 out of 15 patients had stable disease [55].
- Special Considerations in the Treatment of Other Vaginal Cancers

Adenocarcinoma

- Managed similarly to SCC but patients are also younger and therefore every effort should be made to preserve ovarian and vaginal function if possible.
- Risk of pelvic lymph node involvement is 16 % in Stage I and over 30 % in Stage II.
- For early stage tumors involving the upper vagina the preferred treatment is radical hysterectomy, upper vaginectomy, and pelvic lymphadenectomy with ovarian preservation.
- Fertility-sparing local therapy options can be effective in early-stage CCA but may be associated with higher recurrences rates and therefore patients who have completed childbearing should undergo conventional therapy.
- Primary chemoradiation is preferred for advanced disease not amenable to surgical resection.

Melanoma

- Treatment of choice is primarily surgical resection which may or may not require radical procedures such as exenteration for complete resection.
- Lesions located in the lower third of the vagina are managed like vulvar melanomas (vaginectomy, vulvectomy and inguinal lymphadenectomy).
- Recently, more conservative operations with local excision, high-dose pelvic RT, chemotherapy and immunotherapy in various combinations have been utilized to

avoid potentially morbid radical surgeries given the significant risk of distant metastasis and the poor overall prognosis.
  - Interferon therapy has not been studied in this population.

- *Pediatric embryonal rhabdomyosarcoma* is treated with induction multi-agent chemotherapy vincristine, actinomycin-D, and cyclophosphamide (VAC), followed by local resection with or without brachytherapy and reserves radical surgery for persistent or recurrent tumors. On the other hand, adults with vaginal sarcoma are not chemoresponsive and the only reported long-term survivors underwent exenterative procedures [56].

Post-treatment

- The proximity of other pelvic organs to the vagina predisposes them to developing treatment-related complications from both surgery and RT.
- Vaginal atrophy, fibrosis, and stenosis are common following RT.
- Severe adverse events (grade 3–4) occur in 10–13 % of patients after primary RT including proctitis, vaginal necrosis, intestinal obstruction, or fistula formation.
- Patients are at risk for sexual dysfunction and body-image issues requiring regular monitoring and preventive measures (vaginal dilators or regular vaginal intercourse with topical estrogen if needed should be encouraged).
- Surveillance:
  - Treatment failure usually occurs within 2 years of primary therapy.
  - Close clinical follow-up is performed every 3 months for 2 years, then visits every 6 months for 5 years, and annually thereafter.

Prognosis/Survival

- Stage is the most important prognostic factor in vaginal cancers and survival rates for SCC of the vagina are consistently worse than those reported for cervical and vulvar cancers at each stage.

- Beyond stage—tumor size greater than 4 cm, histology subtype, and treatment modality were the most significant prognostic factors [53].
- Five-year overall survival data for SCC by FIGO stage are presented in Table 3.4.

References

1. Society AC. American Cancer Society Key Statistics http://www.cancer.org. Detailed guide to vaginal and vulvar cancer, 2013.
2. Kosary CL. Cancer of the Vulva. In: Ries LAG, Young JL, Keel GE, Eisner MP, Lin YD, Horner M-J, editors. SEER Survival monograph: cancer survival among adults: U.S. SEER Program, 1988–2001, Patient and tumor characteristics. National Cancer Institute, SEER Program, NIH Pub. No. 07-6215, Bethesda, MD, 2007.
3. Trimble CL, Hildesheim A, Brinton LA, Shah KV, Kurman RJ. Heterogeneous etiology of squamous carcinoma of the vulva. Obstet Gynecol. 1996;87(1):59–64. PubMed PMID: 8532267.
4. Sideri M, Jones RW, Wilkinson EJ, Preti M, Heller DS, Scurry J, et al. Squamous vulvar intraepithelial neoplasia: 2004 modified terminology, ISSVD Vulvar Oncology Subcommittee. J Reprod Med. 2005;50(11):807–10. PubMed PMID: 16419625.
5. Hacker NF. Revised FIGO staging for carcinoma of the vulva. Int J Gynaecol Obstet. 2009;105(2):105–6. PubMed PMID: 19329116.
6. Berek JS, Hacker NF. Berek & Hacker's gynecologic oncology. 5th ed. Philadelphia: Wolters Kluwer/Lippincott Williams & Wilkins Health; 2010. xv, 895 p.
7. Gonzalez Bosquet J, Magrina JF, Magtibay PM, Gaffey TA, Cha SS, Jones MB, et al. Patterns of inguinal groin metastases in squamous cell carcinoma of the vulva. Gynecol Oncol. 2007;105(3):742–6. PubMed PMID: 17379281.
8. Clark Jr WH, Mihm Jr MC. Lentigo maligna and lentigo-maligna melanoma. Am J Pathol. 1969;55(1):39–67. PubMed PMID: 5776171, Pubmed Central PMCID: 2013384.
9. Chung AF, Woodruff JM, Lewis Jr JL. Malignant melanoma of the vulva: a report of 44 cases. Obstet Gynecol. 1975;45(6):638–46. PubMed PMID: 1143724.

10. Breslow A. Thickness, cross-sectional areas and depth of invasion in the prognosis of cutaneous melanoma. Ann Surg. 1970; 172(5):902–8. PubMed PMID: 5477666, Pubmed Central PMCID: 1397358.
11. Karlan BY, Bristow RE, Li AJ. Gynecologic oncology: clinical practice and surgical atlas. 1st ed. New York: McGraw-Hill; 2012.
12. Balch CM, Gershenwald JE, Soong SJ, Thompson JF, Atkins MB, Byrd DR, et al. Final version of 2009 AJCC melanoma staging and classification. J Clin Oncol. 2009;27(36):6199–206. PubMed PMID: 19917835, Pubmed Central PMCID: 2793035.
13. Trimble EL, Lewis Jr JL, Williams LL, Curtin JP, Chapman D, Woodruff JM, et al. Management of vulvar melanoma. Gynecol Oncol. 1992;45(3):254–8. PubMed PMID: 1612500.
14. Fanning J, Lambert HC, Hale TM, Morris PC, Schuerch C. Paget's disease of the vulva: prevalence of associated vulvar adenocarcinoma, invasive Paget's disease, and recurrence after surgical excision. Am J Obstet Gynecol. 1999;180(1 Pt 1):24–7. PubMed PMID: 9914572.
15. Horowitz IR. Female genital system. In: Wood WC, Skandalakis JE, Staley CA, editors. Berlin: Springer; 2010, pp 637–678.
16. Berman ML, Soper JT, Creasman WT, Olt GT, DiSaia PJ. Conservative surgical management of superficially invasive stage I vulvar carcinoma. Gynecol Oncol. 1989;35(3):352–7. PubMed PMID: 2599471.
17. Farias-Eisner R, Cirisano FD, Grouse D, Leuchter RS, Karlan BY, Lagasse LD, et al. Conservative and individualized surgery for early squamous carcinoma of the vulva: the treatment of choice for stage I and II (T1-2 N0-1 M0) disease. Gynecol Oncol. 1994;53(1):55–8. PubMed PMID: 8175023.
18. Heaps JM, Fu YS, Montz FJ, Hacker NF, Berek JS. Surgical-pathologic variables predictive of local recurrence in squamous cell carcinoma of the vulva. Gynecol Oncol. 1990;38(3):309–14. PubMed PMID: 2227541.
19. Hacker NF, Van der Velden J. Conservative management of early vulvar cancer. Cancer. 1993;71 Suppl 4:1673–7. PubMed PMID: 8431905.
20. Stehman FB, Bundy BN, Thomas G, Varia M, Okagaki T, Roberts J, et al. Groin dissection versus groin radiation in carcinoma of the vulva: a Gynecologic Oncology Group study. Int J Radiat Oncol Biol Phys. 1992;24(2):389–96. PubMed PMID: 1526880.
21. Levenback CF, Ali S, Coleman RL, Gold MA, Fowler JM, Judson PL, et al. Lymphatic mapping and sentinel lymph node

biopsy in women with squamous cell carcinoma of the vulva: a gynecologic oncology group study. J Clin Oncol. 2012;30(31):3786–91. PubMed PMID: 22753905, Pubmed Central PMCID: 3478573.
22. Coleman RL, Ali S, Levenback CF, Gold MA, Fowler JM, Judson PL, et al. Is bilateral lymphadenectomy for midline squamous carcinoma of the vulva always necessary? An analysis from Gynecologic Oncology Group (GOG) 173. Gynecol Oncol. 2013;128(2):155–9. PubMed PMID: 23201592, Pubmed Central PMCID: 3638213.
23. Oonk MH, van Hemel BM, Hollema H, de Hullu JA, Ansink AC, Vergote I, et al. Size of sentinel-node metastasis and chances of non-sentinel-node involvement and survival in early stage vulvar cancer: results from GROINSS-V, a multicentre observational study. Lancet Oncol. 2010;11(7):646–52. PubMed PMID: 20537946.
24. Zhang SH, Sood AK, Sorosky JI, Anderson B, Buller RE. Preservation of the saphenous vein during inguinal lymphadenectomy decreases morbidity in patients with carcinoma of the vulva. Cancer. 2000;89(7):1520–5. PubMed PMID: 11013366.
25. Dardarian TS, Gray HJ, Morgan MA, Rubin SC, Randall TC. Saphenous vein sparing during inguinal lymphadenectomy to reduce morbidity in patients with vulvar carcinoma. Gynecol Oncol. 2006;101(1):140–2. PubMed PMID: 16364412.
26. Geisler JP, Manahan KJ, Buller RE. Neoadjuvant chemotherapy in vulvar cancer: avoiding primary exenteration. Gynecol Oncol. 2006;100(1):53–7. PubMed PMID: 16257042.
27. Montana GS, Thomas GM, Moore DH, Saxer A, Mangan CE, Lentz SS, et al. Preoperative chemo-radiation for carcinoma of the vulva with N2/N3 nodes: a gynecologic oncology group study. Int J Radiat Oncol Biol Phys. 2000;48(4):1007–13. PubMed PMID: 11072157.
28. Homesley HD, Bundy BN, Sedlis A, Adcock L. Radiation therapy versus pelvic node resection for carcinoma of the vulva with positive groin nodes. Obstet Gynecol. 1986;68(6):733–40. PubMed PMID: 3785783.
29. Kunos C, Simpkins F, Gibbons H, Tian C, Homesley H. Radiation therapy compared with pelvic node resection for node-positive vulvar cancer: a randomized controlled trial. Obstet Gynecol. 2009;114(3):537–46. PubMed PMID: 19701032.
30. Moore DH, Ali S, Koh WJ, Michael H, Barnes MN, McCourt CK, et al. A phase II trial of radiation therapy and weekly cisplatin chemotherapy for the treatment of locally-advanced squamous cell carcinoma of the vulva: a gynecologic oncology group study. Gynecol Oncol. 2012;124(3):529–33. PubMed PMID: 22079361.

31. Helm CW, Hatch KD, Partridge EE, Shingleton HM. The rhomboid transposition flap for repair of the perineal defect after radical vulvar surgery. Gynecol Oncol. 1993;50:164–7.
32. John HE, Jessop ZM, Di Candia M, et al. An algorithmic approach to perineal reconstruction – experience from two international centers. Ann Plast Surg. 2013;71:96–102.
33. Burke TW, Morris M, Roh MS, et al. Perineal reconstruction using single gracilis myocutaneous flaps. Gynecol Oncol. 1995; 57:221–5.
34. Fowler JM. Incorporating pelvic/vaginal reconstruction into radical pelvic surgery. Gynecol Oncol. 2009;115:154–61.
35. Maggino T, Landoni F, Sartori E, Zola P, Gadducci A, Alessi C, et al. Patterns of recurrence in patients with squamous cell carcinoma of the vulva. A multicenter CTF Study. Cancer. 2000;89(1):116–22. PubMed PMID: 10897008.
36. Origoni M, Sideri M, Garsia S, Carinelli SG, Ferrari AG. Prognostic value of pathological patterns of lymph node positivity in squamous cell carcinoma of the vulva stage III and IVA FIGO. Gynecol Oncol. 1992;45(3):313–6. PubMed PMID: 1612509.
37. van Seters M, van Beurden M, ten Kate FJ, Beckmann I, Ewing PC, Eijkemans MJ, et al. Treatment of vulvar intraepithelial neoplasia with topical imiquimod. N Engl J Med. 2008;358(14):1465–73. PubMed PMID: 18385498.
38. Gurumurthy M, Cruickshank ME. Management of vaginal intraepithelial neoplasia. J Lower Genital Tract Dis. 2012;16(3):306–12. PubMed PMID: 22460272.
39. Buck HW, Guth KJ. Treatment of vaginal intraepithelial neoplasia (primarily low grade) with imiquimod 5 % cream. J Lower Genital Tract Dis. 2003;7(4):290–3. PubMed PMID: 17051086.
40. Di Saia PJ, Di Saia PJ, Creasman WT, Di Saia PJ. Clinical gynecologic oncology. 8th ed. Philadelphia, PA: Elsevier/Saunders; 2012. xii, 708 p.
41. Creasman WT. Vaginal cancers. Curr Opin Obstet Gynecol. 2005;17(1):71–6. PubMed PMID: 15711415.
42. Hacker NF, Eifel PJ, van der Velden J. Cancer of the vagina. Int J Gynaecol Obstet. 2012;119 Suppl 2:S97–9. PubMed PMID: 22999510.
43. Frank SJ, Deavers MT, Jhingran A, Bodurka DC, Eifel PJ. Primary adenocarcinoma of the vagina not associated with diethylstilbestrol (DES) exposure. Gynecol Oncol. 2007;105(2):470–4. PubMed PMID: 17292459.
44. Ball HG, Berman ML. Management of primary vaginal carcinoma. Gynecol Oncol. 1982;14(2):154–63. PubMed PMID: 7129211.

45. Davis KP, Stanhope CR, Garton GR, Atkinson EJ, O'Brien PC. Invasive vaginal carcinoma: analysis of early-stage disease. Gynecol Oncol. 1991;42(2):131–6. PubMed PMID: 1894171.
46. Stock RG, Chen AS, Seski J. A 30-year experience in the management of primary carcinoma of the vagina: analysis of prognostic factors and treatment modalities. Gynecol Oncol. 1995;56(1):45–52. PubMed PMID: 7821847.
47. Tjalma WA, Monaghan JM, de Barros LA, Naik R, Nordin AJ, Weyler JJ. The role of surgery in invasive squamous carcinoma of the vagina. Gynecol Oncol. 2001;81(3):360–5. PubMed PMID: 11371123.
48. Creasman WT, Phillips JL, Menck HR. The National Cancer Data Base report on cancer of the vagina. Cancer. 1998;83(5):1033–40. PubMed PMID: 9731908.
49. Benedetti Panici P, Bellati F, Plotti F, Di Donato V, Antonilli M, Perniola G, et al. Neoadjuvant chemotherapy followed by radical surgery in patients affected by vaginal carcinoma. Gynecol Oncol 2008;111(2):307–311.
50. Chyle V, Zagars GK, Wheeler JA, Wharton JT, Delclos L. Definitive radiotherapy for carcinoma of the vagina: outcome and prognostic factors. Int J Radiat Oncol Biol Phys. 1996;35(5):891–905. PubMed PMID: 8751398.
51. Perez CA, Grigsby PW, Garipagaoglu M, Mutch DG, Lockett MA. Factors affecting long-term outcome of irradiation in carcinoma of the vagina. Int J Radiat Oncol Biol Phys. 1999;44(1):37–45. PubMed PMID: 10219792.
52. Frank SJ, Jhingran A, Levenback C, Eifel PJ. Definitive radiation therapy for squamous cell carcinoma of the vagina. Int J Radiat Oncol Biol Phys. 2005;62(1):138–47. PubMed PMID: 15850914.
53. Shah CA, Goff BA, Lowe K, Peters 3rd WA, Li CI. Factors affecting risk of mortality in women with vaginal cancer. Obstet Gynecol. 2009;113(5):1038–45. PubMed PMID: 19384118, Pubmed Central PMCID: 2746762.
54. Di Donato V, Bellati F, Fischetti M, Plotti F, Perniola G, Panici PB. Vaginal cancer. Crit Rev Oncol Hematol. 2012;81(3):286–95. PubMed PMID: 21571543.
55. Thigpen JT, Blessing JA, Homesley HD, Berek JS, Creasman WT. Phase II trial of cisplatin in advanced or recurrent cancer of the vagina: a Gynecologic Oncology Group Study. Gynecol Oncol. 1986;23(1):101–4. PubMed PMID: 3943746.
56. Barakat RR, Markman M, Randall M. Principles and practice of gynecologic oncology. 5th ed. Philadelphia: Wolters Kluwer Health/Lippincott Williams & Wilkins; 2009. xv, 1072 p., 16 p. of plates p.

Chapter 4
Uterine Corpus Cancers

Kristy K. Ward and Michael T. McHale

Epidemiology

Worldwide, cancers of the uterine corpus are the sixth most common cancer in women, with over 218,100 new cases diagnosed each year. Uterine cancer is ten times more common in developed countries and is the most common malignancy of the female genital tract in North America and Europe. In the USA and Europe, it is the fourth overall most common cancer diagnosed in women and the eighth most likely cause of cancer death [1]. It is estimated that 52,630 US women will be diagnosed with uterine cancer in 2014 and 8,590 will die [2]. Uterine malignancies can be divided into endometrial carcinomas (arising from the epithelial cells of the endometrium) and uterine sarcomas (arising from the muscle and connective tissue of the myometrium).

K.K. Ward, M.D., M.A.S. • M.T. McHale, M.D. (✉)
Department of Reproductive Medicine, UC San Diego
Moores Cancer Center, 3855 Health Sciences Drive #0987,
La Jolla, CA 92093-0987, USA
e-mail: Kristy.Kay.Ward@gmail.com; mtmchale@ucsd.edu

R.N. Eskander and R.E. Bristow (eds.), *Gynecologic Oncology: A Pocketbook*, DOI 10.1007/978-1-4939-1976-5_4,

Endometrial Cancer

- Approximately 95 % of cancers of the uterine corpus are endometrial in origin.
  - The mean age of diagnosis with uterine cancer is 60, [3] with the majority of patients being over the age of 50 [4].
  - The greatest risk factor for endometrial cancer is hyperestrogenic states including:
    - Estrogen producing tumors.
    - Unopposed exogenous estrogen.
    - Increased adiposity (obesity).
  - Early menarche, late menopause, and nulliparity are also associated with an increased risk of uterine cancer.
  - Among obesity related cancers in women, endometrial cancer is most strongly associated with increasing body mass, with 49 % of cases in the USA attributable to obesity [5].
  - Conversely, smoking, physical activity, oral contraceptive usage, physical activity, and multiparity decrease the risk.
- Base on clinic-pathological characteristics, Bokhman devised a dualistic classification of endometrial cancers.
  - *Type 1 lesions* are the most common, comprising 80 % of endometrial cancers.
    - They include endometrioid cell type or variants (including squamous differentiation, villoglandular, secretory), are usually well to moderately differentiated, and are less likely to metastasize outside of the uterus.
    - These tumors often occur in women with a history of anovulatory uterine bleeding and can be found in a background of endometrial hyperplasia.
    - Women with a biopsy of complex endometrial hyperplasia with atypia have a 40 % likelihood of having malignancy found in the hysterectomy specimen [6].

  - Conversely those with simple hyperplasia have a 1 % chance of progressing to cancer, simple hyperplasia with atypia 3 % chance and complex hyperplasia without atypia 10 % chance.
- *Type II lesions* are not associated with hyperestrogenism.
  - Clear cell, serous adenocarcinoma, and carcinosarcoma are considered type II tumors.
  - These tumors are poorly differentiated and more aggressive; deep myometrial invasion and metastatic disease are more common than with type I tumors.
  - Recurrence is more likely and survival is worse.
  - Serous carcinoma is characterized by papillae and has highly pleiomorphic tumor cells with necrosis and many mitoses. Endometrial intraepithelial carcinoma (EIC) is a rare finding, but it is thought to be the precursor lesion in serous tumors of the uterus. It involves pleiomorphic but noninvasive tumor cells [7].
  - Carcinosarcoma, also known as malignant mixed mullerian tumors (MMMT), arise from organs of mullerian origin, most commonly the uterus. Once classified as sarcomas, there is evidence to suggest that this tumor type originates from an epithelial-cell precursor. As the names suggest, they contain mixed components of sarcoma and adenocarcinoma.

Uterine Sarcomas

- Uterine sarcomas make up 2–5 % of uterine cancers and less than 1 % of all gynecologic malignancies. In the USA, approximately 1,500 uterine sarcomas were diagnosed in 2013.
  - They primarily include leiomyosarcomas, sarcomas arising from the endometrial stroma, and undifferentiated sarcomas.

  - Risk factors include:
    - A history of pelvic irradiation.
    - Black race.
    - Usage of tamoxifen for treatment or prevention of breast cancer.

- Leiomyosarcomas make up 30 % of all uterine sarcomas.
  - The peak incidence is at age 50.
- Sarcomas arising in the endometrial stroma account for 15 % of all uterine sarcomas.
- Low-grade tumors are more common before menopause while high-grade tumors peak after menopause.
- Other sarcomas include:
  - Mixed endometrial stromal and smooth muscle tumors.
  - Adenosarcomas.
  - Embryonal botryoides or rhabdomyosarcomas.
  - Perivascular epithelial-cell tumors (PEComas) [8].

Diagnosis/Screening

- Clinical features associated with uterine cancer include:
  - Abnormal uterine bleeding.
  - Glandular cells on a pap of a postmenopausal woman.
  - Pelvic pain.
  - Enlarging pelvic mass.
- Approximately 90 % of women with endometrial cancer present with uterine bleeding. The diagnosis is obtained by pathological review of tissue, preferably obtained by endometrial biopsy, dilation and curettage, or hysteroscopy and biopsy.
- While these methods are very efficacious for detecting uterine cancers, leiomyosarcoma may only diagnosed after hysterectomy or myomectomy if the lesion does not invade into the endometrial cavity.
- Screening of asymptomatic women is not recommended [9].
- Ultrasound can be used to assess the endometrial stripe. In women with EMS <4 mm the risk of malignancy is <1 %.

Staging

- Per NCCN guidelines, initial workup for uterine cancer includes:
  - History and physical examination.
  - Chest X-ray.
  - Endometrial sampling and current cervical cytology.
- Traditionally, staging of endometrial cancer involves exploratory laparotomy, total abdominal hysterectomy, bilateral oophorectomy, and pelvic and para-aortic lymph node dissections where appropriate [9].
- *Grade 1 tumors* are well differentiated, with formed glands and no more than 5 % of non-squamous, non-morular solid components.
- *Grade 2* contains 6–50 % solid components
- *Grade 3* has greater than 50 % non-squamous solid components.
- If there is significant cytologic atypia, the tumor should be upgraded.
- Currently, nearly 70 % of patients are diagnosed and treated at early stage with 5-year survival estimated at 95.8 %, and an additional 20 % are diagnosed with only regional disease with a 5-year survival estimated at 67.0 % [2].

Genetics

- The majority of uterine cancers are sporadic with approximately 1 in 10 associated with a genetic syndrome.
- Hereditary non-polyposis colon cancer (HNPCC) syndrome is the most common genetic syndrome associated with endometrial cancer.
  - The NCCN recommends genetic counseling should be considered in women diagnosed under the age of 55 and those who have a family history of colon cancer and endometrial cancer.

  - HNPCC, also known as Lynch Syndrome, is associated with microsatellite instability in the mismatch repair genes MLH1, MSH2, MSH6, PMS2, or EPCAM, leading to cancers including endometrial and colon.
  - Approximately 50 % of women with Lynch syndrome will present with endometrial cancer.
    - Women with Lynch syndrome should receive an endometrial biopsy for abnormal uterine bleeding and consider a risk reducing hysterectomy after child bearing.
    - Colon cancer screening should be stressed in these patients and genetic counseling should be considered for themselves and family members [4, 10].

- *Cowden Syndrome* is associated with multiple hamartomas and increased risk of cancers including endometrial, breast, and thyroid. The most common mutation in Cowden Syndrome is PTEN, but mutations in SDHB, SDHD, and KLLN have also been seen. There is no evidence to support risk reducing hysterectomy, but this should be discussed with women with this syndrome [11].
- Women with a history of retinoblastoma are at an increased risk for leiomyosarcoma. Retinoblastoma is associated with inactivation of the RB1 tumor suppressor gene. When the gene mutation involves all cells, there is increased risk for pinealoma, osteosarcoma, melanoma, and other muscle tumors [12].

Management of Endometrial Cancer

- Multiple controversies regarding the intraoperative and postoperative management of endometrial cancer remain.
  - Currently, the standard surgical management has been defined as hysterectomy as well as bilateral salpingo-oophorectomy.
  - The type of surgical approach, minimally invasive versus traditional open laparotomy, for completing a hysterectomy has been extensively recently addressed.

- Intraoperative assessment for lymphadenectomy and more importantly the significance of a lymphadenectomy remains controversial and has yet to be clearly defined.
- With respect to adjuvant therapy, there are multiple questions and controversies. Identifying the appropriate population for adjuvant therapy, the type of radiotherapy (vaginal versus whole pelvic), the indications for chemotherapy or the combination of chemotherapy and radiotherapy, remain unanswered.
- Many of these controversies have been explored or are currently being assessed in randomized phase III clinical trials. Each of these controversial topics will be addressed.

Surgery

- In 1988 the International Federation of Gynecology and Obstetrics (FIGO), after recognizing the limitations of a clinically based disease assessment, recommended surgical staging for endometrial cancer [13].
- Typically, comprehensive surgical staging has included:
  - Hysterectomy, BSO, bilateral pelvic and para-aortic lymph node "assessment" and peritoneal cytology.
  - Historically this was performed through a laparotomy.
    - In the early 1990s, multiple investigators explored the role of laparoscopy for comprehensive surgical staging. Multiple single institution studies demonstrated many advantages including safety, reduced blood loss and transfusion rates, and shorter hospital stays [14–16].
- In light of these provocative results, the Gynecologic Oncology Group (GOG) designed a randomized trial comparing comprehensive surgical staging with laparotomy to laparoscopy (GOG Lap 2). Eligible patients were clinically Stage I to IIA. The primary outcome measured was recurrence-free survival. Other end points included

operative time, length of hospital stay, conversion rate from laparoscopy to laparotomy, adverse events, quality of life, and survival [16].

- Initially 2,618 patients were randomly assigned with 920 assigned to laparotomy and 1,696 to laparoscopy. Of the 1,682 that were assigned to laparoscopy, 434 patients (25.8 %) were converted to a laparotomy. The most commonly cited reason was poor exposure in 56 % of the patients requiring conversion. Only 11.3 % of those converted were due to excessive bleeding.
- Length of surgery was significantly longer for the laparoscopy group than laparotomy with a median time 204 and 130 min, respectively.
- There were similar intraoperative complications between the two groups; however, laparoscopy had fewer moderate to severe postoperative adverse events than laparotomy (14 % vs. 21 %) respectively.
- Lastly hospital stay was shorter in the laparoscopy cohort compared to laparotomy. As such, the authors concluded that this prospective, randomized trial clearly demonstrated that laparoscopic comprehensive surgical staging is both safe and feasible and that it results in less postoperative complications and shorter hospitals stay than staging completed by laparotomy [17].

- A recent meta analysis, of 8 randomized trials, comparing the safety of a laparoscopic staging to laparotomy demonstrated no difference in intraoperative complications. There were; however, less post-operative complications in the laparoscopy group [18].
- The investigators for the GOG Lap 2 trial recently published the recurrence and survival data for the randomized clinical trial comparing laparoscopic staging to traditional laparotomy [19].
  - Median follow-up for this trial was 59 months. There were 309 recurrences, 350 deaths and a 3-year recurrence rate of 11.4 % for the laparoscopic cohort and 10.2 % for those assigned to laparotomy.

- The estimated 5-year overall survival was 89.8 % for patients assigned to laparoscopy and laparotomy. In summary, the rationale for laparoscopic surgical staging for endometrial cancer is strongly supported by the limited difference in recurrence rates, estimated as 1.14 % at 3 years, coupled with improved quality of life and reduced postoperative complications.

- In 2005, the FDA approved the da Vinci robotic surgical system for gynecology. Since then there have been multiple single institution studies that have demonstrated the safety and feasibility of this approach [20, 21].
  - Boggess and colleagues compared 103 robotically staged endometrial cancer patients to two historical controls, which included 138 patients staged by laparotomy and 81 by laparoscopy.
    - Notable findings from this trial were increased nodal yield, decreased blood loss and shorter hospital stay for the robotic cohort compared to the other two.
    - There was also a reduction in post-operative complication rates when compared to laparotomy (5.85 % vs. 29.7 %, respectively). This cohort was one of the original single institution studies to suggest both the safety and efficacy for robotic surgery.
  - Recently these investigators reported the recurrence free and 5-year survival data from a cohort of women that underwent robotic surgical staging and compared their results with data from the Surveillance Epidemiology and End Result database (SEER) [22].
    - The authors concluded that robotic staging of 499 consecutive patients with endometrial cancer did not adversely affect rates of recurrence or survival.

- In conclusion, although "traditional" comprehensive surgical staging has been completed via laparotomy, there is now sufficient evidence to support a minimally invasive approach by laparoscopy or robotic surgery.

approaches have demonstrated clear benefits including improved quality of life, shorter hospital stay and less blood loss.

- More importantly data now demonstrates that laparoscopy does not impact recurrence rates or survival. Although the data is not as robust for robotic staging, there is a growing body of literature to suggest both the safety and efficacy for robotic staging.
- Some of this data clearly demonstrates a benefit for obese patients that now can be staged minimally invasively utilizing the robotic surgical system [23].

Lymphadenectomy

- Although endometrial cancer remains one of the most common gynecologic malignancies and has been surgical staged since 1988, definitive management remains controversial and highly variable with respect to lymph node assessment.
- There continues to be significant debate regarding what population is at risk for nodal disease and as such warrant a lymphadenectomy. Some have adopted an all or none approach, i.e., complete assessment in all patients or complete omission [24, 25].
- More recent data from the Mayo experience has clearly demonstrated the utility of intraoperative risk assessment utilizing frozen section findings to address indication or lack thereof for a pelvic and para-aortic lymphadenectomy [26, 27].
  - They clearly defined a subgroup of patients (type I endometrial cancer, myometrial invasion <50 %, grades 1 and 2, and primary tumor diameter ≤2 cm, based on intraoperative frozen section) that did not warrant a lymphadenectomy since there was minimal risk for nodal metastasis [25–27].
  - Whether this intraoperative assessment is applicable and generalizable to other institutions remains questionable and needs to be addressed.

- A relatively recent survey of gynecologic oncologist clearly demonstrated the variability in practice patterns amongst gynecologic oncologist with respect to indications for staging and extent of dissection [28].
- The controversy involving lymphadenectomy for endometrial cancer became more complex following the publication of two large, randomized European trials [29, 30]. The purpose of these two trials was to assess in a randomized fashion whether the addition of pelvic lymphadenectomy to a hysterectomy with bilateral salpingo-oophorectomy improved overall and recurrence free survival. These trials are summarized in Table 4.1.
  - Both of these trials failed to demonstrate either an overall survival or recurrence free survival benefit for pelvic lymphadenectomy.
  - Although the investigators should be commended on their efforts to complete a randomized trial assessing the benefits of lymphadenectomy, many questions remain regarding the outcomes and methodologies for both of these trials.
    - Both included a preponderance of low risk patients, which makes identifying a small difference in survival challenging.
    - In the Panici study, there were two significant concerns:
      - Specifically the lack of para aortic node assessment and the lack of standardization for adjuvant therapy.
      - Approximately 22 % of the patients in the no lymphadenectomy arm actually had node sampling or lymphadenectomy.
      - In fact, 7 % had more than 20 nodes excised which was considered the "standard" in the lymphadenectomy arm as an acceptable per protocol node count.
        - With respect to the ASTEC trial, Creasman et al. appropriately summarized some of the confounding factors that "muddy" the investigators conclusions [31].

TABLE 4.1. The lymphadenectomy controversy [62].

	Panici trial	ASTEC trial
#Patients	514	1408
Eligibility	Clinical Stage I, >50 % myometrial invasion (excluded Stage IB grade 1), age <75, good performance status, no prior RT or chemotherapy	Disease clinically confined to corpus
Randomization	Standard treatment[a] with systematic pelvic lymphadenectomy versus Standard treatment and no lymphadenectomy (control)	Hysterectomy, BSO, pelvic node dissection, palpation of para aortic nodes, resection of suspicious nodes at surgeons discretion versus Hysterectomy, BSO, palpation of nodes with removal of suspicious nodes at surgeons discretion (control)
Aortic node dissection required	No	No
Median follow-up	49 months	37 months
Standardized adjuvant therapy	None	Yes-randomized specific cohort of intermediate and high risk, early stage disease defined as Stage IA or B grade 3, pap serous or clear cell and IC or IIA, also included those with positive pelvic nodes. Cohort randomized to external beam RT versus no external beam[b]

Of note: in control arm bulky nodes >1 cm could be excised
[a]Standard Treatment: hysterectomy, BSO, washings
[b]ASTEC Trial: Actually "two trials" intertwined in one cohort attempting to answer two critical questions: benefits of lymphadenectomy and radiation therapy. As such, there were essentially two randomizations designed to answer a surgical and radiation question. The second randomization occurred after surgery

- These include inequitable distribution of high risk factors in the lymphadenectomy arm including 3 % more grade 3 lesions, higher rate of lymphovascular space invasion and more deeply invasive disease.
- In this trial 5 % of those randomized to the no lymphadenectomy group had nodes removed of which 30 % were positive.
- Also 8 % of those randomized to lymphadenectomy had no nodes removed and at least 30 % had less than 9 nodes excised which per GOG standards is considered inadequate.
- More concerning was the second randomization to external beam RT or no RT for those with intermediate or high-risk disease including those with positive nodes. Per the randomization, the cohort of patients that might benefit from lymphadenectomy and adjuvant RT, i.e., those with positive nodes, could be excluded from adjuvant RT at time of second randomization. From a clinical perspective this raises many ethical questions. Although randomized, multi-institutional trials, the flaws in both of these trials make it challenging to modify what has been standard therapy for endometrial cancer.

– Although it may be impossible to design the "perfect" trial to assess the efficacy or therapeutic benefit of lymphadenectomy, it is important to recognize the continued prognostic significance of lymphadenectomy in planning adjuvant therapy.
– The GOG is currently developing a randomized trial to address the questions that still exist with respect to indications and potential benefits from lymphadenectomy.

Risk Assessment

- Following surgery, stage and other significant pathologic risk factors are utilized to determine risk for persistent disease or recurrence. This risk assessment is often utilized to define adjuvant therapy.
- Low Risk: This is typically defined as endometrioid cancers confined to the endometrium, a subset of Stage IA, and grade 1 or 2.
  - Typically these patients are managed with close surveillance alone following surgery.
- Intermediate Risk: This is typically defined as disease confined to the uterus, including the cervix (Stage II) with myometrial invasion (Stage IA or IB).
  - Other prognostic factors such as outer myometrial invasion, grade 2 or 3 and the presence of lymphovascular invasion can further subdivide this group into low or high intermediate risk.
- The Gynecologic Oncology Group defines high intermediate risk based on a combination of age and pathologic factors including deep myometrial invasion, grade 2 or 3 and the presence of lymphovascular invasion [32].
- High intermediate risk is thus defined by the following:
  - Any age with three risk factors.
  - Age 50–69 with two risk factors.
  - 70 or older with one risk factor.
- In contrast, the PORTEC (Post-operative Radiation Therapy in Endometrial Cancer) investigators define high intermediate risk as:
  - Age >60 with two risk factors including outer half myometrial invasion and
  - Grade 3 histology [33].
- Management for intermediate risk category, specifically high intermediate risk remains controversial and will be discussed.

- *High Risk*: This group consists of advanced stage disease, Stage III and uterine serous and clear cell carcinomas of any stage.
  - This category is associated with a high rate of recurrence and death from endometrial cancer. As such, adjuvant chemotherapy is often utilized post-operatively.
  - The role of RT is unclear but is currently being explored in a randomized trial thru the GOG (GOG 258).
    - In GOG 258 eligible patients include surgical Stage III and IVA endometrial cancer as well as early Stage (I and II) serous and clear cell carcinoma.
      - Patients are randomized to cisplatin on days 1 and 29 and volume directed radiation therapy followed then by 4 cycles of carboplatin and paclitaxel versus 6 cycles of carboplatin and paclitaxel.

Adjuvant Therapy

Intermediate "Low and High" Risk

- Two randomized clinical trials would support observation rather than adjuvant radiation therapy for this group.
- The Gynecologic Oncology Group study (GOG 99) was a phase III trial that randomly assigned 448 women with "intermediate-risk" endometrial cancer (defined as Stage IB, IC and occult II, excluding papillary serous and clear cell histologies) following comprehensive surgical staging to whole pelvic radiation versus observation [32].
  - The cumulative incidence of recurrence was higher in the no additional treatment group than the RT (radiation therapy) cohort 12 and 2 %, respectively.
  - The most common site of recurrence in the no RT group was the vagina.
  - There was; however, no statistically significant difference in overall survival between the two groups.

- The estimated 4-year survival for no additional therapy versus RT was 86 and 92 %, respectively.
- Importantly, the investigators identified a subset of patients with "high intermediate risk" that represented 1/3 of the entire cohort but two-thirds of all recurrences. In this population there was a significant benefit from radiation with respect to local recurrence.
- This trial suggested redefining the intermediate risk group, specifically into a low and high risk and reserving radiation therapy for the high intermediate risk patients.

- In comparison, PORTEC I assessed a relatively similar population of patients; however comprehensive surgical staging was not completed [33].
  - Similarly these investigators demonstrated a reduction in pelvic recurrences but no difference in overall survival.
  - Actuarial 5-year loco-regional recurrence rates were 4 % in the radiotherapy group and 14 % for those randomized to observation alone.
  - The overall survival rates were 81 and 85 %, respectively. As in GOG 99, the PORTEC investigators also identified a cohort of patients, based on age and grade 3 histology that accounted for the majority of recurrences.
  - This cohort, like the high intermediate risk subgroup in GOG 99, may actually benefit from adjuvant RT.
  - Table 4.2 summarizes both of these critical trials [34].

- Many have hypothesized that the reason both GOG 99 and PORTEC I failed to demonstrate an improved survival with radiation was due to the preponderance of low risk patients that comprised these cohorts.
- Although both trials failed to demonstrate a survival advantage for external beam radiation, each clearly identified a population of patients defined as "high intermediate risk" that had the most significant reduction in locoregional recurrence after external beam RT.

TABLE 4.2. Intermediate risk endometrial cancer [34].

Trial	Eligibility	# Patients	Surgery	Randomization	Locoregional recurrence	Survival
PORTEC 1	Stage IB, grade 2–3 Stage IC, grade 1–2	714	TAH-BSO	No therapy versus pelvic RT	14 % versus 4 % at 5 years ($p<0.001$)	85 versus 81 % $p=0.31$
GOG 99	Stage IB and IC Occult Stage II	392	TAH-BSO and comprehensive lymphadenectomy (pelvic and para-aortic	No therapy versus pelvic RT	12 % versus 2 % at 2 years ($p<0.01$)	86 versus 92% $p=0.56$

Modified with permission from: Creutzberg C. GOG-99: ending the controversy regarding pelvic radiotherapy for endometrial carcinoma? Gynecol Oncol 2004;92:740–743. Gynecologic oncology by SOCIETY OF GYNECOLOGIC ONCOLOGY Reproduced with permission of ACADEMIC PRESS in the format reuse in a book/textbook via Copyright Clearance Center

- In summary, since the recurrence rates for low intermediate risk endometrial cancer is so low, and prognosis excellent, observation alone may be the most appropriate adjuvant "therapy."
- In comparison, for those with high-intermediate risk, recurrence rates range from 5 to 30 % with or without RT. As such, consideration for adjuvant radiation therapy is warranted.
- Lastly the ASTEC and EN.5 pooled trial demonstrated similar findings in a relatively analogous population of patients [35].
  - This pooled trial raised another important question regarding the role of pelvic radiation in this population but more importantly the type of radiation, specifically vaginal brachytherapy.
  - These initially independent trials sought to assess the benefit of postoperative adjuvant radiation in early staged endometrial cancer with intermediate and high risk of recurrence.
  - Eligible patients include Stage IA and IB grade 3, all IC and all stages of papillary serous and clear cell carcinomas. A lymphadenectomy was not required. Eligible women were randomly assigned to observation or to radiation therapy.
  - Interestingly brachytherapy could be utilized in either arm. In fact 51 % of those randomized to observation alone, received brachytherapy.
  - Overall there was no difference in 5-year survival between the two groups. The rate of locoregional recurrence was 6.1 % in observation arm compared to 3.2 % in RT group.
  - This finding may certainly be due to the extensive use of vaginal brachytherapy in the observation arm.
  - This trial again demonstrated a lack of data to support the use of adjuvant external beam radiation therapy in these intermediate risk patients and high-risk patients with endometrial cancer. As with GOG 99 and PORTEC

1 this trial clearly demonstrated that radiation therapy has no overall effect on distant disease or overall survival. Interestingly, one might conclude from this trial that possibly brachytherapy alone could be used to reduce the risk of local recurrence and in fact may be the preferred strategy.

- Lastly the role of adjuvant therapy for *high intermediate risk* patients recently assessed by a large randomized trial, GOG 249, which recently closed enrollment.
  - GOG 249 is a randomized trial of pelvic radiation versus vaginal cuff brachytherapy followed by paclitaxel/carboplatin in high risk, early stage endometrial cancer. Eligible patients include Stage I with high intermediate risk factors and Stage II as well as Stage I–II serous or clear cell carcinoma with negative cytology. As a review, high intermediate risk categories included patients with:
    - Age ≥70 years with one risk factor.
    - Age ≥50 with 2 risk factors.
    - Age ≥18 years with 3 risk factors.
    - Risk factors were defined as: Grade 2 or 3 tumors, (+) lymphovascular space invasion, and outer 1/2 myometrial invasion. Patients with these risk criteria could be enrolled with either positive or negative cytology.
  - Preliminary results presented at the 2014 SGO Annual Meeting indicated no difference in recurrence free survival at 24 months between the pelvic radiation arm and brachytherapy + chemotherapy arm.
  - OS data was not yet mature.

Vaginal Brachytherapy

- The use of vaginal brachytherapy was addressed indirectly in the ASTEC/EN.5 trial and multiple retrospective studies.

- In light of these data, the PORTEC investigators initiated a trial in high intermediate risk patients to assess whether vaginal brachytherapy was as effective as external beam [36].
  - The primary endpoint for this trial was vaginal recurrence.
  - This non-inferiority randomized trial was undertaken at 19 Dutch centers and enrolled 427 patients with high intermediate risk (age >60 and Stage IC grade 1 or 2, Stage IB, grade 3, Stage IIA, any age.
  - Patients were randomized to vaginal brachytherapy (VBT) and external beam RT (EBRT).
  - At median follow-up of 45 months, there were 3 recurrences in VBT group compared to 4 in the EBRT.
  - The estimated 5 year vaginal recurrence rates were 1.8 % for VBT and 1.6 % for external beam. Other important outcome measures when comparing VBT to external beam included:
    - Similar rate of distant metastasis, 8.3 % versus 5.7 %.
    - No difference in overall survival 84.8 % versus 79.6 %.
    - No difference in disease-free survival 82.7 versus 78.1 %.
    - Rates of GI toxicity lower in VBT compared to external beam 12.6 % versus 53 %.
- Consequently, the PORTEC 2 investigators concluded that vaginal brachytherapy should be recommended for adjuvant therapy in those high-intermediate risk patients since it demonstrated good vaginal control with significantly less GI toxicities than external beam RT.

High Risk Disease

- Women with high-risk endometrial cancer typically have a poor prognosis with surgery alone. As such, adjuvant therapy is typically recommended.

- As mentioned previously, this group typically consists of advanced stage disease, Stage III, and any stage of papillary serous and clear cell carcinoma.
- Currently there is not a "standard" approach for high-risk disease. Often adjuvant therapy is dictated by surgical and pathologic factors, i.e., uterine or extrauterine disease.
- Since multiple questions remain, typically enrollment on a clinical trial may be the most appropriate option for patients in this risk category especially those patients with early stage serous or clear cell carcinoma.

Chemotherapy

- For advanced stage endometrioid cancer, chemotherapy rather than radiation is now typically recommended.
- One of the sentinel trials to support the use of adjuvant chemotherapy as compared to radiation therapy was GOG 122.
  - In this trial patients with Stage III or IV and <2 cm residual disease were randomized to whole abdominal RT versus chemotherapy (doxorubicin plus cisplatin) q 3 weeks for a total of 7 cycles.
  - Overall there was an improvement in PFS and OS in the chemotherapy arm.
  - Five-year survival was 53 and 42 %, respectively.
  - The chemotherapy arm did have a higher pelvic recurrence rate (18 vs. 13 %) and a higher proportion of GI, neurotoxicity and grade 3–4 hematologic toxicity of any type (88 % vs. 14 %) [37].
- In a relatively similar Japanese trial, 385 patients with Stage I–III endometrial cancer were randomized to pelvic RT versus 3 cycles of cyclophosphamide, doxorubicin and cisplatin (CAP).
  - In this trial there was no difference in overall survival or progression free survival. Grade 3–4 toxicity was reported in 4.7 % those receiving chemotherapy versus 1.6 % in the radiation cohort [38].

- The choice of chemotherapy has evolved over the past few decades. Many of the initial phase II and III trials in advanced and recurrent populations demonstrated that taxanes, anthracyclines and platinum compounds are the most active chemotherapeutic agents with response rates ranging from 20 to 35 %.
- Table 4.3 summarizes the Gynecologic Oncology Group's efforts to study chemotherapy in the advanced and recurrent setting.
- The GOG has clearly studied in a progressive and rational fashion the role of chemotherapy for advanced and recurrent disease.
  - Although the triplet of paclitaxel, cisplatin and doxorubicin (TAP) demonstrated an improved PFS and overall survival, widespread acceptance was tempered by the significant peripheral neuropathy and treatment related deaths observed in this trial.
  - Recently, preliminary results from GOG 209 have been presented at the Annual Meeting of the Society of Gynecologic Oncology.
    - At time of presentation it would appear that the carboplatin and paclitaxel arm was not inferior to TAP.
    - As reported, there was a similar overall response rate (51 %), similar PFS (13 months for each arm) and overall survival.
    - The limited toxicity, familiarity, and preliminary findings from GOG 209 has led to an increasing use of this doublet for advanced or recurrent disease.
- With respect to second line therapy, there remains a relative paucity of options. The GOG has conducted multiple phase II trials of single agent therapy with a limited number of objective responses.
  - Some of the agents studied include ifosfamide, topotecan, oxaliplatin, docetaxel, ixabepilone, bevacizumab, and pegylated liposomal doxorubicin [39].

TABLE 4.3. Summary of highlighted GOG trials for advanced and recurrent endometrial cancer [63–65].

Trial	Population	Regimens	RR	PFS	OS	"Winner"
GOG 107 [63]	Stage III/IV or recurrent	Dox versus Dox + Cis	25 % versus 42 %[a]	3.8 versus 5.7 months[a]	9.2 versus 9.0 months	Dox + Cis
GOG 163 [64]	Stage III/IV or recurrent	Dox – Cis versus Dox + Tax	40 % versus 43 %	7.2 versus 6.0 months	12.6 versus 13.6 months	Dox + Tax Not superior
GOG 177 [65]	Stage III/IV or recurrent	Dox + Cis versus Dox + Cis + Tax (TAP)	34 % versus 57 %[a]	5.3 versus 8.3 months[a]	12.3 versus 15.3 months[a]	TAP but significant peripheral neuropathy
GOG 209	Stage III/IV or recurrent	TAP versus Carbo/Taxol	Awaiting results			

RR = response rate; Dox = doxorubicin; Cis = cisplatin; Tax = paclitaxel; TAP = paclitaxel, doxorubicin, cisplatin; Carbo = carboplatin

[a] Statistically significant

Combined Therapy: Chemotherapy and Radiation

- The role for combined therapy, radiation and chemotherapy, has yet to be clearly defined.
- It has been hypothesized that an improved overall survival would be the theoretic benefit of combined therapy by improving both local and distal control. As such, this is currently being explored in three large randomized collaborative group trials:
  - GOG 249, PORTEC 3, and GOG 258. Although the populations being studied in these three trials are similar, there are some essential inclusion criteria differences meant to address different clinical questions.
  - GOG 249 has previously been discussed (with preliminary findings showing no difference in recurrence free survival between arms); however, the population of interest in this trial included women with Stage I disease with high intermediate risk characteristics and early stage papillary serous and clear cell carcinomas with negative cytology.
  - In comparison, PORTEC 3 is an international collaborative trial, that randomizes high-risk patients (Stage IB, grade 3, +LVSI, IC, Stage IIA grade 3, IIB, IIIA, IIIC, and all stages of serous or clear cell) to either pelvic RT versus concurrent cisplatin and pelvic RT followed by 4 cycles carboplatin/paclitaxel.
  - Lastly GOG 258 is a randomized trial comparing cisplatin plus volume directed RT followed by carboplatin plus paclitaxel for 4 cycles versus 6 cycles carboplatin and paclitaxel in patients with Stage III or IVA endometrial carcinoma or Stage I and II clear cell or papillary serous carcinoma with positive cytology.

Recurrent or Metastatic Disease

Chemotherapy

Chemotherapeutic options have been detailed above.

Endocrine Therapy

- For patients in whom radiation or cytotoxic therapy is not a reasonable option, endocrine therapy is an acceptable alternative for recurrent disease.
- Although the published data is not entirely consistent, a favorable response to endocrine therapy is expected in patients that express estrogen and progesterone receptors [40, 41].
  - Additionally hormonal therapy is most effective in well-differentiated tumors.
  - It is recommended that specimen ER and PR receptor staining be performed prior to initiation of therapy.
- Progesterone was one of the original hormone therapies to demonstrate activity in the setting of advanced/recurrent disease. Multiple trials have demonstrated response rates of 15 to 20 %.
- Tamoxifen is currently the only selective estrogen receptor modulator to demonstrate activity [42].
- The combination of the two in a sequential fashion was assessed by the GOG. Megestrol acetate (160 mg orally for 3 weeks) alternating with tamoxifen for 3 weeks demonstrated an overall response rate of 27 % [43].

Special Population: Papillary Serous Carcinoma (UPSC)

- UPSC represents a histologically aggressive subtype of endometrial carcinoma that typically presents with extra-uterine disease.

- Although this histology accounts for 10 % of all endometrial cancers, it accounts for the majority of recurrences.
- The rarity of this histology significantly limits prospective studies. As such, many of the current recommendations are based on small, single institution retrospective studies. Given the paucity of data, enrollment in a clinical trial should be strongly recommended.

Surgery

- In general, either comprehensive surgical staging or optimal cytoreduction is an essential component of the management for UPSC.
  - At many institutions surgical staging for serous uterine cancers mirrors that for serous ovarian cancer.
- The significance for comprehensive staging including pelvic and para aortic lymphadenectomy has been studied in multiple small series.
- It is has been clearly demonstrated that the prognostic factors utilized for endometrioid adenocarcinomas are not predictive for UPSC [44].
  - As such, comprehensive staging for early stage UPSC is recommended in all patients.
- With respect to advanced stage disease multiple studies have demonstrated an improved survival following optimal cytoreductive surgery.
  - In one of the largest series, 79 patients with Stage III–IV disease were taken to the operating room for primary surgical management. Optimal cytoreduction (largest residual tumor <1 cm) was associated with a median survival of 39 months compared to 12 months in those suboptimally debulked [45].
  - In summary, it would appear that optimal resection of metastatic disease confers a survival benefit; as such, it should be the goal at time of primary surgery.

Adjuvant Therapy

- Due to the propensity for this disease to recur distantly, chemotherapy has been considered as an essential component of adjuvant therapy.
- It is important to recognize that the role of chemotherapy in Stage I/II disease is not founded on randomized trials.
  - One of the largest studies of adjuvant therapy for 142 patients with Stage I uterine serous cancer, demonstrated an improved recurrence free and overall survival with the addition of adjuvant platinum/taxane chemotherapy with or without radiation therapy.
  - This study demonstrated a significant reduction in recurrence rate in those receiving adjuvant chemotherapy as compared to those without, 11.2 % compared to 26.9 % [46].
  - It would appear from multiple small series that any myometrial invasion is associated with higher risk of recurrence.
  - Controversy also persists regarding the benefit of adjuvant therapy for disease confined to a polyp. Although the risk of recurrence is low in this population, it is not negligible [47].
- With respect to Stage II disease, one of the largest series reported on the outcomes of 55 patients of which 10 were treated with observation, 26 radiation and 19 with chemotherapy (with or without RT) [48].
  - The risk for recurrence was lowest, 11 %, in those treated with chemotherapy compared to 50 % for those managed with observation or radiation therapy alone.
  - The 5 year progression free survival for those treated with chemotherapy compared to those without was 86 and 41 %, respectively ($p=0.015$).

- For *advanced stage disease*, following optimal cytoreduction, chemotherapy is the recommended adjuvant therapy due to high risk of distant recurrence.
  - As has been discussed previously, the recommended cytotoxic therapy has evolved via progressive randomized trials many of which were completed by the GOG.
  - Currently, the combination of paclitaxel and carboplatin is an appropriate choice of cytotoxic therapy for advanced stage UPSC. The role of radiation therapy is limited and not typically recommended.

Management of Carcinosarcoma

Surgery

- As with endometrial carcinoma, surgery is the primary management for carcinosarcoma.
- Typically surgical staging is recommended which includes:
  - Hysterectomy, bilateral salpingo-oophorectomy, pelvic and para aortic lymphadenectomy, and peritoneal washings.
  - Omentectomy and peritoneal biopsies are often recommended but the value of which is not entirely clear.
  - Lymphadenectomy is recommended to define stage as well as to possibly improve survival.
- In a large query of the SEER database, 1,855 patients with Stage I–III carcinosarcoma were identified [49].
  - For those undergoing a lymphadenectomy compared to those without, the disease free survival and median survival (54 and 25 months, respectively) were significantly improved regardless of adjuvant radiotherapy.
- For advanced stage disease confined to the abdomen, cytoreduction is also recommended; although the data to support this recommendation is limited.
  - One of the larger retrospective studies reviewed the outcomes of 44 patients with Stage III and IV disease.

In this cohort, those that had a complete cytoreduction had a survival advantage compared those with gross residual disease, 52.3 months versus 8.6 months [50].

Adjuvant Therapy

- For *early stage disease*, Stage I and II, there is a relative paucity of quality data to recommend adjuvant therapy.
- In the limited number of trials that do exist, there is a consistent improvement in progression free survival but not overall survival.
  - A multi-institutional retrospective assessment of 111 women with Stages I and II carcinosarcoma assessed outcomes after surgery followed then by observation, radiation, chemotherapy or chemotherapy plus radiation [51].
  - Chemotherapy was associated with improved progression free survival compared to observation or radiation therapy.
  - There was no difference in overall survival between any of the groups. A very early GOG trial demonstrated a lower recurrence rate in patients that received post -operative chemotherapy, Adriamycin, than observation but no improvement in progression free or overall survival [52].
- Lastly, the EORTC assessed the role of adjuvant radiation therapy in a trial of 200 patients with Stage I and II uterine sarcoma [53].
  - This cohort consisted of 91 patients with carcinosarcoma. Patients were randomized to post-operative RT versus observation. Although there was a reduction in local recurrences in the RT cohort compared to observation, 4 % versus 24 %, there was no difference en progression free or overall survival.
- In summary, the role for radiation therapy or chemotherapy is questionable for early stage disease.

- Given the paucity of data, consideration should be given to enrollment on a clinical trial.
  - GOG 261 is currently enrolling patients. This is a randomized trial comparing ifosfamide plus paclitaxel to paclitaxel and carboplatin in newly diagnosed Stage I–IV and recurrent carcinosarcoma. The indications for these chemotherapeutic agents will be discussed below.
- For *advanced stage disease*, Stage III and IV, chemotherapy is recommended as adjuvant therapy. The rational for chemotherapy is best supported by GOG 150.
  - In this trial patients with Stage I–IV carcinosarcoma were randomized to whole abdominal radiation versus 3 cycles of chemotherapy (ifosfamide, mesna, and cisplatin).
  - The overall crude probability of recurring within 5 years was comparable between the groups 58 % in radiation therapy group versus 52 % for the chemotherapy cohort.
  - The risk of recurrence was 21 % lower for the chemotherapy group compared to radiation therapy and the risk of death was also lower for chemotherapy group.
  - Both of these were not statistically significant; however, the observed differences provided the impetus to recommend the use of chemotherapy.
- The GOG has studied multiple chemotherapeutic agents for advanced and recurrent disease.
  - From these trials, ifosfamide, cisplatin, adriamycin and paclitaxel have had the most significant evidence of activity.
  - Thigpen et al. reported in an early phase II trial of cisplatin, a 19 % overall response rate and a median survival of 7 months [54]. In another phase II GOG trial, the overall response rate for ifosfamide was 32 % [55].
- Since these initial trials multiple combinations have been assessed. Table 4.4 summarizes some of the sentinel assessments.
- These trials have provided the background for the currently open GOG trial, 261.

TABLE 4.4. Summary of highlighted GOG trials for carcinosarcoma [66–69].

Trial	Regimens	Response rates	PFS	Survival
GOG 108 [66]	IFX versus IFX + cis	36 % versus 54 %[a]	4 months versus 6 months	No difference
GOG 161 [67]	IFX versus IFX + taxol	29 % versus 45 %	3.6 months versus 5.8 months[a]	8.4 months versus 13.5 months[a]
GOG 232B [68]	Phase II Carbo/taxol	54 %	7.6 months	14.2 months
Japan [69]	Phase II Carbo/taxol	67 %	9.1 months	Pending

IFX ifosfamide, *Taxol*: paclitaxel, *Cis* cisplatin, *Carbo* carboplatin, *RR* response rates

[a]Statistically significant

Eligible patients include newly diagnosed Stage I–IV as well as persistent or recurrent carcinosarcoma. Patients are randomized to carboplatin + paclitaxel versus ifosfamide + paclitaxel.

Leiomyosarcoma

Surgery

- Typically this uterine sarcoma is identified incidentally following a hysterectomy or myomectomy for presumed uterine leiomyomas.
- The standard surgical management for leiomyosarcoma is hysterectomy often coupled with a bilateral salpingo-oophorectomy (BSO) in post-menopausal women.
    - The role of a BSO has been questioned due to a growing body of literature failing to demonstrate a survival benefit.
    - A review of 1396 women in the SEER database, demonstrated the lack of effect of oophorectomy on disease free survival [56].
    - For those with disease outside of the uterus, the role of cytoreduction is controversial and not clearly understood.

- As with cytoreduction, the role of a lymphadenectomy is also controversial. At the time of initial surgery bulky nodes should be removed.
  - Standard staging when disease is confined to the uterus is questionable since the risk of nodal metastasis is low.
  - The GOG studied 59 patients with Stage I and II disease. The rate of lymph node metastasis in this population, all of which had lymph node sampling, was less than 5 % [57].
  - This was supported by a SEER review, in which nodal metastasis were identified in 23 /348 (6.6 %) women that had a lymph node dissection [56].
  - Certainly in patients with an incidental finding of leiomyosarcoma on final histology, a return to the operating room for "staging" is not indicated.
  - Imaging to identify extrauterine disease is recommended however as this can provide prognostic information and guide recommendations for adjuvant therapy.

Adjuvant Therapy

- The role of chemotherapy, radiation therapy or a combination of the two is controversial and evolving.
- Adjuvant therapy for early stage disease is especially controversial since it is uncertain if any adjuvant therapy improves survival compared to observation alone. As such, enrollment on a clinical trial should be recommended.
- From a historical perspective, both chemotherapy and radiotherapy have been explored for Stage I and II disease.
  - In a randomized EORTC trial of adjuvant radiation versus observation for Stage I and II uterine sarcomas, the recurrence rates were comparable in both arms, 50 % [53].

- With respect to chemotherapy, a randomized trial of doxorubicin versus observation was completed by the GOG in patients with Stage I and II uterine sarcoma.
  - For the entire cohort there was no difference in progression free or overall survival.
  - For the subgroup with leiomyosarcoma, the recurrence rate was 61 % for those in the observation arm versus 44 % in the chemotherapy cohort.
- More recently the combination of docetaxel and gemcitabine has been explored with favorable results in completely resected Stages I–IV.
  - Fixed dose gemcitabine (900 mg/m^2 on days 1 and 8) plus docetaxel (75 mg/m^2 on day 8) demonstrated a progression free survival of 59 % at 2 years. This led to a randomized phase III trial [58].
- Lastly, a phase II multi-institutional trial, the SARC 005 trial, enrolled 47 patients with uterine limited leiomyosarcoma [70].
  - Patient received four cycles of fixed dose gemcitabine plus docetaxel followed by doxorubicin.
  - Approximately 78 % of patients were progression free at 2 years and 57 % remained progression free at 3 years.
  - This provided further support for a randomized trial assessing the role of this combination versus observation.
  - As such, the GOG in collaboration with the EORTC is conducting a randomized trial comparing gemcitabine plus docetaxel followed by doxorubicin to observation in patients with uterine limited disease (GOG 277).

Advanced or Recurrent Leiomyosarcoma

- For decades doxorubicin- based therapy has been the standard therapy for advanced, metastatic disease.

- Other agents that have demonstrated efficacy include ifosfamide, gemcitabine and more recently fixed dose gemcitabine plus docetaxel.
- Two GOG trials have clearly demonstrated promising response rates with the combination of fixed dose gemcitabine and docetaxel.
  - The initial phase II trial of 25 patients with Stage I–IV disease was discussed previously.
  - The second phase II trial (GOG 87 L) of 42 patients with advanced stage disease assessed the same combination. This trial demonstrated an overall response rate of 35.8 % and stable disease in 26.2 % [59].
    - The median duration of an objective response was 6 months.
    - These response rates compare favorably to previously evaluated single agents such as doxorubicin, gemcitabine, and ifosfamide.
- With respect to recurrent disease, leiomyosarcoma commonly recurs in the lungs, liver, abdomen, pelvis and retroperitoneal lymph nodes.
- Local recurrences associated with prolonged progression free survival can be managed with surgical intervention.
- For patients with a local recurrence who are not ideal surgical candidates, radiation therapy can be considered.
- For those women with recurrent metastatic disease, chemotherapy is the recommended approach. The combination of fixed dose gemcitabine and docetaxel is supported by multiple clinical trials that have demonstrated efficacy as both first and second line therapy.
  - A phase II GOG trial (GOG 137G) assessed the activity of this combination in patients with recurrent leiomyosarcoma [60].
  - Many of these patients, 90 %, had previously been exposed to doxorubicin. The overall response rate in this cohort was 27 and 52 % were progression free at 6 months.

- As mentioned previously, gemcitabine, doxorubicin and ifosfamide can also be considered for recurrent disease with estimated response rates of 15–20 %.
- Recently a novel oral multi-kinase inhibitor, pazopanib, has been studied in an EORTC phase III trial in patients that failed anthracycline based therapy.
- Compared to placebo, there was a modest improvement in progression free survival of 4.6 months compared to 1.6 months [61].
- In summary, in the setting of recurrent disease, the chemotherapeutic agent of choice is often dictated by performance status, medical history and patient choice. Palliative intent, unfortunately, is the goal of chemotherapy in the setting of recurrent metastatic disease.

References

1. Jemal A, Bray F, Center MM, Ferlay J, Ward E, Forman D. Global cancer statistics. CA Cancer J Clin. 2011;61(2):69–90. doi:10.3322/caac.20107.
2. SEER. Cancer of the endometrium. SEER Stat Fact Sheets. 2013:1–10 http://seer.cancer.gov/statfacts/html/corp.html. Accessed 20 Jan 14.
3. NCI. Endometrial cancer prevention (PDQ®). National Cancer Institute. 2013:1–21.
4. Sorosky JI. Endometrial cancer. Obstet Gynecol. 2012;120(2 Part 1):383–97. doi:10.1097/AOG.0b013e3182605bf1.
5. Renehan AG, Tyson M, Egger M, Heller RF, Zwahlen M. Body-mass index and incidence of cancer: a systematic review and meta-analysis of prospective observational studies. Lancet. 2008;371(9612):569–78. doi:10.1016/S0140-6736(08)60269-X.
6. Trimble CL, Kauderer J, Zaino R, et al. Concurrent endometrial carcinoma in women with a biopsy diagnosis of atypical endometrial hyperplasia. Cancer. 2006;106(4):812–9. doi:10.1002/cncr.21650.
7. Trimble CL, Method M, Leitao M, et al. Management of endometrial precancers. Obstet Gynecol. 2012;120(5):1160. doi:10.1097/AOG.0b013e31826bb121.

8. d'Angelo E, Prat J. Uterine sarcomas: a review. Gynecol Oncol. 2009:1–9. doi:10.1016/j.ygyno.2009.09.023.
9. NCCN. Uterine Neoplasm. 2012:1–63.
10. Lynch syndrome – Genetics Home Reference. 2014:1–7. http://ghr.nlm.nih.gov/condition/lynch-syndrome. Accessed 20 Jan 14.
11. Cowden syndrome – Genetics Home Reference. 2014:1–7. http://ghr.nlm.nih.gov/condition/cowden-syndrome. Accessed 20 Jan 14.
12. Retinoblastoma – Genetics Home Reference. 2014:1–4. http://ghr.nlm.nih.gov/condition/retinoblastoma. Accessed 20 Jan 14.
13. Shepherd JH. Revised FIGO staging for gynaecological cancer. Br J Obstet Gynaecol. 1989;96(8):889–92.
14. Childers JM, Spirtos NM, Brainard P, Surwit EA. Laparoscopic staging of the patient with incompletely staged early adenocarcinoma of the endometrium. Obset Gynecol. 1994;83:597–600.
15. Spirtos NM, Schlaerth JB, Spirtos TW, Schlaerth AC, Indman PD, Kimball RE. Laparoscopic bilateral pelvic and paraaortic lymph node sampling: an evolving technique. Am J Obstet Gynecol. 1995;173(1):105–11.
16. Spirtos NM, Schlaerth JB, Gross GM, Spirtos TW, Schlaerth AC, Ballon SC. Cost and quality-of-life analyses of surgery for early endometrial cancer: laparotomy versus laparoscopy. Am J Obstet Gynecol. 1996;174(6):1795–9.
17. Walker JL, Piedmonte MR, Spirtos NM, Eisenkop SM, Schlaerth JB, Mannel RS, Spiegel G, Barakat R, Pearl ML, Sharma SK. Laparoscopy compared with laparotomy for comprehensive surgical staging of uterine cancer: Gynecologic Oncology Group Study LAP2. J Clin Oncol. 2009;27(32):5331–6.
18. Zullo F, Falbo A, Palomba S. Safety of laparoscopy vs laparotomy in the surgical staging of endometrial cancer: a systematic review and metaanalysis of randomized controlled trials. Am J Obstet Gynecol. 2012;207(2):94–100.
19. Walker JL, Piedmonte MR, Spirtos NM, Eisenkop SM, Schlaerth JB, Mannel RS, Barakat R, Pearl ML, Sharma SK. Recurrence and survival after random assignment to laparoscopy versus laparotomy for comprehensive surgical staging of uterine cancer: Gynecologic Oncology Group LAP2 Study. J Clin Oncol. 2012;30(13):695–700.
20. Boggess JF, Gehrig PA, Cantrell L, Shafer A, Ridgway M, Skinner EN, Fowler WC. A comparative study of 3 surgical methods for hysterectomy with staging for endometrial cancer: robotic assistance, laparoscopy, laparotomy. Am J Obstet Gynecol. 2008;199(4):360e1–e9.

21. Seamon LG, Cohn DE, Henretta MS, Kim KH, Carlson MJ, Phillips GS, Fowler JM. Minimally invasive comprehensive surgical staging for endometrial cancer: robotics or laparoscopy? Gynecol Oncol. 2009;113(1):36–41.
22. Kilgore JE, Jackson AL, Ko EM, Soper JT, Van Le L, Gehrig PA, Boggess JF. Recurrence-free and 5-year survival following robotic-assisted surgical staging for endometrial carcinoma. Gynecol Oncol. 2013;129(1):49–53.
23. Gehrig PA, Cantrell LA, Shafer A, Abaid LN, Mendivil A, Boggess JF. What is the optimal minimally invasive surgical procedure for endometrial cancer staging in the obese and morbidly obese woman? Gynecol Oncol. 2008;111(1):41–5.
24. Mariani A, Sebo TJ, Katzmann JA, Keeney GL, Roche PC, Lesnick TG, Podratz KC. Pretreatment assessment of prognostic indicators in endometrial cancer. Am J Obstet Gynecol. 2000;182(6):1535–44.
25. Frederick PJ, Straughn JM. The role of comprehensive surgical staging in patients with endometrial cancer. Cancer Control. 2009;16(1):23–9.
26. Kumar S, Medeiros F, Dowdy SC, Keeney GL, Bakkum-Gamez JN, Podratz KC, Cliby WA, Mariani A. A prospective assessment of the reliability of frozen section to direct intraoperative decision making in endometrial cancer. Gynecol Oncol. 2012;127:525–31.
27. Dowdy SC, Borah BJ, Bakkum-Gamez JN, Weaver AL, McGree ME, Haas LR, Keeney GL, Mariani A, Podratz KC. Prospective assessment of survival, morbidity, and cost associated with lymphadenectomy in low-risk endometrial cancer. Gynecol Oncol. 2012;127(1):5–10.
28. Soliman PT, Frumovitz M, Spannuth W, Greer MJ, Sharma S, Schmeler KM, Ramirez PT, Levenback CF, Ramondetta LM. Lymphadenectomy during endometrial cancer staging: practice patterns among gynecologic oncologists. Gynecol Oncol. 2010;119(2):291–4.
29. Panici PB, Basile S, Maneschi F, Alberto LA, Signorelli S, Scambia G, et al. Systematic pelvic lymphadenectomy vs. no lymphadenectomy in early-stage endometrial carcinoma: randomized clinical trial. J Natl Cancer Inst. 2008;100(23):1707–16.
30. ASTEC Study Group, Kitchener H, Swart AM, Qian Q, Amos C, Parmar MK. Efficacy of systematic pelvic lymphadenectomy in endometrial cancer (MRC ASTEC trial): a randomised study. Lancet. 2009;373:125–36.

31. Creasman WT, Mutch DE, Herzog TJ. ASTEC lymphadenectomy and radiation therapy studies: are conclusions valid? Gynecol Oncol. 2010;116:293–4.
32. Keys HM, Roberts JA, Brunetto VL, Zaino RJ, Spirtos NM, Bloss JD, Pearlman A, Bell JG. A phase III trial of surgery with or without adjunctive external pelvic radiation therapy in intermediate risk endometrial adenocarcinoma: a Gynecologic Oncology Group study. Gynecol Oncol. 2004;92(3):744–51.
33. Creutzberg CL, van Putten WL, Koper PC, Lybert ML, et al. Surgery and postoperative radiotherapy versus surgery alone for patients with stage-1 endometrial carcinoma: multicentre randomised trial. PORTEC Study Group. Post operative radiation therapy in endometrial carcinoma. Lancet. 2000;355:1404–11.
34. Creutzberg C. GOG-99: ending the controversy regarding pelvic radiotherapy for endometrial carcinoma? Gynecol Oncol. 2004;92:740–3.
35. The ASTEC/EN.5 Writing Group. Adjuvant external beam radiotherapy in the treatment of endometrial cancer (MRC ASTEC and NCIC CTG EN.5 randomised trials): pooled trial results, systemic review, and meta-analysis. Lancet. 2009;373:137–46.
36. Nout RA, et al. Lancet. 2010;375:816–23.
37. Randall ME, Filiaci VL, Muss H, et al. Randomized phase III trial of whole-abdominal irradiation versus doxorubicin and cisplatin chemotherapy in advanced endometrial carcinoma: a Gynecologic Oncology Group Study. J Clin Oncol. 2006;24:36–44.
38. Susumu N, Sagae S, Udagawa Y, et al. Randomized phase III trial of pelvic radiotherapy versus cisplatin-based combined chemotherapy in patients with intermediate- and combined chemotherapy in patients with intermediate- and high-risk endometrial cancer: a Japanese Gynecologic Oncology Group study. Gynecol Oncol. 2008;108:226–33.
39. Dizon DS. Treatment options for advanced endometrial carcinoma. Gynecol Oncol. 2010;117:373–81.
40. Decruze SB, Green JA. Hormone therapy in advanced and recurrent endometrial cancer: a systematic review. Int J Gynecol Cancer. 2007;17:964.
41. Singh M, Zaino RJ, Filiaci VJ, Leslie KK. Relationship of estrogen and progesterone receptors to clinical outcome in metastatic endometria carcinoma: a Gynecologic Oncology Group Study. Gynecol Oncol. 2007;106:325.
42. Thigpen T, Brady MF, Homesley HD, et al. Tamoxifen in the treatment of advanced or recurrent endometrial carcinoma: a Gynecologic Oncology Group Study. J Clin Oncol. 2001;19:364.

43. Fiorica JV, Brunetto VL, Hanjani P, et al. Phase II tial of alternating courses of megestrol acetate and Tamoxifen in advanced endometrial carcinoma: a Gynecologic Oncology Group study. Gynecol Oncol. 2004;92:10.
44. Growden WB, Rauh-Hain AJ, Cordon A, Garrett LA, Schorge JO, Goodman AK, et al. Prognostic determinants in patients with stage I uterine papillary serous carcinoma: a 15 year multi-institutional review. Int J Gynecol Oncol. 2012;22:417–24.
45. Rauh-Hain JA, Growdon WB, Schorge JO, Goodman AK, Boruta DM, McCAnn C, et al. Prognsotic determinants in patients with stage IIIC-Iv uterine papillary serous carcinoma. Gynecol Oncol. 2010;299–304.
46. Fader AN, Drake RD, O'Malley DM, Gibbons HE, Huh WK, Havrilesky LJ, et al. Platinum/taxane based chemotherapy with or without radiotherapy favorably impacts survival outcomes in stage I uterine papillary serous carcinoma. Cancer. 2009;115:2119–27.
47. Boruta DM, Gehrig PA, Groben PA, Bae-jump V, Boggess JF, Fowler WC, et al. Uterine serous and grade 3 endometrioid carcinomas: is there a survival difference? Cancer. 2004;101:2214–21.
48. Fader AN, Nagel C, Axtell AE, Zanotti KM, Kelley JL, Moore KN, Walsh CS, Huh WK, Gehrig PA, Gibbons H, Rose PG, Havrilesky LJ, Tuller E, Drake RD, Bottsfored-Miller J, O'Malley DM. Stage II uterine papillary serous carcinoma: carboplatin/paclitaxel chemotehrap improves recurrence and survival outcomes. Gynecol Oncol. 2009;112(3):558.
49. Nemani D, Mitra N, Guo M, Lin L. Assessing the effects of lymphadenectomy and radiation therapy in patients with uterine carcinosarcoma: a SEER analysis. Gynecol Oncol. 2008;111(1):82–8.
50. Tanner EJ, Leitao Jr MM, Garg K, Chi DS, Sonoda Y, Gardner GJ, Barakat RR, Jewell EL. The role of cytoreductive surgery for newly diagnosed advanced-stage uterine carcinosarcoma. Gynecol Oncol. 2011;123(3):548–52.
51. Cantrell LA, Havrilesky L, Moore DT, O'Malley D, Liotta M, Secord AA, Nagel CI, Cohn DE, Fader AN, Wallace AH, Rose P, Gehrig PA. A multi-institutional cohort study of adjuvant therapy in stage I-II uterine carcinosarcoma. Gynecol Oncol. 2012;127(1):22.
52. Omura GA, Blessing JA, Major F, Lifshitz S, Ehrlich CE, Mangan C, Beecham J, Park R, Silverberg S. A randomized clinical trial of adjuvant adriamycin in uterine sarcomas: a Gynecologic Oncology Group Study. J Clin Oncol. 1985;3(9):1240.

53. Reed NS, Mangioni C, Malmström H, Scarfone G, Poveda A, Pecorelli S, Tateo S, Franchi M, Jobsen JJ, Coens C, Teodorovic I, Vergote I, Vermorken JB, European Organisation for Research and Treatment of Cancer Gynaecological Cancer Group. Phase III randomised study to evaluate the role of adjuvant pelvic radiotherapy in the treatment of uterine sarcomas stages I and II: an European Organisation for Research and Treatment of Cancer Gynaecological Cancer Group Study (protocol 55874). Eur J Cancer. 2008;44(6):808.
54. Thigpen J, Blessing JA, Orr Jr JW, DiSaia PJ. Phase II trial of cisplatin in the treatment of patients with advanced or recurrent mixed mesodermal sarcomas of the uterus: a Gynecologic Oncology Group study. Cancer Treat Rep. 1986;70:271–4.
55. Sutton GP, Blessing JA, Rosenshein N, Photopulos G, DiSaia PJ. Phase II trial of ifosfamide and mesna in mixed mesodermal tumors of the uterus (a Gynecologic Oncology Group Study). Am J Obstet Gynecol. 1989;161:309–12.
56. Kapp DS, Shin JY, Chan JK. Prognostic factors and survival in 1396 patients with uterine leiomyosarcomas: emphasis on impact of lymphadenectomy and oophorectomy. Cancer. 2008;112(4):820.
57. Major FJ, Blessing JA, Silverberg SG, Morrow CP, Creasman WT, Currie JL, Yordan E, Brady MF. Prognostic factors in early-stage uterine sarcoma. A Gynecologic Oncology Group study. Cancer. 1993;71 Suppl 4:1702.
58. Hensley ML, Ishill N, Soslow R, Larkin J, Abu-Rustum N, Sabbatini P, Konner J, Tew W, Spriggs D, Aghajanian CA. Adjuvant gemcitabine plus docetaxel for completely resected stages I-IV high grade uterine leiomyosarcoma: Results of a prospective study. Gynecol Oncol. 2009;112(3):563.
59. Hensley ML, Blessing JA, Mannel R, Rose PG. Fixed-dose rate gemcitabine plus docetaxel fas first-line therapy for metastatic uterine leiomyosarcoma: A Gynecologic Oncology Group phase II trial. Gynecol Oncol. 2008;109:329.
60. Hensley ML, Blessing JA, Degeest K, Abulafia O, Rose PG, Homesley HD. Fixed-dose rate gemcitabine plus docetaxel as second-line therapy for metastatic uterine leiomyosarcoma: a Gynecologic Oncology Group phase II study. Gynecol Oncol. 2008;109(3):323.
61. van der Graaf WT, Blay JY, Chawla SP, Kim DW, Bui-Nguyen B, Casali PG, Schöffski P, Aglietta M, Staddon AP, Beppu Y, Le Cesne A, Gelderblom H, Judson IR, Araki N, Ouali M, Marreaud S,

Hodge R, Dewji MR, Coens C, Demetri GD, Fletcher CD, Dei Tos AP, Hohenberger P, EORTC Soft Tissue and Bone Sarcoma Group, PALETTE Study Group. Pazopanib for metastatic soft-tissue sarcoma (PALETTE): a randomised, double-blind, placebo-controlled phase 3 trial. Lancet. 2012;379(9829):1879.

62. Seamon LG, Fowler JM, Cohn DE. Lymphadenectomy for endometrial cancer: the controversy. Gynecol Oncol. 2010;117(1):6–8.
63. Thigpen JT, Brady MF, Hmoesley HD, Malfetano J, Dubeshter B, Burger RA, Liao S. Phase III trial of doxorubicin with or without cisplatin in advanced endometrial carcinoma: a gynecologic oncology group study. J Clin Oncol. 2004;22:3902–8.
64. Fleming GF, Filiaci VL, Bentley RC, Herzog T, Sorosky J, Vaccarello L, Gallion H. Phase III randomized trial of doxorubicin and cisplatin versus doxorubicin and 24-h paclitaxel and filgrastim in endometrial carcinoma: a Gynecologic Oncology Group study. Ann Oncol. 2004;15:1173–8.
65. Fleming GF, Brunetto VL, Cella D, Look KY, Reid GC, Munkarah AR, Kline R, Burger RA, Goodman A, Burks RT. Phase III trial of doxorubicin plus cisplatin with or without paclitaxel plus filgrastim in advanced endometrial carcinoma: a gynecologic oncology group study. J Clin Oncol. 2004;22:2159–66.
66. Sutton GP, Brunetto VL, Kilgore L, et al. A phase III trial of ifosfamide with or without cisplatin carcinosarcoma of the uterus: A Gynecologic Oncology Group Study. Gynecol Oncol. 2001;79:147–53.
67. Homesley HD, Filiaci V, Markman M, et al. A Gynecologic Oncology Group Phase III trial of ifosfamide versus ifosfamide plus paclitaxel as first-line treatment of advanced or recurrent uterine carcinosarcoma (mixed mesodermal tumors): a Gynecologic Oncology Group study. J Clin Oncol. 2007;25(5):526–31.
68. Powell MA, Filiaci VL, Rose PG, Mannel RS, Hanjani P, Degeest K, Miller BE, Susumu N, Ueland FR. Phase II evaluation of paclitaxel and carboplatin in the treatment of carcinosarcoma of the uterus: a Gynecologic Oncology Group study. J Clin Oncol. 2010;28:2727–31.
69. Takano T, Otsuki T, Tokunaga H, Toyoshima M, Utsunomiya H, Nagase S, Niikura H, Ito K, Yaegashi N, Yamada H, Tase T, Kagabu M, Shoji T, Sugiyama T, Sato N, Fujimoto T, Terada Y, Nakahara K, Kurachi H, Yokoyama Y, Mizunuma H, Soeda S, Nishiyama H, Matsumoto T, Sato S, Shimada M, Kigawa J.

Paclitaxel-carboplatin for advanced or recurrent carcinosarcoma of the uterus: the Japan Uterine Sarcoma Group and Tohoku Gynecologic Cancer Unit Study. Int J Clin Oncol 2014 (epub ahead of print).

70. Hensley ML, Wathen JK, Maki RG, Araujo DM, Sutton G, Priebat DA, George S, Soslow RA, Baker LH. Adjuvant therapy for high-grade, uterus-limited leiomyosarcoma: results of a phase 2 trial (SARC 005). Cancer. 2013;119(8):1555.

Chapter 5
Gestational Trophoblastic Disease

Elizabeth L. Dickson and Sally A. Mullany

Epidemiology

Incidence

- Difficult to determine true incidence due to uncommon diagnosis of GTD and inaccuracy of documentation of pregnancy loss [2].
- North America, Australia, New Zealand, and Europe incidence ranges from 0.57 to 1.1 per 1,000 pregnancies; Southeast Asia and Japan 2.0 per 1,000 [2].
- In Europe and North America, incidence of CCA estimated at 1 in 40 hydatidiform moles and 1 in 160,000 term pregnancies [3].
- In Southeast Asia and Japan, incidence of CCA is higher, ranging from 3.3 to 9.2 per 40,000 term pregnancies [3].
- Incidence rates of CCA and hydatidiform moles have declined over past 30 years [3].

E.L. Dickson, M.D. (✉) • S.A. Mullany, M.D.
Division of Gynecologic Oncology, Department of Obstetrics, Gynecology and Women's Health, University of Minnesota Medical Center, Fairview, 420 Delaware Street SE, MM395, Minneapolis, MN 55455, USA
e-mail: dilla026@umn.edu; smullany@umn.edu

R.N. Eskander and R.E. Bristow (eds.), *Gynecologic Oncology: A Pocketbook*, DOI 10.1007/978-1-4939-1976-5_5,

- Most consistent *risk factors* for GTD:
  - Extremes of reproductive age (RR 1–5).
  - History of prior molar pregnancy (RR 10–40) [4].
- Only consistent environmental association: Inverse relationship between β carotene and dietary animal fat intake [5].
- CCA risk factors: Prior complete hydatidiform mole, ethnicity, advanced maternal age.
  - Invasive mole or CCA: follows complete molar pregnancy in 15–20 % of cases [6].
  - CCA has never been confirmed after partial mole [6].
  - CCA is 1,000 times more likely after complete mole than any other pregnancy event [4].

Pathology

- All GTD originate from placental trophoblast.
  - Normal trophoblast includes: cytotrophoblast, syncytiotrophoblast, intermediate trophoblast [7].
    - Cytotrophoblast: supplies syncytium with cells and becomes chorionic villi.
      - Basalis layer of endometrium and villous chorion adjacent to endometrium form functional placenta [4].
    - Syncytiotrophoblast: Invades endometrial stroma and produces hCG.
    - Intermediate trophoblast: Located in villi, implantation site, and chorionic sac [7].
  - Hydatidiform moles and CCA from villous trophoblast (Fig. 5.1a).
  - PSTT from intermediate trophoblast.
- Hydatidiform moles: Varying degrees of trophoblastic proliferation.
  - Complete moles: Absence of fetus or embryo.
    - Trophoblast is hyperplastic.

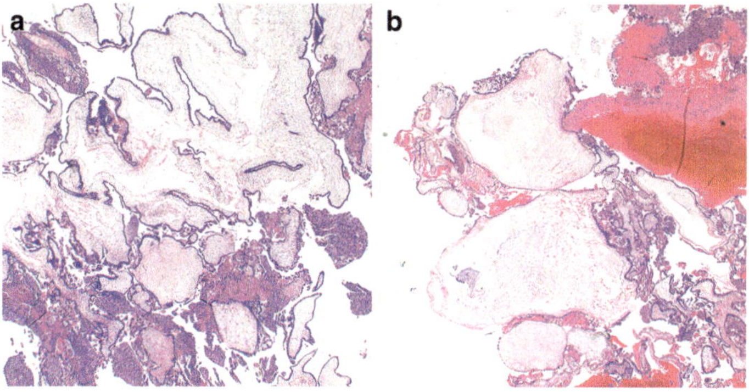

FIG. 5.1. (**a**) Complete hydatidiform mole. All chorionic villi are enlarged and have abnormal shapes. There is marked hyperplasia of the trophoblast. Circumferential proliferation of the trophoblast around the villi is also noted, best seen in the upper left corner. Hematoxylin and eosin, original magnification 20×. (**b**) Partial hydatidiform mole. A few markedly enlarged chorionic villi containing central fluid-filled spaces (cisterns) are interspersed with smaller villi, creating a dimorphic population of villi. There is hyperplasia of the trophoblast, best seen in the upper right corner. Hematoxylin and eosin, original magnification 20×

- Partial moles: Identifiable fetal tissue (Fig. 5.1b).
  - Villi with focal edema [7].
- 10–17 % of hydatidiform moles become invasive mole: Myometrial invasion of hydatidiform mole via direct extension through tissue or venous channels [7].
- 15 % of invasive moles metastasize: Lung and vagina most common.
  - Clinically diagnosed with persistently elevated hCG levels.
    - CCA: Abnormal trophoblastic hyperplasia and anaplasia, absence of chorionic villi, hemorrhage, and necrosis [4] (Fig. 5.2).

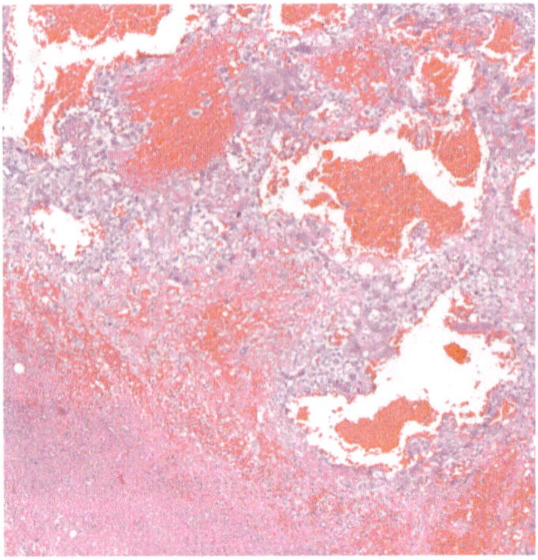

Fig. 5.2. Choriocarcinoma. The tumor is highly hemorrhagic. Necrosis is seen in the lower left corner. The tumor is composed of neoplastic cytotrophoblast (clear cells) and syncytiotrophoblast (purple-staining cells with multiple nuclei). Hematoxylin and eosin, original magnification 100×.

- PSTT: From placental implantation site with mononuclear intermediate trophoblasts without chorionic villi.
  - More lymphatic metastasis.
    - Diffuse cytokeratin and human placental lactogen (HPL) staining [9] (Fig. 5.3).
- Matrix metalloproteinases (MMPs): Involved in metabolism of extracellular matrix, needed for invasion of maternal tissues [10].
  - CCA: high levels of MMP 1, 2, 21, and 28 [11].
    - Low expression of inhibitors of MMPs.
  - PSTT low expression of MMPs.
  - Non-responsive CCA: treated with MMP inhibitors [12].

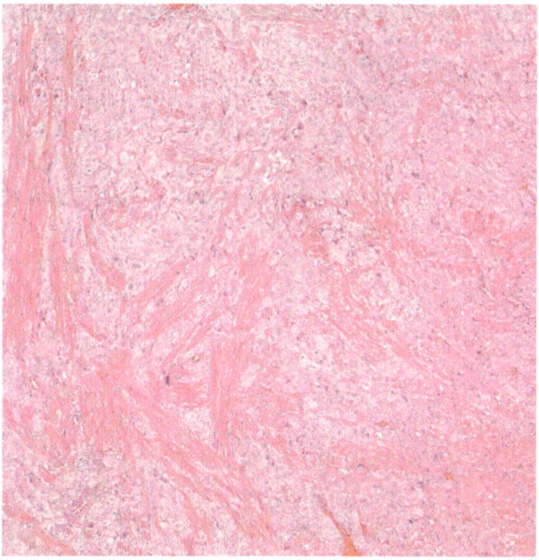

FIG. 5.3. Placental site trophoblastic tumor. The tumor is composed of masses of atypical intermediate trophoblast (pale-staining cells) infiltrating between the bundles of myometrium (staining bright pink). Hematoxylin and eosin, original magnification 100×.

Genetics

- Partial moles typically are triploid in nature (69 XXX or 69 XXY) (Table 5.1) [8].
  - Normal ovum with two spermatozoa [13].
- Complete moles are diploid with all chromosomes from paternal origin (46 XX or XY).
  - Paternally imprinted, maternally expressed genes are not expressed in complete moles [14].
  - $p57^{KIP2}$ is a maternally expressed gene that is absent in complete moles [15].

TABLE 5.1. Characteristics of complete and partial moles [8].

Feature	Partial mole	Complete mole
Karyotype	Triploid (90 %) 69XXX or 69XXY Usually fertilization of normal ovum by 2 sperm	Diploid; 46XX (90 %) or 46XY (10 %) Usually ovum without maternal chromosomes or inactive chromosomes and fertilized by 1 sperm that duplicates
Pathology	–	–
Fetus	Often present	Absent
Amnion, fetal red blood cells	Usually present	Absent
Villous edema	Variable, focal	Diffuse
Trophoblastic proliferation	Focal, slight to moderate	Diffuse, slight to severe
Clinical presentation	–	–
Diagnosis	Missed abortion	Molar gestation
Uterine size	Small for gestational age	50 % larger for gestational age
Theca lutein cysts	Rare	15–25 %
Medical complications	Rare	Less than 25 %
Postmolar malignant sequelae	<5 %	6–32 %

Modified and printed with permission from Soper JT, Lewis JL, Hammond CB. Gestational trophoblastic disease. In: Hoskins WJ, Perez CA, Young RC, editors. Principals and practice of gynecologic oncology. 2nd ed. Philadelphia (PA): Lippincott-Raven; 1997. pp 1039–7 [8]

- Recurrent molar pregnancies have biparental rather than androgenic complete moles [16].
  - Associated with a strong family history, with imprinting abnormalities noted that resemble fully paternal chromosomes [17].
  - Affected chromosome noted in familial cases: 19q13.3–13.4 with mutations in NLRP7 [18].
  - NLRP7 is a cytoplasmic protein, with members of the NLRP family associated with inflammatory processes and apoptosis [15].

Diagnosis

Symptoms

- Complete hydatidiform moles:
  - Present with vaginal bleeding 80–90 % of the time between weeks 6 and 16 of gestation [19].
  - Characterized by uterine size greater than gestational dates, hyperemesis gravidarum, pregnancy induced hypertension, theca lutein cysts, and hyperthyroidism [19].
- Partial moles:
  - Present with incomplete or missed abortion 90 % of the time, followed by vaginal bleeding (75 %) [20].

Imaging

- Ultrasound has replaced any other diagnostic tool to diagnose complete or partial moles [21].
- Complete moles are characterized by a heterogenous mass (snowstorm pattern) without fetus.
  - Ultrasound can demonstrate cystic spaces in the placenta and vesicular pattern of multiple echoes [22].
  - Only 40–60 % of complete moles are detected as molar on ultrasound.
  - American Congress of Obstetrics and Gynecology (ACOG) recommends pathologic evaluation of tissue after spontaneous and therapeutic abortions to confirm diagnosis [23].
  - Presentation of gestational trophoblastic neoplasia is dependent on the antecedent pregnancy event, extent of disease, and histopathology [19].
  - Postmolar GTN presents with enlarged irregular uterus, persistent ovarian enlargement, and irregular bleeding [19].
  - GTN can be diagnosed after metastases are found, and these metastases can bleed.

HCG Levels in GTD

- hCG is composed of an α- subunit, and β-subunit; the β-subunit is specific to the placenta.
- hCG is hyperglycosylated in the first trimester of normal pregnancies; in GTD there are other subunits, such as β core, free β-hCG, nicked free β, or c-terminal peptide [24].
- Hydatidiform moles have markedly elevated hCG levels above normal pregnancy.
  - Complete moles pre-evacuation have hCG levels >100,000 [25].
  - Less than 10 % of partial moles have pre-evacuation hCG levels >100,000.
- Postmolar GTN is diagnosed with rising or plateauing hCG levels after evacuation. CCA is diagnosed with elevated hCG levels after other pregnancy event, likely associated with metastatic disease. PSTT only associated with slight elevation of hCG, but elevated human placental lactogen.
- Postmolar GTN diagnosed by one of the following [26].
  - hCG level plateau of 4 values plus or minus 10 % recorded over a 3-week period (days 1, 7, 14, and 21).
  - hCG level increase of more than 20 % of 3 values recorded over a 2-week period (days 1, 7, and 10).
  - Persistence of detectable hCG for more than 6 months after molar evacuation.
  - Histopathologic diagnosis of CCA.
  - Presence of metastatic disease.
  - New pregnancy must be excluded prior to diagnosis.
- Important to use an assay that can detect intact hCG molecules, but also H-hCG and H-freeβ, as well as degradation products.
  - Different assays can have up to 58-fold variation of hCG results [27].
- Diagnosis of GTD confirmed by cervical dilation and suction curettage; [28]. GOG 242 (results discussed below) illustrated utility of second D&C as a curative measure.

Persistently Low Levels of hCG

- Multiple conditions can cause low levels of hCG.
  - Pregnancy, GTD, false positive or phantom hCG, other malignancies, pituitary hCG.
  - High proportion of women with persistent hCG, without findings of pregnancy or GTD, can go on to unnecessary chemotherapy or hysterectomy [29].
  - Guidelines recommended by the USA hCG reference service for persistent hCG values include ruling out pregnancy, determining if hCG values are real, and determining if active GTN, PSTT, or non-trophoblastic malignancy is present.
    - Serum should be sent to special laboratories to check for H-hCG and free βhCG [29].
  - Phantom or false hCG values can be present in 3–4 % of healthy women [30].
  - Caused by cross-reactivity with heterophilic antibodies in the serum.
    - Product of "sandwich" assays that measure mixtures of hCG.
  - Not present in urine hCG tests; and thus negative urine hCG can be used to confirm false positive [31].
  - Serum can be diluted serially and run through assays to check for false positives (dilution does not affect false titers), or sent for additional tests (see above) [32].
  - No treatment is required for false positive hCG results [32].

Diagnostic Evaluation

- When GTN diagnosed or greatly suspected, patient should undergo thorough evaluation for assessment of extent of disease prior to initiation of therapy.
  - Blood work: Hepatic function, renal function, baseline serum hCG, blood count (CBC), thyroid function tests, blood type.

- Pelvic imaging: By ultrasound or CT to assess for residual disease within uterus, evidence of pelvic spread.
- Chest imaging: Can be performed via Chest X-ray or CT scan. While there is a higher sensitivity for detection of pulmonary metastasis with Chest CT (as high as 40 % in patients with negative Chest X-ray) compared to Chest X-ray, mandatory Chest CT is not necessary if detection of occult pulmonary metastasis does not change treatment protocol [33].
- Patients who are asymptomatic with normal pelvic and chest imaging do not require any additional radiologic imaging [23].
- In all patients with choriocarcinoma or in those patients with vaginal or lung metastasis, Brain MRI should be obtained.
- If lesion in vagina suggestive of GTN present, biopsy is not recommended due to severe bleeding risk [34].

Staging

- FIGO Committee on Gynecologic Oncology in 2000 set forth a staging and classification system for Gestational Trophoblastic Neoplasia [35].
- The staging system is used in combination with the World Health Organization risk-factor scoring system for GTN [36] (see Tables 5.2 and 5.3).

TABLE 5.2. FIGO anatomic staging for gestational trophoblastic neoplasia [36].

FIGO stage	
Stage I	Disease confined to the uterus
Stage II	GTN extending outside of the uterus but limited to genital structures (adnexa, vagina, broad ligament)
Stage III	GTN extending to the lungs with or without genital tract involvement
Stage IV	GTN involving all other metastatic sites

Modified with permission from FIGO committee on Gynecologic Oncology report—Ngan HY, Kohorn EI, Cole LA, et al. Trophoblastic disease. Int J Gynaecol Obstet. 2012; 119S2: S130–6 with permission from Elsevier [36]

TABLE 5.3. Modified WHO prognostic scoring system as adapted by FIGO [36].

	Score			
Risk factor	0	1	2	4
Age	<40	≥40		
Antecedent pregnancy	Mole	Abortion	Term	
Pregnancy event to treatment interval (months)	< 4	4–6	7–12	>12
Pretreatment hCG (mIU/mL)	$< 10^3$	10^3–$<10^4$	10^4–$<10^5$	$\geq 10^5$
Largest tumor size (including uterus)	–	3–<5 cm	≥5 cm	–
Site of metastases	Lung	Spleen, kidney	Gastrointestinal	Liver, brain
Number of metastases	–	1–4	5–8	≥8
Previous failed chemotherapy	–	–	Single drug	2 or more drugs

Modified with permission from FIGO committee on Gynecologic Oncology report—Ngan HY, Kohorn EI, Cole LA, et al. Trophoblastic disease. Int J Gynaecol Obstet. 2012; 119S2: S130–6 with permission from Elsevier [36]

- The FIGO staging system is anatomically based.
- Diagnosis should be presented with Stage (denoted by roman numerals I–IV), followed by the sum of actual risk factors (in Arabic numerals) separated by a colon. For example, II: 4 [35].
- Non metastatic and low risk metastatic GTN (Stage I and Stages II–III with scores <7) can be treated with single agent chemotherapy (see Sect. 6) [4].
- High risk metastatic disease (Stage IV and Stages II–III with scores ≥7) should be treated with multi-agent chemotherapy (see Sect. 6) [4].

Treatment

- Pretreatment workup includes: CBC including platelet count, clotting studies, renal and liver function tests, blood type with antibody screen, hCG level, and chest X-ray (pre-evacuation) [23].

- Prior to suction evacuation and curettage, include possible cross match of 2 units.
- Suction evacuation and curettage is standard of care for those who desire fertility; hysterectomy is appropriate for those who do not [37].
- The largest cannula that can be introduced through the cervix should be utilized to facilitate rapid evacuation [23].
- Intraoperative ultrasound can be used to decrease risk of uterine perforation.
- Oxytocin IV should be used at the start of evacuation to increase uterine contractility and minimize blood loss [23].
- Rh negative patients should be given rhesus immunoglobulin at the time of the evacuation; Rh is expressed on the trophoblast [38].
- Medical induction of labor, or hysterotomy is not recommended as they can increase the risk of postmolar GTN and maternal morbidity [39].
- Prophylactic administration of methotrexate or actinomycin-D chemotherapy should be used only in those with greater than normal risk of postmolar GTN; associated with increased morbidity, and those developing postmolar GTN can be cured with chemotherapy [40].
- No clear guidelines of management for twin pregnancies with molar and normal fetal pregnancy; may continue pregnancy if desired after close evaluation, although risk of persistent or invasive mole approaches 50 % [23, 41].
- Close monitoring of patients after evacuation is essential. Serial hCG should be obtained within 48 h of evacuation, followed by weekly assessments during evaluation (until 3 normal values), and at monthly intervals for at least 6 months [23].
- Contraception recommended for 6–12 months after 1st normal value.
- Future pregnancies should have first trimester ultrasound, pathologic examination of placenta and other products of conception, and 6 week postpartum hCG value [19].

- *LOW RISK GTN:* Stage I, Stage II, or Stage III with score <7, can be treated with single agent Methotrexate (MTX) or actinomycin D chemotherapy [42].
  - Weekly IM or IV MTX, biweekly single dose actinomycin D, 5 day MTX or actinomycin D, and 8 day MTX plus folinic acid can be used (see Treatment Algorithms).
  - hCG levels should be monitored weekly during treatment and consolidation chemotherapy continued for 1–2 cycles after three negative weekly hCG levels have been achieved [4].
- *GOG protocol 242* (initially presented at SGO in March 2014).
  - Evaluated the utility of second curettage in the management of persistent GTN.
  - Low risk patients (WHO score 0–6); nonmetastatic disease; excluded CCA and PSTT.
  - 64 patients enrolled, 59 eligible for assessment. 39 % surgical cure with secondary curettage—efficacy in those with WHO score 0–4.
- *High risk GTN:* Stage II or III with score ≥7, or Stage IV should be treated with multi agent chemotherapy with or without adjuvant surgery and radiotherapy.
  - Etoposide, high dose methotrexate with folinic acid, actinomycin D, cyclophosphamide, and vincristine (EMA-CO) as primary therapy for high risk GTD [43].
  - Chemotherapy should be used for 2–3 courses after first normal hCG evaluation.
  - Whole brain radiation can be used for brain metastasis; surgery can be used for chemotherapy resistant disease or to control for bleeding metastasis [44].
  - 30 % of high risk GTN patients will have an incomplete response to chemotherapy or relapse [45].
    - Salvage chemotherapy with platinum based drugs or surgical resection can treat resistant tumors [46].

- Patients with high risk GTN who have high risk prognostic factors can be treated with EP (etoposide-cisplatin induction therapy) [47].
  - High risk features: High thoracic burden of disease, concerns for respiratory compromise, FIGO score greater than 12, hemorrhage, and rapid tumor destruction.
  - Low dose induction with etoposide and cisplatin reduced the number of deaths from 11 of 140 patients (7.8 %) to 1 of 140 patients (0.7 %) [47].
- PSTT are relatively resistant to chemotherapy, and treatment should begin with hysterectomy and lymph node dissection [48].
- Chemotherapy for PSTT should be limited to metastatic disease or nonmetastatic disease with adverse prognostic factors [48].
  - Chemotherapy regimens include paclitaxel/cisplatin-paclitaxel/etoposide doublet or EMA-EP [49].
- In patients with GTN, after hCG is returned to normal, quantitative hCG levels should be evaluated monthly for 12 months.
- 3 % of patients will relapse in 1st year, and less than 1 % in subsequent years [34].
- Contraception in cases of GTN should continue for 12 months.
- Similar subsequent pregnancy evaluation as to molar pregnancy should be utilized.

Clinical Trials

- GOG 57: Poor prognosis GTD received methotrexate, dactinomycin, and chlorambucil (MAC) or methotrexate, dactinomycin, cyclophosphamide, doxorubicin, melphalan, hydroxyurea, vincristine (CHAMOMA).
  - MAC equally effective and much less toxic than CHAMOMA regimen [50].

- GOG 69: Phase 2 study of nonmetastatic gestational trophoblastic disease patients given Actinomycin-D.
- ACT-D efficacy and toxicity comparable to conventional nonmetastatic GTD therapy [51].
- GOG 79: Study of nonmetastatic GTD patients to determine efficacy, toxicity, and cost-effectiveness of weekly IM methotrexate.
  - Weekly IM methotrexate found to be efficacious, minimally toxic, and cost-effective [52].
  - In GOG 79 follow-up study, 40 mg/m^2 weekly IM methotrexate therapy had comparable efficacy and had similar toxicity to the 30 mg/m^2 weekly dosing.
- GOG 26U: Phase II study of refractory malignant GTD.
  - Ifosfamide (IFX) has activity against choriocarcinoma; addition of etoposide and cisplatin (known as VIP) had significant response in hCG levels and may be curative [53].
- GOG 174: Phase 3 trial of the GOG, JGOG, NCIC, and ECOG in patients with low risk GTN.
  - Compared biweekly intravenous actinomycin-D to weekly IM methotrexate. The remission rate with Actinomycin D was 69 %, compared to 53 % in the methotrexate arm. In the low-risk GTN population, RR with act-D was 73 and 58 % with MTX. No differences in toxicity were reported [54].
- GOG 275 (currently enrolling): Phase 3 randomized trial of the GOG in patients with low risk GTN.
  - Comparing pulsed actinomycin D (1.25 mg/m^2) every 14 days versus IV methotrexate (0.4 mg/kg) daily for 5 days every 14 days versus IM methotrexate (50 mg) on days 1, 3, 5, 7 (4 doses per cycle) with leucovorin (15 mg) on days 2, 4, 8, repeated every 14 days.

- Thailand trial: Randomized controlled trial of actinomycin D versus MTX-folinic acid in Stage I low risk GTN patients.
  - Complete remission achieved in 74 % of MTX therapy, and 100 % of actinomycin D arm [55].
- Brazil trial: Retrospective analysis of low risk GTD patients treated with 5 day regimen of single agent MTX or single agent actinomycin D or combination of MTX and actinomycin.
  - Response rates were not statistically significantly different.
  - Adverse side effects increased with combination therapy (62 %) versus single agent MTX (29 %) or actinomycin D (19 %) [56].
- Northwestern trial: Prospective single institution trial of patients with high risk gestational trophoblastic tumors treated with EMA-CO.
  - EMA-CO therapy was well tolerated and had 71 % complete response rate and 91 % survival rate [57].
- Dutch working party on GTD trial: Randomized controlled trial of EMA-CO versus EMA-CP (cisplatin based combination therapy).
  - Remission rates were similar with only slightly shorter duration of treatment [58].

Treatment Algorithms

Figure 5.4 shows treatment algorithms [59].

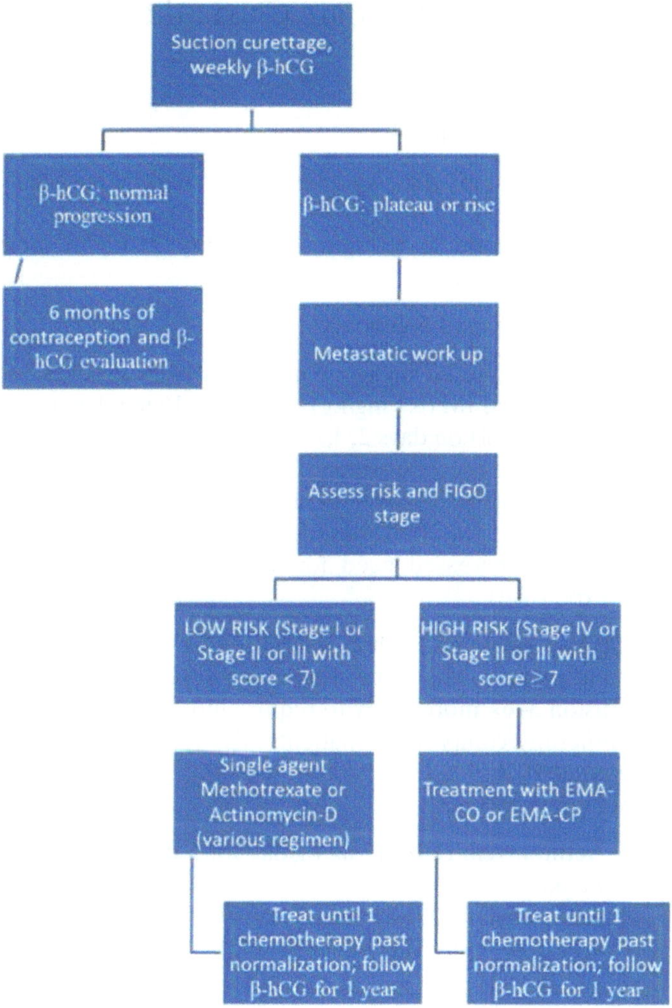

FIG. 5.4. Treatment Algorithm [59]. Adapted with permission from Reynolds, RK. Overview of Gynecologic Oncology: The Blue Book. University of Michigan Gynecologic Oncology handbook. 11th ed. Ann Arbor; 2010. pp 24–8 [59]

Current Standard of Care Chemotherapy

Low Risk GTN [4]

- Methotrexate alone:
  - Methotrexate 0.4 mg/kg (maximum 25 mg) IV push daily for 5 days every 14 days (89 % primary remission).
  - Methotrexate 30–50 mg/m^2 IM weekly (30 mg/m^2 most commonly used).
- Methotrexate and Folinic Acid:
  - Methotrexate 1.0 mg/kg–1.5 mg/kg IM or IV days 1, 3, 5, 7.
  - Folinic acid IM (0.1 mg/kg) or po (7.5–15 mg depending on protocol) on days 2, 4, 6, 8.
  - High dose Methotrexate (100 mg/m^2 IV push followed by 200 mg/m^2 IV over 12 h) with Folinic acid rescue. Treatment interval based on post-treatment hCG trends (increased need for second line therapy and expensive).
- The New England Trophoblastic Disease Center (NETDC) found patients who received the high dose IV MTX 1 day infusion 3–6× more likely to require more courses of chemotherapy compared to patients who received the 8-day regimen [60].
- Actinomycin D.
  - Actinomycin D 10–12 μg/kg/day for 5 days every other week.
  - Actinomycin D 1.25 mg/m^2 IV every 2 weeks (2 mg max dose; more side effect profile).

Conclusions Regarding Treatment of Low-Risk GTN

- No consensus of optimal first line chemotherapy regimen for low risk GTN [61].
- 8 day Methotrexate most cost-effective when compared to weekly methotrexate or pulsed actinomycin D [62]. Active area of investigation in GOG 275.

- hCG levels should be followed on a weekly basis during treatment until negative. Once normalization of hCG has been achieved, an additional 2–3 cycles of consolidation therapy should be administered. Lybel et al. showed a significantly higher relapse rate (8.3 %) in patients treated with two courses of consolidation MTX compared to those treated with three courses (4.0 %) [63].

High Risk GTN

- EMA-CO regimen: Current treatment of choice [58].
  - Day 1: Etoposide 100 mg/m^2 IV over 30 min, Methotrexate 100 mg/m^2 IV push followed by 200 mg/m^2 IV over 12 h, Actinomycin D 0.5 mg IV bolus.
  - Day 2: Etoposide 100 mg/m^2 IV over 30 min, Actinomycin D 0.5 mg IV bolus.
  - Day 8: Cyclophosphamide 600 mg/m^2 IV, Vincristine 1 mg/m^2.
  - Folinic Acid: 15 mg po every 12 h × 4 doses, starting 24 h after initiation of MTX.
  - Cycle repeated every 2 weeks until normalization of hCG and then continued for an additional three cycles (6 weeks).
  - In resistant cases, cisplatin 80 mg/m^2 IV can be added on day 8 and etoposide 100 mg/m^2 to cyclophosphamide and vincristine portions of protocol [64].
- EMA-CP regimen [58]:
  - Day 1: Etoposide 100 mg/m^2, Methotrexate 300 mg/m^2, Cyclophosphamide 600 mg/m^2.
  - Day 2: Etoposide 100 mg/m^2, Actinomycin D 0.6 mg.
  - Day 3: Etoposide 100 mg/m^2.
  - Day 4: Etoposide 100 mg/m^2, Cisplatin 60 mg/m^2.
  - Day 5: Etoposide 100 mg/m^2.
  - Comparable remission rate to EMA-CO, but not more effective [58].

- *Low dose induction chemotherapy with EP*: Patients with high risk GTN who were at high risk of death during EMA/CO chemotherapy can be treated with EP (etoposide-cisplatin) induction therapy [47].
  - Patients with high thoracic burden of disease, concerns for respiratory compromise, FIGO score more than 12, hemorrhage, as well as rapid tumor destruction all at increased risk of early death when treatment initiated with standard EMA/CO regimen [47].
  - Giving patients low dose induction with etoposide 100 mg/m^2 and cisplatin 20 mg/m^2 (for 1–2 cycles) greatly reduced the number of deaths from 11 of 140 patients (7.8 %) to 1 of 140 patients (0.7 %) [47].

Treatment of Specific Metastatic Lesions

- Surgical procedures to resect isolated metastasis can help to reach curative states, especially in cases with concern for hemorrhage [44].
- Central Nervous System.
  - Whole brain irradiation performed, 3,000 cGy at 200 cGy fractions can achieve cure rates of 50–80 % [65].
  - Stereotactic radiosurgery for isolated lesions (oligometastasis), selected patients.
- Lung.
  - Surgical resection especially in setting of resistant disease, isolated lung nodule.
  - Study by Tomodo et al. identified criteria for appropriate patient selection:
    - Good surgical candidate, controlled primary malignancy, no other evidence of metastatic disease, pulmonary metastasis confined to one lung, and hCG <1,000.
    - If all 5 criteria met, complete remission achieved in 93 % [66].

- Liver [61].
  - Surgical resection for isolated lesions or acute bleeding [67].
  - Embolization for bleeding.

Chemoresistant and/or Recurrent GTN

- Of the high risk GTN patients treated with EMA/CO, 30 % will either have an incomplete response or relapse [68].
  - Metastasis to other sites common in these patients.
  - Chemotherapy can be combined with surgical excision to reach cure [44].
- EMA-EP: Can be used for plateauing low levels of hCG or rising levels after complete response to EMA-CO [69].
  - Day 1: Etoposide 100 mg/m^2 IV over 30 min, Methotrexate 100 mg/m^2 IV push followed by 200 mg/m^2 IV over 12 h, Actinomycin D 0.5 mg IV bolus.
  - Day 8: Etoposide 150 mg/m^2 IV, Cisplatin 75 mg/m^2.
  - Folinic Acid: 15 mg po every 12 h × 4 doses, starting 24 h after start of methotrexate.
- Other salvage regimens can include paclitaxel, etoposide, cisplatin, ifosfamide, vinblastine, and bleomycin [70, 71].
  - 82 % of patients with failure of initial chemotherapy who were treated with etoposide-platinum based salvage chemotherapy as well as surgical and radiotherapy techniques were able to achieve cure [70].

Survival

- Cure rates for both low risk and non metastatic disease states approach 100 %.
- 20 % of low risk patients will develop initial resistance, but will reach 90 % cure rate with single agent chemotherapy [19].
- 10 % of low risk patients will require multi-agent chemotherapy.

- 80–90 % of high risk GTN patients will have curative therapy.
- 30 % of high risk patients will relapse or fail first line therapy.
- Gastrointestinal tract metastasis has lowest survival rates at 50 % [72].
- Curative rates for PSTT 50–60 % for metastatic disease [48].

References

1. Sebire NJ, Seckle MJ. Gestational trophoblastic disease: current management of hydatidiform mole. BMJ. 2008;227:A1193.
2. Palmer JR. Advances in the epidemiology of gestational trophoblastic disease. J Repro Med. 1994;39(3):155–62.
3. Smith HO. Gestational trophoblastic disease epidemiology and trends. Clin Obstet Gynecol. 2003;46(3):541–56.
4. Singh DK. Gestational trophoblastic disease. In: Karlan BY, Brostow RE, Li AJ, editors. Gynecologic oncology: clinical practice and surgical atlas. 1st ed. New York, NY: Mc Graw Hill; 2012. p. 157–71.
5. Parazzini F, La Vecchia C, Mangili G, et al. Dietary factors and risk of trophoblastic disease. Am J Obstet Gynecol. 1988;158(1):93–9.
6. Berkowitz RS, Im SS, Bernstein MR, et al. Gestational trophoblastic disease: subsequent pregnancy outcome, including repeat molar pregnancy. J Reprod Med. 1998;43:81–6.
7. Bentley RC. Pathology of gestational trophoblastic disease. Clin Obstet Gynecol. 2003;46(3):513–22.
8. Soper JT, Lewis JL, Hammond CB. Gestational trophoblastic disease. In: Hoskins WJ, Perez CA, Young RC, editors. Principals and practice of gynecologic oncology. 2nd ed. Philadelphia, PA: Lippincott-Raven; 1997. p. 1039–77.
9. Tang X, Yang F, Jia L, et al. Placental site trophoblastic tumor in the pelvic wall: a case report and review of literature. Indian J Pathol Microbiol. 2013;56(3):300–2.
10. Kessenbrock K, Plaks V, Werb Z. Matrix metalloproteinases: regulators of the tumor microenvironment. Cell. 2010;141: 52–67.
11. Singh M, Kindelberger D, Nagymanyoki Z, et al. Matrix metalloproteinases and their inhibitors and inducers in gestational

trophoblastic disease and normal placenta. Gynecol Oncol. 2011;122:178–82.

12. Butler GS, Dean RA, Tam EM, et al. Pharmacoproteiomics of metalloproteinase hydroxamate inhibitor in breast cancer cells: dynamics of membrane type 1 matrix metalloproteinase-mediated membrane protein shedding. Mol Cell Biol. 2008;28:4896–914.
13. Szulman AE, Surti U. The syndromes of hydatidiform mole I and II. Am J Obstet Gynecol. 1978;132(1):20–7.
14. Fukanaga M. Immunohistochemical characterization of p57 (KIP2) expression in early hydatidiform moles. Hum Pathol. 2002;33(12):1188–92.
15. Hoffner L, Surti U. The genetics of gestational trophoblastic disease: a rare complication of pregnancy. Cancer Genet. 2012;205(3):63–77.
16. Fisher RA, Hodges MD, Newlands ES. Familial recurrent hydatidiform mole: a review. J Reprod Med. 2004;49(8):595–601.
17. Kou YC, Shao L, Peng HH, et al. A recurrent intragenic genomic duplication, other novel mutations in NLRP7 and imprinting defects in recurrent biparental hydatidiform moles. Mol Hum Reprod. 2008;14(1):33–40.
18. Moglabey YB, Kircheisen R, Seoud M, et al. Genetic mapping of a maternal locus responsible for familial hydatidiform moles. Hum Mol Genet. 1999;8(4):667–71.
19. Lurain JR. Gestational trophoblastic disease I: epidemiology, pathology, clinical presentation and diagnosis of gestational trophoblastic disease, and management of hydatidiform mole. Am J Obstet Gynecol. 2010;203(6):531–9.
20. Berkowitz RS, Goldstein DB, Bernstein MR. Natural history of partial molar pregnancy. Obstet Gynecol. 1985;66(5):677–81.
21. Benson CB, Genest DR, Bernstein MR, et al. Sonographic appearance of first trimester complete hydatidiform moles. Ultrasound Obstet Gynecol. 2000;16(2):188–91.
22. Reid MH, McGahan JP, Oi R. Sonographic evaluation of hydatidiform mole and its look-alikes. AM J Roentgenol. 1983;140(2): 307–11.
23. Committee on Practice Bulletins-Gynecology. American College of Obstetricians and Gynecologists. ACOG Practice Bulletin 53. Diagnosis and treatment of gestational trophoblastic neoplasms. Obstet Gynecol 2004;103:1365–73.
24. Mitchell H, Seckl MJ. Discrepancies between commercially available immunoassays in the detection of tumour-derived hCG. Mol Cell Endocrinol. 2007;260–262:310–3.

25. Genest DR, Laborde O, Berkowitz RS, et al. A clinicopathologic study of 153 cases of complete hydatidiform mole (1980–1990): histologic grade lacks prognostic significance. Obstet Gynecol. 1991;78:402–9.
26. Kohorn EL. The new FIGO 2000 staging and risk factor scoring system for gestational trophoblastic disease: description and critical assessment. Int J Gynecol Cancer. 2001;11(1):73–7.
27. Cole L, Shahabi S, Butler S, et al. Utility of commonly used commercial human chorionic gonadotropin immunoassays in the diagnosis and management of trophoblastic diseases. Clin Chem. 2001;47(2):308–15.
28. Garner EI, Feltmate CM, Goldstein DP, et al. The curative effect of a second curettage in persistent trophoblastic disease: a retrospective cohort survey. Gynecol Oncol. 2005;99(1):3–5.
29. Cole L, Khanlian SA, Giddings A, et al. Gestational trophoblastic diseases: 4. Presentation with persistent low positive human chorionic gonadotropin test results. Gynecol Oncol. 2006;102:165–72.
30. Palmieri C, Dhillon T, Fisher RA, et al. Management and outcome of healthy women with a persistently elevated beta-hCG. Gynecol Oncol. 2007;106(1):35–43.
31. Rotmensch S, Cole LA. False diagnosis and needless therapy of presumed malignant disease in women with false-positive human chorionic gonadotropin concentrations. Lancet. 2000;355(9205): 712–5.
32. Cole L, Khanian S. Inappropriate management of women with persistent low hCG results. J Reprod Med. 2004;49(6):423–32.
33. El G, Garrett A, Goldstein DP, et al. Significance of chest computed tomography findings in the evaluation and treatemtn of persistent gestational trophoblastic neoplasia. J Reprod Med. 2004;49(6):411–4.
34. Berry E, Hagopian GS, Lurain JR. Vaginal metastases in gestational trophoblastic neoplasia. J Reprod Med. 2006;53(7):487–92.
35. Ngan HY, Bender H, Benedet JL, et al. Gestational trophoblastic neoplasia, FIGO 2000 staging and classification. Int J Gynaecol Obstet. 2003;83 suppl 1:175–7.
36. Ngan HY, Kohorn EI, Cole LA, et al. Trophoblastic disease. Int J Gynaecol Obstet. 2012;119S2:S130–6.
37. Berkowitz RS, Goldstein DP. Molar pregnancy. N Engl J Med. 2009;360:1639–45.
38. Hancock BW, Tidy JA. Current management of molar pregnancy. J Reprod Med. 2002;47(5):347–54.

39. Tidy JA, Gillespie AM, Bright N, et al. Gestational trophoblastic disease: a study of mode of evacuation and subsequent need for treatment with chemotherapy. Gynecol Oncol. 2000;78(3 pt 1): 309–12.
40. Limpongsanurak S. Prophylactic actinomycin D for high risk complete hydatidiform mole. J Reprod Med. 2001;46(2): 110–6.
41. Steller MA, Genest DR, Bernstein MR, et al. Natural history of twin pregnancy with complete hydatidiform mole and coexisting fetus. Obstet Gynecol. 1994;83:35–42.
42. Alazzam M, Tidy J, Hancock BW, et al. First line chemotherapy in low-risk gestational trophoblastic neoplasia. Cochrane Database Syst Rev. 2009;(1):CD007102.
43. Turan T, Karacay O, Tulunay G, et al. Results with EMA/CO (etoposide, methotrexate, actinomycin D, cyclophosphamide, vincristine) chemotherapy in gestational trophoblastic neoplasia. Int J Gynecol Cancer. 2006;16(3):1432–8.
44. Feng F, Xiang Y. Surgical management of chemotherapy-resistant gestational trophoblastic neoplasia. Expert Rev Anticancer Ther. 2010;10(1):71–80.
45. Powles T, Savage PM, Stebbing J, et al. A comparison of patients with relapsed and chemo-refractory gestational trophoblastic neoplasia. Br J Cancer. 2007;96(5):732–7.
46. Wang J, Short D, Sebire NJ, et al. Salvage chemotherapy of relapsed or high-risk gestational trophoblastic neoplasia (GTN) with paclitaxel/cisplatin alternating with paclitaxel/etoposide (TP/TE). Ann Oncol. 2008;19(9):1578–83.
47. Alifrangis C, Agarwal R, Short D, et al. EMA/CO for high risk gestational trophoblastic neoplasia: good outcomes with induction low-dose etoposide-cisplatin and genetic analysis. J Clin Oncol. 2013;31(2):280–6.
48. Hassadia A, Gillespie A, Tidy J, et al. Placental site trophoblastic tumour: clinical features and management. Gynecol Oncol. 2005;99(3):603–7.
49. Lurain JR. Gestational trophoblastic disease II: classification and management of gestational trophoblastic neoplasia. Am J Obstet Gynecol. 2011;204(1):11–8.
50. Curry SL, Twiggs L, Slayton R, et al. Preliminary report of toxicity in a randomized comparison of methotrexate, actinomycin D, and chlorambucil (MAC) vs modified bagshawe regimen in "poor prognosis4" gestational trophoblastic disease. Obstet Gynecol. 1989;73(3):357–62.

51. Petrilli ES, Twiggs LB, Blessing JA, et al. Single dose actinomycin-D treatment for nonmetastatic gestational trophoblastic disease: a prospective phase II trial of the Gynecologic Oncology Group. Cancer. 1987;60:2173–6.
52. Homesley HD, Blessing JA, Rettenmaier M, et al. Weekly intramuscular methotrexate for nonmetastatic gestational trophoblastic disease (A Gynecologic Oncology Group Study). Obstet Gynecol. 1988;72(3-I):413–8.
53. Sutton GP, Soper JT, Blessing JA, et al. Ifosfamide alone and in combination in the treatment of refractory malignant gestational trophoblastic disease. Am J Obstet Gynecol. 1992;167(2):489–95.
54. Osborne RJ, Filiaci V, Schink JC, et al. Phase III trial of weekly methotrexate or pulsed dactinomycin for low-risk gestational trophoblastic neoplasia: a gynecologic oncology group study. J Clin Oncol. 2011;19(7):825–31.
55. Lertkhachonsuk AA, Isranqura N, Wilailak S, et al. Actinomycin d vs. methotrexate-folinic acid as the treatment of stage I, low-risk gestational trophoblastic neoplasia: a randomized controlled trial. Int J Gynecol Cancer. 2009;19(5):985–8.
56. Abrao RA, de Andrade JM, Tiezzi DG, et al. Treatment for low-risk gestational trophoblastic disease: comparison of single-agent methotrexate, dactinomycin and combination regimens. Gynecol Oncol. 2008;108(1):149–53.
57. Escobar PF, Lurain JR, Singh DK, et al. Treratment of high-risk gestational trophoblastic neoplasia with etoposide, methotrexate, actinomycin D, cyclophosphamide, and vincristine chemotherapy. Gynecol Oncol. 2003;91(3):552–7.
58. Lybol C, Thomas CM, Blanken EA, et al. Ccomparin cisplatin-based combination chemotherapy with EMA/CO chemotherapy for the treatment of high risk gestational trophoblastic neoplasia. Eur J Cancer. 2013;49(4):860–7.
59. Reynolds, RK. Overview of gynecologic oncology. University of Michigan Gynecologic Oncology handbook. 11th ed. Ann Arbor; 2010. pp 24–8.
60. Growden WB, Wolfberg AJ, Goldstein DP, et al. Evaluating methotrexate treatment in patients with low-risk postmolar gestational trophoblastic neoplasia. Gynecol Oncol. 2009;112:353–7.
61. Berkowitz RS, Goldstein DP. Current advances in the management of gestational trophoblastic disease. Gynecol Oncol. 2013;128(1):3–5.
62. Shah NT, Barroilhet L, Berkowitz RS, et al. A cost analysis of first-line chemotherapy for low-risk gestational trophoblastic neoplasia. J Reprod Med. 2012;57(5–6):211–8.

63. Lybol C, Sweep FC, Harvey R, et al. Relapse rates after two vs. three consolidation coursres of methotrexate in the treatment of low-risk gestational trophoblastic neoplasia. Gynecol Oncol. 2012;125:576–9.
64. Ghaemmaghami F, Behtash N, Soleimani K, et al. Management of patients with metastatic gestational trophoblastic tumor. Gynecol Oncol. 2004;94(1):1870190.
65. Newlands ES, Holden L, Seckl MJ, et al. Management of brain metastases in patients with high-risk gestational trophoblastic tumors. J Reprod Med. 2002;47(6):465–71.
66. Tomoda Y, Arii Y, Kaseki S, et al. Surgical indications for resection in pulmonary metastasis of choriocarcinoma. Cancer. 1980;46(12):2723–30.
67. Grumbine FC, Rosenshein NB, Brereton HD, et al. Management of liver metastasis from gestational trophoblastic neoplasia. Am J Obstet Gynecol. 1980;137:959–96.
68. Yang J, Xiang Y, Wan X, et al. The prognosis of gestational trophoblastic neoplasia patient with residual lung tumor after completing treatment. Gynecol Oncol. 2006;103(2):479–82.
69. Mao Y, Wan X, Lv W, et al. Relapsed or refractory gestational trophoblastic neoplasia treated with the etoposide and cisplatin/etoposide, methotrexate, and actinomycin D (EP-EMA) regimen. Int J Gynaecol Obstet. 2007;98(1):44–7.
70. Lurain JR, Schink JC. Importance of salvage therapy in the management of high risk gestational trophoblastic neoplasia. J Reprod Med. 2012;57(5–6):219–24.
71. Osborne R, Covens A, Mirchandani D, et al. Successful salvage of relapsed high-risk gestational trophoblastic neoplasia patients using a novel paclitaxel-containing doublet. J Reprod Med. 2004;49(8):655–61.
72. Hoekstra AV, Lurain JR, Rademaker AW, et al. Gestational trophoblastic neoplasia: treatment outcomes. Obstet Gynecol. 2008;112(2 Pt 1):251–8.

Section 2
Chemotherapy

Chapter 6 Chemotherapy for Gynecologic Cancer

Quan Li and Jack L. Watkins

Chemotherapeutic Agents in Gynecologic Oncology

Introduction

The most commonly used agents in the treatment of gynecologic cancers are the platinums (carboplatin and cisplatin) and taxanes (paclitaxel and docetaxel). While these agents are used frequently, there are a number of other drugs employed in the recurrent setting and in the treatment of rare diseases.

Q. Li, Pharm.D. (✉)
Department of Pharmacy, The James Cancer Hospital, The Ohio State University, 410 West 10th Avenue, Doan Room 110, Columbus, OH 43210, USA
e-mail: Quan.Li@osumc.edu

J.L. Watkins, Pharm.D., B.C.O.P.
Department of Clinical Effectiveness, University of Texas MD Anderson Cancer Center, 1515 Holcombe Blvd. T. Boone Pickens Academic Tower (FCT6.6006), Unit 1425, Houston, TX 77030, USA
e-mail: jlwatkins@mdanderson.org

R.N. Eskander and R.E. Bristow (eds.), *Gynecologic Oncology: A Pocketbook*, DOI 10.1007/978-1-4939-1976-5_6,

Pharmacology and Clinical Pearls

Mechanism of action, common and severe toxicities, and clinical pearls of each agent used in the treatment of gynecologic malignancies are outlined in Table 6.1.

Treatment Regimens

Regimens used for the treatment of gynecologic cancers including the drugs, dosage, and frequency are detailed in Table 6.2.

Chemotherapy-Induced Nausea and Vomiting (CINV)

Background [154–157]

Nausea /Vomiting (N/V) are two of the most feared adverse effects of chemotherapy. 70–90 % of patients will experience some form of N/V during their treatment. Since the advent of 5-Hydroxytryptamine-3 (5HT3) antagonists the incidence of vomiting has been decreased to 30 %. However, nausea still remains a significant adverse effect that can have a major impact on the treatment of gynecologic cancers.

Definitions [155, 158]

- Nausea—a feeling of sickness in the stomach characterized by an urge to vomit.
- Vomiting—an expulsion of gastrointestinal contents through the mouth.
- Acute emesis—occurs in the first 24 h after chemotherapy.
- Delayed emesis—takes place 24 h or more after chemotherapy administration.
- Anticipatory emesis—result of a learned response to chemotherapy.

TABLE 6.1. Mechanism of action, common and severe toxicities, and clinical pearls of agents used in the treatment of gynecologic malignancies.

Agent	Mechanism of action	Toxicities	Clinical pearls
Paclitaxel [1, 2]	Antimicrotuble agent; stabilizes microtubules inhibiting interphase and mitosis	• Myelosuppression • Nausea/vomiting (low risk) • Peripheral neuropathy • Arthralgia/myalgia • Hypersensitivity • Alopecia • Vascular irritant	• Should be administered prior to platinum derivatives (to avoid toxicity due to decreased paclitaxel clearance) • Premedicate with corticosteroid, H2 and H1 antagonist • Infuse through 0.22 μm in-line filter and nonsorbing administration set • Myelosuppression increased with higher doses, more frequent doses, and longer infusion times • Peripheral neuropathy increased with more frequent dosing and shorter infusion times • Dose adjust for hepatic toxicity • Drug interactions 1. Anthracyclines 2. CYP2C8, CYP3A4 inducers and inhibitors 3. P-glycoprotein inducers/inhibitors
Docetaxel [2, 3]	Antimicrotubule agent, stabilizes microtubules inhibiting interphase and mitosis	• Myelosuppression • Nausea/vomiting (low) • Peripheral neuropathy • Arthralgia/myalgia • Oncholysis, Alopecia • Hypersensitivity reactions • Fluid retention • Vascular irritant	• Should be administered prior to platinum derivatives (to avoid toxicity due to decreased clearance) • Premedicate with corticosteroid for 3 days starting the day prior to treatment to help with edema • Infuse with nonsorbing polyethylene lined (non-DHEP) tubing • Dose adjust for hepatic toxicity • Drug interactions 1. Anthracyclines 2. CYP3A4 inducers and inhibitors 3. P-glycoprotein inducers/inhibitors

(continued)

TABLE 6.1. (continued)

Agent	Mechanism of action	Toxicities	Clinical pearls
Cisplatin [2, 4]	Alkylating agent, forms DNA intrastrand and interstrand cross-links inhibiting DNA function and synthesis	• Nausea/vomiting (high risk) • Nephrotoxicity • Electrolyte depletion (potassium, magnesium) • Ototoxicity • Peripheral neuropathy • Myelosuppression • Vesicant at higher concentrations (> 0.4 mg/mL)	• Hypersensitivity may develop with prolonged (> 6 cycles) or prior exposure • Administer after taxanes • Adequate hydration prior to (1–2 L) and post infusion is recommended to prevent nephrotoxicity • Do not administer with aluminum needles or IVs • Dose adjust for renal impairment • Drug interactions 1. Aminoglycosides 2. Renal eliminated drugs 3. Loop diuretics
Carboplatin [2, 5]	Alkylating agent, forms DNA interstrand cross-links inhibiting DNA function and synthesis	• Nausea/vomiting (moderate risk) • Peripheral neuropathy • Myelosuppression • Electrolyte depletion (potassium, magnesium) • Nephrotoxicity	• Hypersensitivity may develop with prolonged (>6 cycles) or prior exposure • Administer after taxanes • Do not administer with aluminum needles or IVs • If dose calculated using estimated GFR consider capping estimated GFR at 125 mL/min to avoid toxicity • Doses calculated by target AUC via the Calvert Formula [Total dose = Target AUC × (GFR + 25)] • Drug interactions 1. Aminoglycosides 2. Renally eliminated drugs

Oxaliplatin [2, 6]	Alkylating agent, forms DNA intrastrand and interstrand cross-links inhibiting DNA function and synthesis	• Nausea/vomiting (moderate risk) • Myelosuppression • Peripheral neuropathy (acute and chronic) • Fatigue • *Vesicant*	• Hypersensitivity may develop with prolonged (>6 cycles) or prior exposure • Must be administered via central vein • Do not administer with aluminum needles or IVs • Counsel patients to avoid cold to prevent worsening of acute neuropathies/paresthesia
Irinotecan [2, 7]	Topoisomerase I inhibitor, reversibly binds to topoisomerase I stabilizing the cleavable complex resulting in double-strand DNA breaks and cell death. *S-phase specific*	• Fatigue • Nausea/vomiting (moderate risk) • Myelosuppression • Diarrhea (early and late) • Cholinergic toxicity • Alopecia • Hyperbilirubinemia	• Cholinergic symptoms and early diarrhea may be treated/prevented with atropine 0.25–1 mg • Treat late diarrhea with loperamide 4 mg PO at onset followed by 2 mg every 2 h until no bowel movement for 12 h • Patients with homozygous UGT1A1*28 allele are at increased risk for toxicity • Dose adjust for hepatic impairment • Drug interactions 1. Azole antifungals 2. Carbamazepine 3. CYP2B6, CYP3A4 inducers/inhibitors 4. Conivaptan 5. Fosphenytoin/phenytoin 6. Grapefruit juice 7. P-glycoprotein inducers/inhibitors 8. St. John's Wort

(continued)

TABLE 6.1. (continued)

Agent	Mechanism of action	Toxicities	Clinical pearls
Topotecan [2, 8]	Topoisomerase I inhibitor, binds to topoisomerase I and stabilizing the cleavable complex resulting in single-strand DNA breaks. *S-phase cell cycle specific*	• Myelosuppression • Alopecia • Fatigue • Nausea/vomiting (low risk) • Constipation • Diarrhea • Stomatitis • Vascular irritant	• Dose adjust for renal impairment • Drug interactions 1. Clozapine 2. Fosphenytoin/phenytoin 3. P-glycoprotein inhibitors
Liposomal doxorubicin [2, 9]	Topoisomerase II inhibitor; intercalates between DNA base pairs causing disruption of topoisomerase II. Chelates with iron forming complex which can produce free radicals that cause damage to DNA and cell membranes. Liposomal formulation is pegylated which increases blood circulation time	• *Palmar-plantar erythrodysesthesia* (*Hand-foot syndrome*) • Nausea/vomiting (Low risk) • Stomatitis/mucositis • Diarrhea • Myelosuppression • Discolored urine/body fluids • Infusion reaction • Vascular irritant	• Do not infuse with in-line filter • Associated with less cardiotoxicity than doxorubicin but cumulative lifetime dose should be considered • Monitor cardiac function (LVEF) at baseline and periodically during treatment • May cause radiation recall • Dose adjust for hepatic impairment • Drug interactions 1. Clozapine 2. CYP2B6 substrates 3. CYP2D6, CYP3A4 inhibitors/inducers 4. Taxanes

Doxorubicin [2, 10]	Topoisomerase II inhibitor; intercalates between DNA base pairs causing disruption of topoisomerase II. Chelates with iron forming complex which can produce free radicals that cause damage to DNA and cell membranes	• *Cardiotoxicity (acute and delayed)* • Myelosuppression • Nausea/vomiting (moderate risk) • Diarrhea • Mucositis • Alopecia • Discolored urine/body fluids • Photosensitivity • Radiation recall • Infertility • Secondary malignancy • *Vesicant*	• Increased risk of cardiotoxicity with lifetime cumulative dose >500 mg/m^2 • Baseline and periodic LVEF monitoring is recommended • Prolonging infusion time decreases risk of cardiotoxicity • Dexrazoxane may be used at a 10:1 ratio to decrease risk of cardiotoxicity • If administering continuous infusion use of a central venous line is recommended • Dose adjust for hepatic impairment. • Drug interactions 1. Clozapine 2. CYP2B6 substrates 3. CYP2D6, CYP3A4 inhibitors/inducers 4. Taxanes
Epirubicin [2, 11]	Topoisomerase II inhibitor; intercalates between DNA base pairs causing disruption of topoisomerase II. Chelates with iron forming complex which can produce free radicals that cause damage to DNA and cell membranes	• Nausea/vomiting (moderate risk) • Cardiotoxicity • Alopecia • Myelosuppression • Infertility • Mucositis • Secondary malignancy • *Vesicant*	• Increased risk of cardiotoxicity with lifetime cumulative dose >900 mg/m^2 • Baseline and periodic LVEF monitoring is recommended • Dose adjust for hepatic impairment and severe renal impairment • Drug interactions 1. Cimetidine 2. Taxanes

(continued)

TABLE 6.1. (continued)

Agent	Mechanism of action	Toxicities	Clinical pearls
Gemcitabine [2, 12]	Pyrimidine antimetabolite inhibits DNA synthesis in *S-phase*. Phosphorylated intracellularly to its active metabolites, gemcitabine diphosphate and gemcitabine triphosphate	• Myelosuppression • Nausea/vomiting (low risk) • Rash • Diarrhea • Alopecia • Transient flu-like symptoms • *Hemolytic uremic syndrome*	• Increasing infusion time >60 min increases toxicity • Drug interactions 1. Bleomycin 2. Fluorouracil
Vinorelbine [2, 13]	Antimicrotubule agent; inhibits the formation of microtubules preventing cell replication. *M phase specific*	• Myelosuppression • Peripheral neuropathy • Constipation • *Paralytic ileus/intestinal obstruction* • Fatigue • Nausea/vomiting (minimal risk) • Alopecia • *Vesicant*	• Consider placing patient on bowel regimen • Dose adjust for hepatic impairment • Drug interactions 1. Substrates of CYP3A4 2. Azole antifungals 3. Phenytoin
Vinblastine [2, 14]	Antimicrotubule agent; inhibits the formation of microtubules preventing cell replication. *M phase specific*	• Myelosuppression • Hypertension • Alopecia • *Constipation* • Peripheral neuropathy • Nausea/vomiting (minimal risk) • *Vesicant*	• Dose adjust for hepatic impairment • Consider placing patient on bowel regimen • Drug interactions 1. CYP3A4 and P-glycoprotein substrates 2. Induces P-glycoprotein 3. Itraconazole 4. Voriconazole 5. Erythromycin

Vincristine [2, 15]	Antimicrotubule agent; inhibits the formation of microtubules preventing cell replication. M and S phase specific	• Alopecia • Myelosuppression • Nausea/vomiting (minimal risk) • Cranial nerve dysfunction • *Constipation* • *Paralytic ileus/intestinal perforation* • Peripheral neuropathy • Foot drop/gait changes • *Vesicant*	• Consider placing patient on bowel regimen • Drug Interactions 1. CYP3A4 and P-glycoprotein substrates 2. Itraconazole 3. Voriconazole
Methotrexate [2, 16]	Folate antimetabolite; binds to and inhibits dihydrofolate reductase decreasing formation of reduced folates and thymidylate synthetase inhibiting DNA synthesis, repair and cell replication. *S phase specific*	• Myelosuppression • Alopecia • Nausea/vomiting (low to minimal risk) • Mucositis	• Leucovorin given with some regimens to mitigate hematologic and gastrointestinal side effects • *Elimination reduced in patients with ascites and/or pleural effusions* • Dose adjust for renal and hepatic impairment • Drug interactions 1. Substrates of P-glycoprotein 2. Probenecid 3. Salicylates 4. Hydantoin anticonvulsants 5. Nonsteroidal anti-inflammatory drugs (NSAIDs)
Dactinomycin [2, 17]	Binds to guanine DNA base inhibiting DNA, RNA, and protein synthesis	• Alopecia • Nausea/vomiting (moderate risk) • Increased pigmentation • Rash • Myelosuppression • *Vesicant*	• Adjust dose for hepatic impairment • Drug interactions 1. NSAIDs 2. Salicylates

(continued)

TABLE 6.1. (continued)

Agent	Mechanism of action	Toxicities	Clinical pearls
Cyclophosphamide [2, 18]	Alkylating agent; forms cross-links between strands of DNA inhibiting DNA synthesis. Prodrug that requires activation by liver	• Nausea/vomiting (moderate risk) • Alopecia • *Secondary malignancy* • Infertility • *Hemorrhagic cystitis* (rare at doses use for gynecologic malignancy) • Myelosuppression	• Increase fluid intake during treatment to prevent bladder toxicity • Mesna may be given with higher doses (≥1,000 mg/m^2) to prevent/treat hemorrhagic cystitis • Oral doses should be taken in morning with plenty of fluid • Drug interactions 1. CYP2B6 substrates 2. Nalidixic acid
Altretamine [2, 19]	Alkylating agent; not fully characterized	• Myelosuppression • Peripheral neuropathy • Nausea/vomiting (moderate risk)	• Available as 50 mg capsule • Drug interactions 1. Monoamine oxidase inhibitors 2. NSAIDs 3. Pyridoxine
Capecitabine [2, 20]	Pyrimidine antimetabolite; Prodrug of fluorouracil, activated by liver and tissue to active form which inhibits thymidylate synthetase inhibiting DNA and RNA synthesis. *G1 and S phase specific*	• Nausea/vomiting (low risk) • Myelosuppression • Mucositis • Diarrhea • *Palmar plantar erythrodysesthesia (Hand-foot syndrome)* • Photosensitivity	• Take within 30 min of meal • Swallow tablets whole • Contraindicated in known deficiency of dihydropyrimidine dehydrogenase (DPD) • Not recommended for CrCl <30 mL/min • Dose adjust for renal and hepatic impairment • Drug interactions 1. CYP2C9 inhibitor 2. Warfarin 3. Folic acid 4. Leucovorin

Fluorouracil [2, 21]	Pyrimidine antimetabolite; inhibits thymidylate synthetase inhibiting DNA and RNA synthesis. *G1 and S phase specific*	• Vascular irritant • *Palmar-plantar erythrodysesthesia* • Nausea/vomiting (Low risk) • Photosensitivity • Myelosuppression	• Contraindicated in known deficiency of dihydropyrimidine dehydrogenase (DPD) • Drug interactions 1. Inhibits CYP2CP 2. Dapsone 3. Trimethoprim 4. Hydantoin anticonvulsants 5. Levamisole
Ifosfamide [2, 22]	Alkylating agent; cross-linking strands of DNA inhibiting protein and DNA synthesis	• *Hemorrhagic cystitis* • Alopecia • Nausea/vomiting (High to moderate risk) • Myelosuppression • Encephalopathy (confusion, somnolence, dizziness) • Infertility • Secondary malignancy	• Must be administered with Mesna (at least 60 % of ifosfamide dosage) to prevent hemorrhagic cystitis • Adequate hydration, dose fractionation may be used to decrease hemorrhagic cystitis • Neurotoxicity increased in patients with hypoalbuminemia, renal dysfunction, and history ifosfamide induced encephalopathy • Neurotoxicity may be treated with methylene blue • Dose adjust for renal impairment • Drug interactions 1. CYP2A6, CYP2C19, and CYP3A4 substrates 2. CYP2C9 inducer 3. Conivaptan 4. St. John's wort 5. Telithromycin

(continued)

TABLE 6.1. (continued)

Agent	Mechanism of action	Toxicities	Clinical pearls
Melphalan [2, 23]	Alkylating agent; Cross-links strands of DNA inhibiting DNA and RNA synthesis	• Myelosuppression • Nausea/vomiting (minimal risk) • Secondary malignancy (risk as high as 11 %)	• Administer oral formulation on empty stomach • Dose adjust for renal impairment
Pemetrexed [2, 24]	Folate antimetabolite, inhibits folate dependent enzymes involved in DNA and RNA function and synthesis, thus inhibiting cell function and replication	• Fatigue • Nausea/vomiting • Myelosuppression	• Do not give when CrCl <45 mL/min • Must give with vitamin B12 1,000 mcg subQ every 9 weeks and folic acid 400–1,000 mcg PO daily started 1 week prior to initial dose • Give dexamethasone 4 mg PO BID for 3 days starting 24 h prior to each dose • Drug interactions 1. NSAIDs
Dacarbazine [2, 25]	Exact mechanism unknown, suggested to have alkylating effect as well as antimetabolite activity	• Nausea/vomiting (High risk) • Diarrhea • Flu-like syndrome • Alopecia • Photosensitivity • Rash • Vascular irritant	• Dose adjust for renal impairment • Drug interactions 1. CYP1A2 and CYP2E1 substrates
Temozolomide [2, 26]	Prodrug which is nonenzymaticaly converted to alkylating agent. Bonds to DNA leading to double strand breaks and cell death	• Nausea/vomiting (moderate risk) • Myelosuppression • Fatigue • Alopecia • Constipation	• Capsules should be taken with a full glass of water • Food decreases absorption • Do not crush, break or chew capsule • Administer on empty stomach at bedtime to avoid nausea/vomiting

Pazopanib [2, 27]	Tyrosine kinase inhibitor, decreases activity of vascular endothelial growth factors (VEGF), platelet-derived growth factor receptors, cytokine receptor, interleukin-2 receptor inducible T-cell kinase, leukocyte-specific protein tyrosine kinase, and transmembrane glycoprotein receptor tyrosine kinase	• Hypertension • Fatigue, insomnia, hemiparesis • Hair color change • Hand-foot skin reaction • Rash/skin depigmentation • Diarrhea • Nausea/vomiting (minimal risk) • Myelosuppression • Hepatotoxicity	• Administer 1 h before or 2 h after a meal • Do not crush or chew tablet • If receiving steroids monitor for *Pneumocystis Jiroveci* and consider prophylaxis • Dose adjust for hepatic impairment • Drug interactions 1. CYP3A4 and P-glycoprotein substrates 2. CYP3A4 strong inhibitors—consider decreasing dose by at least 50 % 3. CYP3A4 strong inducers - do not use 4. Avoid grapefruit juice
Etoposide [2, 28, 29]	Topoisomerase II inhibitor, activity results in DNA strand breaks. *S-phase specific*	• Nausea/vomiting (low risk) • Myelosuppression • Alopecia • *Secondary malignancy* • Infusion reaction/hypersensitivity • Vascular irritant	• Do not crush, open or chew capsules • Dose adjust for renal impairment • Drug interactions 1. CYP3A4 and P-glycoprotein substrates
Bleomycin [2, 30]	Antitumor antibiotic, binds to DNA leading single and double strand breaks and decreased DNA, RNA, and protein synthesis	• Vascular irritant • Hypersensitivity reaction • *Pulmonary dysfunction* • Hyperpigmentation • Mucositis • Acute febrile reaction	• Complete pulmonary function tests prior to initiation and consider monitoring every 2 cycles or as clinically indicated • Risk factors for pulmonary toxicity include smoking, prior radiation, and concurrent oxygen administration • Dose adjust for renal impairment

TABLE 6.2. Common gynecologic oncology treatment regimens [31–153].

Chemotherapy regimen	Chemotherapy regimens details	References
Cervical cancer: locally advanced		
Cisplatin + RT	Cisplatin 40 mg/m^2 IV day 1 Q1 week × 6 weeks Concurrent radiotherapy 55–75 Gy	[31–34]
Cisplatin + 5-FU + RT	Cisplatin 70 mg/m^2 IV day 1 5-FU 1,000 mg/m^2/day continuous IV days 1–4 Q3w × 2 cycles Concurrent radiotherapy 49.3 Gy Followed by cisplatin 70 mg/m^2 IV day 1 5-FU 1,000 mg/m^2/day continuous IV days 1–4 Q3w × 2 more cycles	[35]
Cervical cancer: recurrent or metastatic first line		
Cisplatin + paclitaxel	Cisplatin 50 mg/m^2 IV day 1 Paclitaxel 135 mg/m^2 IV day 1 Q3w	[36, 37]
Carboplatin + paclitaxel	Carboplatin AUC = 6 IV day 1 Paclitaxel 175 mg/m^2 IV day 1 Q3w	[38]
Cisplatin + topotecan	Cisplatin 50 mg/m^2 IV day 1 Topotecan 0.75 mg/m^2/day IV days 1–3 Q3w × 6 cycles	[37, 39]
Cisplatin + paclitaxel + bevacizumab	Cisplatin 50 mg/m^2 IV day 1 Paclitaxel 135–175 mg/m^2 IV day1 Bevacizumab 15 mg/kg IV day 1 Q3w	[40]

Cisplatin + gemcitabine	Cisplatin 50 mg/m² IV day 1 Gemcitabine 1,000 mg/m²/day IV days 1, 8 Q3w	[37]
Cisplatin	Cisplatin 50 mg/m² IV day 1 Q3w	[39]
Carboplatin	Carboplatin AUC = 5–7.5 IV day 1 Q3w	[41]
Paclitaxel	Paclitaxel 135–175 mg/m² IV day 1 Q3w	[42]
Cervical cancer: recurrent or metastatic second line		
Bevacizumab	Bevacizumab 15 mg/kg IV day 1 Q3w	[43]
Docetaxel	Docetaxel 75 mg/m² IV day 1 Q3w	[44]
5-FU	5-FU 370 mg/m²/day IV push days 1–5 Leucovorin 200 mg/m² IV push days 1–5 Q4w OR 5-FU 1,000 mg/m²/day continuous IV infusion days 1–5 Q4w	[45]
Gemcitabine	Gemcitabine 800 mg/m² IV days 1, 8, 15 Q4w	[46]
Ifosfamide	1.5 g/m²/day IV days 1-5 Mesna 300 mg/m² IV 0 h, 4 h, 8 h, d1–5 Q4w	[47, 48]
Irinotecan	Irinotecan 125 mg/m² IV days 1, 8, 15 & 22 Q6w	[49]
Mitomycin	Mitomycin 10–15 mg/m² IV push day 1 Q4-6w	[50]
Topotecan	Topotecan 1.5 mg/m²/day IV days 1–5 Q3–4w or Topotecan 3–4 mg/m²/d IV days 1, 8, 15 Q4w	[51, 52]

(continue

Table 6.2. (continued)

Cervical cancer: locally advanced		
Chemotherapy regimen	Chemotherapy regimens details	References
Endometrial cancer: hormonal therapy for recurrent, metastatic, or high-risk endometrial cancer		
Hormonal regimen	Hormonal regimen details	References
Medroxyprogesterone	Medroxyprogesterone 200–1,000 mg po daily days 1–14 Q28d	[53]
Tamoxifen	Tamoxifen 20 mg po bid	[54]
Megestrol acetate	Megestrol 80 mg po bid OR Megestrol 800 mg po daily in divided doses	[55, 56]
Megestrol/tamoxifen	Megestrol 80 mg po bid × 3 weeks alternative with tamoxifen 20 mg po bid	[57]
Letrozole	Letrozole 2.5 mg po daily	[58]
Anastrozole	Anastrozole 1 mg po daily	[59]
Endometrial cancer: adjuvant for recurrent, metastatic, or high-risk endometrial cancer		
Cisplatin + doxorubicin	Doxorubicin 60 mg/m^2 IV day 1 Cisplatin 50 mg/m^2 IV day 1 Q3w	[60, 61]
Cisplatin + doxorubicin + paclitaxel	Doxorubicin 45 mg/m^2 IV day 1 Cisplatin 50 mg/m^2 IV day 1 Paclitaxel 160 mg/m^2 IV day 2 Q3w	[62]
Carboplatin + paclitaxel	Paclitaxel 175 mg/m^2 IV day 1 Carboplatin AUC 5-7 IV day 1 Q4w	[63–65]
Weekly paclitaxel + carboplatin	Paclitaxel 80 mg/m^2 IV days 1, 8, 15 Carboplatin AUC = 2 IV days 1, 8, 15 Q3w	[66]

Carboplatin + docetaxel	Carboplatin ACU = 6 IV day 1 Docetaxel 60 mg/m² IV day 1 Q3w Carboplatin AUC = 6 IV day 1 Docetaxel 75 mg IV day 1 followed by radiation Q3w	[65, 67, 68]
Cisplatin	Cisplatin 50–60 mg/m² IV day 1 Q3w	[69, 70]
Carboplatin	Carboplatin 350–400 mg/m² IV Q3-4w	[71, 72]
Doxorubicin	Doxorubicin 45–60 mg/m² IV day 1 Q3w	[73]
Liposomal doxorubicin	Liposomal doxorubicin 40–50 mg/m² IV day 1 Q3w	[74]
Paclitaxel	Paclitaxel 175–250 mg/m² IV day 1 Q3w	[75, 76]
Weekly docetaxel	Docetaxel 36 mg/m² IV days 1, 8, 15 Q3w	[77]
Bevacizumab	Bevacizumab 15 mg/kg IV day 1 Q3w	[78]
Cisplatin + ifosfamide (for carcinosarcoma)	Cisplatin 20 mg/m²/day IV days 1–4 Ifosfamide 1.5 g/m²/day IV days 1–4 Mesna 120 mg/m² IV loading dose followed by 1.5 g/m²/day IV days 1–4 Q3w	[79, 80]
Ifosfamide + paclitaxel (for carcinosarcoma)	Ifosfamide 1.6 g/m²/day (1.2 g/m²/day if patients received prior radiation) IV days 1–3 Paclitaxel 135 mg/m² IV over 3 h day 1 Mesna 2 g IV over 12 h days 1–3 Q3w × 8 cycles	[81]

(continued)

Table 6.2. (continued)

Cervical cancer: locally advanced		
Chemotherapy regimen	Chemotherapy regimens details	References
Ifosfamide (for carcinosarcoma)	Ifosfamide 2.0 g/m²/day (1.2 g/m²/day if patients received prior radiation) IV days 1–3 Mesna 2 g IV over 12 h days 1–3 Q3w × 8 cycles	[81]
Uterine sarcoma: hormonal therapy for endometrial stromal sarcoma		
Hormonal regimen	Hormonal regimen details	References
Medroxyprogesterone	Medroxyprogesterone 500–1,000 mg po daily	[82]
Megestrol acetate	Megestrol 160 mg po daily	[83, 84]
Letrozole	Letrozole 2.5 mg po daily	[85]
Anastrozole	Anastrozole 1 mg po daily	[85]
GnRH analog	Optimal dose unknown	
Uterine sarcoma: chemotherapy		
Gemcitabine + docetaxel	Gemcitabine 900 mg/m² IV over 90 min days 1, 8 Docetaxel 75–100 mg/m² IV day 8 Q3w Dose reduced by 25 % for patients with prior history of pelvic radiation	[86–89]
Doxorubicin + ifosfamide	Doxorubicin 50–75 mg/m² IV day 1 Ifosfamide 5 g/m² IV over 24 h day 1 Mesna 6 g/m² IV over 36 h day 1 Q3w Dose reduced by 25 % for patients with prior history of pelvic radiation	[90, 91]

Doxorubicin + dacarbazine	Doxorubicin 60 mg/m² IV day 1 Dacarbazine 250 mg/m² IV days 1–5 Q3w Dose reduced by 25 % for patients with prior history of pelvic radiation	[92]
Gemcitabine + dacarbazine	Gemcitabine 1,800 mg/m² IV over 180 min day 1 Dacarbazine 500 mg/m² IV Q2w	[93, 94]
Gemcitabine + vinorelbine	Vinorelbine 25 mg/m² IV day 1 Gemcitabine 800 mg/m² IV over 90 min days 1, 8 Q3w	[95]
Doxorubicin	Doxorubicin 60 mg/m² IV day 1 Q3w	[92]
Epirubicin	Epirubicin 75 mg/m² IV day 1 Q3w	[96]
Gemcitabine	Gemcitabine 1,000 mg/m² IV days 1, 8, 15 Q4w	[97]
Ifosfamide	Ifosfamide 1.5 g/m²/day IV days 1–5 Q3w	[98]
Liposomal doxorubicin	Liposomal doxorubicin 50 mg/m² IV day 1 Q4w	[99]
Paclitaxel	Paclitaxel 175 mg/m² IV day 1 Q3w	[100, 101]
Temozolomide	Temozolomide 50–75 mg/m² po daily week 1–6 Q8w	[102]
Dacarbazine	Dacarbazine 1,200 mg/m² IV day 1 Q3w	[94]

(continued)

Table 6.2. (continued)

Cervical cancer: locally advanced		
Chemotherapy regimen	Chemotherapy regimens details	References
Vinorelbine	Vinorelbine 30 mg/m^2 IV day 1 Q2w	[103]
Pazopanib	Pazopanib 800 mg po daily	[104]
Ovarian, fallopian tube, or primary peritoneal carcinoma: primary chemotherapy for Stage II–IV		
Paclitaxel + carboplatin	Paclitaxel 175 mg/m^2 IV over 3 h day 1 Carboplatin AUC = 5–7.5 IV day 1 Q3w × 6 cycles	[105]
Docetaxel + carboplatin	Docetaxel 60–75 mg/m^2 IV day 1 Carboplatin AUC = 5–6 IV day1 Q3w × 6 cycles	[106]
Paclitaxel + cisplatin	Paclitaxel 135 mg/m^2 IV over 24 h day 1 Cisplatin 75–100 mg/m^2 IV day 2 Q3w × 6 cycles	[107]
Paclitaxel IV + cisplatin IP + paclitaxel IP	Paclitaxel 135 mg IV over 3 h or 24 h day 1 Cisplatin 75–100 mg/m^2 IP day 2 Paclitaxel 60 mg/m^2 IP day 8 Q3w × 6 cycles	[108]
Paclitaxel D1,8, 15 + carboplatin	Paclitaxel 80 mg/m^2 IV over 1 h days 1, 8, 15 Carboplatin AUC = 6 IV day 1 Q3w × 6 cycles	[109]
Paclitaxel + carboplatin + bevacizumab	Paclitaxel 175 mg/m^2 IV day 1 Carboplatin AUC = 5–7.5 IV day 1 Q3w × 6 cycles + Bevacizumab 15 mg/kg IV day 1 (C2–22)	[110]

Paclitaxel + carboplatin + bevacizumab	Paclitaxel 175 mg/m^2 IV day 1 Carboplatin AUC = 5–7.5 IV day 1 Q3w × 6 cycles + Bevacizumab 15 mg/kg IV day 1 (C2-18)	[111]
Ovarian, fallopian tube, or primary peritoneal carcinoma: platinum-sensitive, first-relapse		
Paclitaxel + carboplatin	Paclitaxel 175 mg/m^2 IV day 1 Carboplatin AUC = 5–6 IV day 1 Q3w	[112, 113]
Gemcitabine + carboplatin	Gemcitabine 1,000 mg/m^2 IV days 1, 8 Carboplatin AUC = 4 IV day 1 Q3w	[114]
Gemcitabine + carboplatin + bevacizumab	Gemcitabine 1,000 mg/m^2 IV days 1, 8 Carboplatin AUC = 4 IV day 1 Bevacizumab 15 mg/kg IV day 1 Q3w	[115]
Gemcitabine + cisplatin	Gemcitabine 600–750 mg/m^2 IV days 1, 8 Cisplatin 30 mg/m^2 IV days 1, 8 Q3w	[116, 117]
Docetaxel + carboplatin	Docetaxel 75 mg/m^2 IV day 1 Carboplatin AUC = 5 IV day 1 Q3w	[118]
Paclitaxel D1,8, 15 + carboplatin	Paclitaxel 80 mg/m^2 IV over 1 h days 1, 8, 15 Carboplatin AUC = 6 IV day 1 Q3w	[109]
Docetaxel D1,8,15 + carboplatin	Docetaxel 35 mg/m^2 IV days 1, 8, 15 Carboplatin AUC = 2 IV days 1, 8, 15 Q4w	[119]

(continued)

TABLE 6.2. (continued)

Chemotherapy regimen	Chemotherapy regimens details	References
Cervical cancer: locally advanced		
Liposomal doxorubicin + carboplatin	Liposomal doxorubicin 30 mg/m² IV day 1 Carboplatin AUC = 5 IV day 1 Q4w	[120]
Carboplatin	Carboplatin AUC = 5–6 IV day 1 Q3w	[112, 114, 121]
Bevacizumab	Bevacizumab 15 mg/kg IV day 1 Q3w	[122]
Ovarian, fallopian tube, or primary peritoneal carcinoma: platinum-resistant or subsequent recurrence		
Docetaxel	Docetaxel 75–100 mg/m² IV day 1 Q3w Or Docetaxel 30 mg/m² IV days 1, 8, 15 Q4w	[123, 124]
Weekly paclitaxel	Paclitaxel 80 mg/m² IV days 1, 8, 15 Q4w	[125]
Gemcitabine	Gemcitabine 600–1,000 mg/m² IV days 1,8, 15 Q4w	[126–128]
Etoposide (oral)	Etoposide 50 mg/m² po days 1–21 Q4w	[129]
Altretamine	Altretamine 260 mg/m² po days 1–14 Q4w	[130]
Bevacizumab	Bevacizumab 15 mg/kg IV day 1 Q3w	[122, 131, 132]
Nab-paclitaxel	Nab-paclitaxel 260 mg/m² IV day 1 Q3w	[133]

Oxaliplatin	Oxaliplatin 130 mg/m² IV day 1 Q3w	[134]
Liposomal doxorubicin	Pegylated liposomal doxorubicin 40 mg/m² IV day 1 Q4w	[135–137]
Topotecan	Topotecan 1.25 mg/m² IV days 1–5 Q3–4w Or Topotecan 3–4 mg/m² IV days 1, 8, 15 W3-4w	[135, 138–140]
Vinorelbine	Vinorelbine 30 mg/m² IV days 1, 8 Q3w	[141]
Pemetrexed	Pemetrexed 900 mg/m² IV day 1 Q3w	[142]
Ifosfamide	Ifosfamide 1,000–1,200 mg/m²/day IV days 1–5 Mesna 200 mg/m²/day IV 0 h, 4 h, 8 h, days 1–5 Q4w	[143]
Capecitabine	Capecitabine 2,000 mg/m²/day po in two divided doses, days 1–14 Q3w	[144]
Irinotecan	Irinotecan 250–300 mg/m² IV day 1 Q3w	[145]
Tamoxifen	Tamoxifen 20 mg po bid	[146]
Anastrozole	Anastrozole 1 mg po daily	[147]
Letrozole	Letrozole 2.5 mg po daily	[148–150]
Leuprolide acetate	Leuprolide 3.75 mg im Q4w	[151]
Megestrol acetate	Megestrol 800 mg po daily × 28 days followed by 400 mg po daily	[152, 153]

- Breakthrough emesis occurs despite prophylactic antiemetics.
- Refractory emesis failure to respond to prevention or intervention in the previous cycle.

Alternative Etiologies [159]

- Medications (opioids, antimicrobials).
- Surgery/radiation.
- Electrolyte imbalances/dehydration.
- Gastrointestinal: obstruction, gastroparesis, constipation.
- Psychological (anxiety, anticipatory).
- Brain metastasis.

Complications [157, 158]

- Metabolic imbalances.
- Decreased performance status.
- Nutrient depletion/Anorexia.
- Wound dehiscence.
- Esophageal tears.
- Noncompliance with treatment.
- Aspiration.
- Decreased quality of life.

Risk Factors [154, 157, 158, 160, 161]

Patient Related

- Age—increased risk in younger patients.
- Gender—increased risk for females.
- History of alcohol use—decreased with prior use.
- History of CINV.
- History of vertigo/motion sickness.
- Non-chemotherapy related etiologies.
- History of nausea/vomiting with pregnancy.

Chemotherapy Related

- >90 % = High risk.
- 31–90 % = Moderate risk.
- 10–30 % = Low risk.
- <10 % = Minimal risk.

See Table 6.3 for CINV risk for agents used to treat gynecologic cancers.

Table 6.3. Chemotherapy induced nausea/vomiting (CINV) risk by agent.

Risk category	Agents
High risk (>90 %)	Cisplatin
	Dacarbazine
	Doxorubicin >60 mg/m^2
	Ifosfamide ≥2 g/m^2/dose
Moderate risk (31–90 %)	Carboplatin
	Dactinomycin
	Doxorubicin <60 mg/m^2
	Epirubicin ≤90 mg/m^2
	Ifosfamide <2 g/m^2/dose
	Irinotecan
	Melphalan
	Methotrexate ≥250 mg/m^2
	Oxaliplatin
	Temozolomide
Low risk (10–30 %)	Docetaxel
	Liposomal doxorubicin
	Etoposide
	Fluorouracil
	Gemcitabine
	Mitomycin
	Paclitaxel
	Pemetrexed
	Topotecan
Minimal risk (<10 %)	Bevacizumab
	Bleomycin
	Vinblastine
	Vincristine
	Vinorelbine

Therapeutic Options [2, 160, 168]

High Therapeutic Index Agents

Used primarily for prevention first line breakthrough. Dosing outlined in Table 6.4.

- 5HT3 receptor antagonists:

  Agents: Ondansetron, Palonosetron, Granisetron, Dolasetron.
  Adverse effects: headache, constipation, QT prolongation.

- Corticosteroids.

  Agents: Dexamethasone, Prednisone, Methylprednisolone.
  Adverse effects: hyperglycemia, insomnia, hypertension, immunosuppression.

TABLE 6.4. High therapeutic index antiemetic common dosing.

Agent	Pre-chemotherapy	Post-chemotherapy
Ondansetron	8–16 mg IV/PO 30 min prior to	8 mg PO TID × 3 days
Dolasetron	100 mg IV/PO 30 min prior to	100 mg PO daily × 3 days
Granisetron	1 mg IV/PO 30 min prior to; 34.3 mg transdermal patch applied 24–48 h prior to	1–2 mg PO BID × 3 days
Palonosetron	0.25 mg IV 30 min prior to	
Dexamethasone w/ aprepitant 125 mg PO	12 mg IV/PO 30 min prior to	8 mg PO daily × 3 days
Dexamethasone w/ fosaprepitant 150 mg IV	12 mg IV/PO 30 min prior to	8 mg day 2, 8 mg PO BID days 3 and 4
Dexamethasone w/o aprepitant	8-20 mg IV/PO 30 min prior to	8 mg PO BID × 3 days
Aprepitant	125 mg PO 1 h prior to	80 mg PO × 2 days
Fosaprepitant	150 mg IV 30 min prior to	

- Neurokinin-1 receptor antagonists.

  Agents: Aprepitant, Fosaprepitant.
  Adverse effects: headache, hiccups, fatigue.
  Moderate inhibitor and inducer of CYP3A4, weak inducer of CYP2C9.

Low Therapeutic Index Agents

Used primarily for breakthrough N/V. Dosing outlined in Table 6.5.

- Phenothiazines.

  Agents: Prochlorperazine, Promethazine.
  Adverse effects: sedation, anticholinergic effects, extrapyramidal side effects.

- Metoclopramide.

  Adverse effects: sedation, extrapyramidal side effects, diarrhea.

TABLE 6.5. Low therapeutic index antiemetic common dosing.

Agent	Dosing
Promethazine	6.25–25 mg IV/PO q6h prn 25 mg PR q6h prn
Prochlorperazine	5–10 mg IV/PO q6h prn 25 mg PR q6h prn
Metoclopramide	0.5–2 mg/kg IV q4h prn (must give w/diphenhydramine 25 mg IV q6h to prevent extrapyramidal side effects) 10–40 mg PO q6h prn
Olanzapine	2.5–5 mg PO qHS
Alprazolam	0.5–2 mg PO prior to chemotherapy
Lorazepam	1–2 mg IV/PO prior to chemotherapy 0.5–2 mg PO q4h prn N/V
Haloperidol	1 mg IV q4h PRN
Dronabinol	5–10 mg PO q3h prn
Nabilone	1–2 mg PO q12h prn

- Olanzapine.

  Adverse effects: sedation, weight gain.

- Benzodiazepines.

  Drug of choice for anticipatory N/V.
  Agents: Lorazepam, Alprazolam.
  Adverse effects: sedation, amnesia.

- Butyrophenones.

  Agents: Haloperidol
  Adverse effects: sedation, constipation, arrhythmias, extra-pyramidal side effects.

- Cannabinoids.

  Agents: Dronabinol, Nabilone.
  Adverse effects: sedation, abnormal thinking, palpitations, tachycardia, euphoria.

General Principles of Treatment [155, 160, 161, 165]

- Primary goal is prevention of CINV.
- Agents are chosen based upon chemotherapy regimen.
- Consider toxicity of antiemetics used.
- Always provide "rescue" medication for breakthrough CINV.

Treatment Recommendations [160, 161, 165, 169, 170]

High Risk Chemotherapy

- Acute Emesis Prevention.

  5HT3 antagonist + Dexamethasone + Neurokinin 1 antagonist +/− lorazepam +/− H2 blocker or proton pump inhibitor.

- Delayed Emesis Prevention.

  If fosaprepitant 150 mg: dexamethasone 8 mg PO day 2 then 8 mg PO BID days 3–4.
  If aprepitant day 2–3: dexamethasone 8 mg PO days 2–4.

Moderate Risk Chemotherapy

- Acute Emesis Prevention.

  5HT3 antagonist + dexamethasone +/– Neurokinin 1 antagonist +/– lorazepam +/– H2 blocker or proton pump inhibitor.

- Delayed Emesis Prevention.

  5HT3 antagonist monotherapy for 2–3 days, OR.
  Dexamethasone monotherapy for 2–3 days, OR.
  Neurokinin 1 antagonist (if used day 1) + dexamethasone.

Low Risk

- Prior to chemotherapy.
  Dexamethasone PO/IV, OR.
  Metoclopramide PO/IV, OR.
  Prochlorperazine PO/IV, OR.
  +/– Lorazepam and/or H2 blocker or proton pump inhibitor.

Minimal Risk

- No prophylaxis recommended.

Multiday Chemotherapy Regimens

- Consider emetogenic potential of each day.
- 5-HT3 antagonist should be administered daily for moderately or highly emetogenic chemotherapy.

- Dexamethasone should be given daily prior for moderately or highly emetogenic chemotherapy.
- Prevent delayed emesis with 2–3 days of prophylaxis following chemotherapy.
- Palonosetron or transdermal granisetron may be used in lieu of daily 5HT3 dosing.
- Dosing of Aprepitant beyond 3 days has been shown to be safe and effective in phase II trials.
- Repeat doses of palonosetron have been studied and shown to reduce CINV.

Breakthrough Emesis

- Add agent from different class.
- PO administration often unfeasible due to emesis.
- Routine administration of "rescue" medication should be considered.
- Multiple concurrent agents in alternating schedules.
- Reevaluate for alternative etiologies.
- Change regimen for next cycle.

Chemotherapy-Induced Diarrhea

Introduction [171–173]

Many chemotherapy agents can cause damage to the intestinal mucosa ultimately resulting in diarrhea. If not managed properly chemotherapy-induced diarrhea can result in treatment delays, dose reductions, and serious complications that may be fatal. Most agents for the primary treatment of gynecologic oncology do not commonly cause diarrhea but a number of agents used for recurrence or rare tumor types are known to cause diarrhea.

Pathogenesis [171–178]

- Direct damage to intestinal mucosa (fluorouracil, capecitabine, Irinotecan late-onset, doxorubicin, gemcitabine, dacarbazine).
- Cholinergic stimulation (Irinotecan acute-onset).
- Inhibition of vascular endothelial growth factor (pazopanib).
- Dihydropyrimidine dehydrogenase (DPD) deficiency and thymidylate synthetase gene (TYMS) polymorphism can increase severity of diarrhea with fluorouracil and capecitabine.
- Irinotecan is metabolized by the enzyme uridine diphospho-glucuronosyltransferase 1A1 (UGT1A1).
- Patients that are heterozygous or homozygous for UGT1A1*28 may be at increased risk for diarrhea.

Signs and Symptoms [171–173, 179]

- Increase in number of stools or ostomy output.
- Dehydration.
- Renal insufficiency.
- Electrolyte abnormalities (hypokalemia, metabolic acidosis, hyponatremia, or hypernatremia).
- Fatigue.
- Decreased quality of life.
- Noncompliance with treatment.

Evaluation [171–173, 179]

- Determine onset and duration.
- Assess for alternative etiologies (infection, medication, radiation, diet, colitis, etc.).
- Consider testing for DPD deficiency, TYMS variants, or UGT1A1 polymorphism.
- Determine severity (Table 6.6).
- Identify causative agent.

TABLE 6.6. Severity/grade of chemotherapy-induced diarrhea.

	Grade 1	Grade 2	Grade 3	Grade 4	Grade 5
Diarrhea	Increase of <4 stools per day over baseline; mild increase in ostomy output compared to baseline	Increase of 4–6 stools per day over baseline; moderate increase in ostomy output compared to baseline	Increase of >6 stools per day over baseline; incontinence; severe increase in ostomy output compared to baseline; limiting self-care ADL	Life-threatening consequences; urgent intervention indicated	Death

Therapeutic Options [2, 162–164, 167, 171–173, 179, 180]

General Principles

- Treat any alternative/underlying etiologies.
- Provide supportive care in the form of hydration and electrolyte repletion.
- Severe cases may require delays or dose reduction of chemotherapy.
- Scheduled doses of antidiarrheal are usually necessary to control symptoms.
- Once controlled medications can be titrated to maintain control.

Nonpharmacologic Treatment

- Avoid diarrhea inducing foods (dairy, spicy foods, alcohol, caffeine, high fiber).
- Discontinue all laxative, stool softeners, or promotility agents.
- Aggressive oral hydration (8–10 glasses per day).
- Small frequent meals.

Pharmacologic Treatment

- Loperamide.
  - Rapid onset of action.

Formulation

Tablet: 2 mg.
Capsule: 2 mg.
Solution: 1 mg/7.5 mL, 1 mg/5 mL.
Suspension: 1 mg/7.5 mL.

Dose

Standard dose: 4 mg PO after initial loose stool, 2 mg PO every 4 h or after subsequent loose stool.
High dose: 4 mg PO after initial loose stool, 2 mg PO every 2 h until diarrhea free for 12 h.
Maximum dose (16 mg/day) listed in drug references may be exceeded.

- Diphenoxylate and atropine.
  - Rapid onset of action.

Formulation

Tablet: diphenoxylate 2.5 mg/atropine 0.025 mg.
Solution diphenoxylate 2.5 mg/atropine 0.025 mg per 5 mL.

Dose: 5 mg diphenoxylate every 6 h until diarrhea controlled.

- Deodorized tincture of opium.
  - Contains 10 mg/mL of morphine.
  - Doses are expressed in milligrams of morphine.
  - Dose: 6 mg (0.6 mL) PO every 6 h.
  - Use with caution.

- Paregoric.
  - Contains 0.4 mg/mL of morphine.
  - Dose: 5–10 mL PO every 6 h.
- Octreotide.
  - Somatostatin analog.
  - Best used for complicated or refractory chemotherapy induced diarrhea.

Dose

100–150 mcg subQ three times daily; may increase dose up to 500 mcg three times daily.
25–50 mcg/h IV infusion.

Treatment Recommendations [172, 173, 180]

Uncomplicated Diarrhea

- Grade 1–2 with no complicating signs or symptoms.
- Nonpharmacologic therapy.
- Hold chemotherapy for grade 2 until symptoms resolve.
- Initiate standard dose loperamide and reevaluate in 12–24 h.
- If symptoms resolve you may discontinue treatment after 12 h with no loose stool.
- If symptoms persist increase to high dose loperamide, consider antibiotics, and reevaluate in 12–24 h.
- If diarrhea persists discontinue loperamide, complete more comprehensive workup and begin octreotide or other second line agent.
- If at any time the patients show worsening diarrhea or develop complication, they should be treated as such.

Complicated Diarrhea

- Grade 3–4 or Grade 1–2 with cramping, nausea/vomiting, decrease performance status, fever, sepsis, neutropenia, bleeding, or dehydration.
- Admit patient to hospital.

- Give supportive care (IV hydration/electrolytes) and non-pharmacologic treatment.
- Start octreotide and antibiotics as needed.
- Hold all chemotherapy until symptoms resolve, restart at a reduced dose.

Peripheral Neuropathy

Introduction [181–183]

Peripheral neuropathy is an often overlooked but serious adverse effect that is common in patients with gynecologic cancers. Over 2/3 of gynecologic oncology patients my experience some form of peripheral neuropathy. Onset may result in the need for dose reductions or treatment delays potentially effecting treatment outcomes as well as patient's quality-of-life.

Risk Factors [1–6, 15, 182–186]

- Diabetes.
- Preexisting neuropathy.
- History of alcohol abuse.
- Nutritional deficiencies.
- Metabolic abnormalities.
- Paraneoplastic disorders.
- Tumor compression or infiltration.
- Chemotherapy use (Table 6.7).

Definitions [179]

- Peripheral neuropathy: a disorder characterized by inflammation or degeneration of the peripheral sensory nerves.
- Paresthesia: abnormal cutaneous sensations of tingling, numbness, pressure, cold and warmth experienced in the absence of stimulus.

TABLE 6.7. Chemotherapy agents commonly causing peripheral neuropathy.

Drug	Onset dosage	Incidence	Notes
Cisplatin	300 mg/m^2	28–100 %	Worsens in combination with taxane May progress after discontinuation
Oxaliplatin	Acute: any Persistent: 500 mg/m^2	Acute: 65–80 % Persistent: 43 %	Acute neuropathy, transient and triggered by cold Persistent neuropathy similar to cisplatin
Carboplatin	600–800 mg/m^2	6–42 %	Less neurotoxic than other platinums Worsens in combination with taxane
Paclitaxel	100–1,000 mg/m^2	57–83 %	Worsens in combination with platinum Increased incidence with short/frequent infusions
Docetaxel	400 mg/m^2	11–64 %	Less severe neurotoxicity compared to paclitaxel Worsens in combination with platinum
Vincristine	Onset: 4 mg/m^2 Motor dysfunction: >6 mg/m^2		May cause autonomic neuropathy Motor neuropathy more common
Altretamine		31 %	Generally reversible upon discontinuation

- Instrumental activities of daily living (ADL): preparing meals, shopping, using the telephone, etc.
- Self-care ADL: bathing, dressing and undressing, feeding self, using toilet, taking medications, not bedridden.

Clinical Manifestations [181–184, 186, 187]

- Sensory symptoms (paresthesia, numbness, pain) are most common.
- Motor symptoms (weakness, loss of tendon reflexes) are uncommon.

- Autonomic symptoms are rare (typically caused by vinca alkaloids).
- Symmetrical "glove and stalking" distribution.
- Starts distally in fingers and toes and moves proximally.
- Symptoms may progress after discontinuation of offending agent.
- Resolution usually occurs within 3 months but may persist.

Evaluation [179, 182, 183, 185]

- Patients receiving neurotoxic agents should be questioned on the presence of peripheral neuropathy at each encounter.
- Grade severity of symptoms and effect on functioning (Table 6.8).
- Evaluate for the presence of pain.
- Neurophysiologic testing is inconsistent and often unnecessary.
- Need for interventions should be based upon severity of symptoms, and patient preference.
- Referral to neurologist, physical/occupational therapy, or pain specialist may be needed.

Prevention [2, 182–190]

Chemotherapy Selection

- For patients at high risk avoid chemotherapy regimens commonly associated with peripheral neuropathy.
- Use docetaxel instead of paclitaxel.
- Carboplatin use is preferred over cisplatin.
- Avoid dose-dense paclitaxel.
- Extend duration of paclitaxel infusion.
- Avoid vinca alkaloids.

TABLE 6.8. Peripheral neuropathy severity/grading.

	Grade 1	Grade 2	Grade 3	Grade 4	Grade 5
Paresthesia	Mild symptoms	Moderate symptoms; limiting instrumental ADL	Severe symptoms; limiting self-care ADL	–	–
Peripheral neuropathy	Asymptomatic; observation; intervention not indicated	Moderate symptoms; limiting instrumental ADL	Severe symptoms; limiting self-care ADL; assistive device indicated	Life-threatening consequences; urgent intervention indicated	Death

Pharmacologic Prevention

- No treatment is proven to prevent the onset of chemotherapy-induced peripheral neuropathy.
- Use of prophylactic medications cannot be recommended for routine use.
- Amifostine.
  - Multiple randomized trials and a meta-analysis failed to show benefit.
  - Not recommended due to lack of evidence and potential toxicity.
- Glutathione.
  - Meta-analysis of five trials showed no benefit for cisplatin-induced peripheral neuropathy.
  - Small trial of patient receiving oxaliplatin showed decreased grade II–IV neuropathy with glutathione use.
- Vitamin E.
  - Patients having received 300 mg/m^2 of cisplatin or more have shown decreased incidence and severity of peripheral neuropathy with vitamin E 400 international units daily during and 3 months following discontinuation of cisplatin.
  - Due to antioxidant effect there is theoretical concern about potential to decrease chemotherapy efficacy.
  - Further study evaluating efficacy and safety is needed.
- Erythropoietin.
  - Animal studies suggest potential for prevention with cisplatin and docetaxel-induced peripheral neuropathy.
  - Study of patients receiving paclitaxel and erythropoietin for anemia suggests decreased peripheral neuropathy.
  - Risks of erythropoietin currently outweigh potential benefits for prophylaxis in patients being treated with curative intent or those without anemia.

- IV calcium and magnesium.
  - Early trials in patient receiving infusion of calcium and magnesium with oxaliplatin showed potential benefit.
  - Randomized placebo controlled trial of 353 patients showed no difference in acute or cumulative neurotoxicity.
  - Expert consensus is to avoid use.
- Glutamine and acetyl-L-carnitine.
  - Conflicting data from small trials with a variable design.
  - Further study needed to determine benefit.
- Serotonin-norepinephrine reuptake inhibitors.
  - Venlafaxine has been shown to decrease oxaliplatin-induced acute peripheral neuropathy.
  - No information regarding efficacy for chronic neuropathy.
  - Not recommended due to limited evidence.

Treatment

General Principles [2, 182, 183, 185, 187]

- Treat any underlying neuropathy or metabolic abnormalities that may cause neuropathy.
- Chemotherapy may be switched to an agent that causes less CIPN (i.e., paclitaxel to docetaxel) if clinically appropriate.
- Dose reduction or discontinuation of offending agent may be necessary.

Pharmacologic Treatment

- There are no approved medications for the treatment of CIPN.
- Most medications available have been approved based upon their ability to treat pain in patients with diabetic neuropathy.
- A variety of agents have been used (Table 6.9).

TABLE 6.9. Agents commonly used for chemotherapy-induced peripheral neuropathy pain.

Drug	Dose	Adverse effects
Duloxetine	Starting: 20–30 mg/day Maximum: 120 mg/day	Nausea, xerostomia, constipation, diarrhea
Gabapentin	Starting: 100–300 mg nightly Maximum: 1,200 mg TID	Somnolence, dizziness, nausea, diarrhea, edema, discoordination
Lidocaine 5 % patch	3 Patches daily	Rash
Opioids	Variable	Constipation, nausea, vomiting, sedation, respiratory depression
Pregabalin	Starting: 25–50 mg TID Maximum: 200 mg TID	Dizziness, somnolence, xerostomia, edema, blurred vision, decreased concentration
Tramadol	Starting: 50 mg 1–2/day Maximum: 100 mg q6h or q8h for elderly	Dizziness, constipation, nausea, somnolence, seizure, serotonin syndrome
Tricyclic antidepressants	Variable	Anticholinergic effects, cardiovascular effects, dizziness, somnolence

- Motor weakness and loss of light touch and proprioception are not treatable with medication.
- Start with low dose and titrate to doses that maximize symptom control while limiting side effects.
- A trial of 2–8 weeks should be given to determine efficacy.
- Addition of a second agent with a different mechanism of action may be necessary.
- Dietary supplements such as acetyl-L-carnitine, glutamine, vitamin E, and glutathione have been studied but efficacy has not been established.

Nonpharmacologic Treatment

- Acupuncture.
- Neurostimulation.
- Massage.
- Meditation.
- Occupational/physical therapy.

Febrile Neutropenia

Introduction [191, 192]

Febrile neutropenia (FN) is one of the major dose-limiting toxicities of chemotherapy regimens used in patients with gynecologic oncology. It often requires hospitalization and broad spectrum antibiotics. Without prompt recognition and treatment, FN is associated with substantial morbidity, mortality, and cost. This section reviews some key points of management of FN and common drugs used in the clinical practice.

Definitions [193]

- Neutropenia: absolute neutrophil count (ANC) $<0.5 \times 10^9$/L or ANC $<1 \times 10^9$/L with predicted decrease to $\leq 0.5 \times 10^9$/L with the next 48 h.
- Febrile neutropenia: ANC $<0.5 \times 10^9$/L and a single oral temperature of ≥38.3 °C (101 °F) or ≥38.0 °C (100.4 °F) for at least an hour.

Risk Factors [194]

- Patient related.
  - Neutropenia.
  - Type of malignancy (hematologic malignancies have higher risk).
  - Asplenic.
  - Genetic factors.
- Chemotherapy regimen related.
- Immune system dysfunction.
- Corticosteroids and other lymphotoxic agents.
- Other defects in host defense.

Microbiology [193, 195]

- Bacterial infection (80–85 %).
- Most common bacterial pathogen for febrile neutropenia has changed over the past two decades from gram-negative to gram-positive organisms.
- Extended-spectrum β-lactamase (ESBL)-producing *E. coli* and Klebsiella species are emerging.
- Gram-negative organisms:
  - *E. coli.*
  - Klebsiella spp.
  - "SPICE" organisms: Serratia, Pseudomonas spp, indole-positive Proteus species, *Citrobacter freundii, Enterobacter cloacae.*
- Gram-positive organisms:
  - Staphylococcus species (most coagulase negative).
  - Streptococcus species.
  - Enterococci.
- Polymicrobial.
- Fungal infection.
  - Candida species.
  - Aspergillus species.
  - Others.
- Other infections: viral.

Diagnosis and Workup [193, 195]

- Diagnosis: Fever and ANC <0.5 × 109/L.
- Workup:
- History.
- Complete physical exam (rectal exam not recommended due to a risk of transient bacteremia).
- Two sets of blood cultures and any site-specific culture (i.e., port-a-cath, PICC line; results often negative).
- Chest X-ray.

- CBC with differential.
- Chemistry including liver and renal function.

Initial Risk Assessment [193, 194, 196]

Low Risk

Outpatient status at time of development of fever.

- No acute comorbidity.
- Anticipated short duration of profound neutropenia.
- Good performance status (PS 0–1).
- No hepatic insufficiency.
- No renal insufficiency
  OR
- MASCC Risk index score ≥21 (see Table 6.10).

High Risk

Inpatient status at time of development of fever.

- Significant medical comorbidity or clinically unstable.
- Anticipated prolonged profound neutropenia (ANC ≤0.1 × 109/L and ≥7 days).
- Hepatic insufficiency (AST/ALT ≥5 × UNL).
- Renal insufficiency (CrCL <30 ml/min).
- Uncontrolled/progressive cancer.
- Pneumonia or other complex complications.
- Alemtuzumab.
- Mucositis grade 3–4.
  OR
- MASCC Risk index score <21 (see Table 6.10).

Primary Prophylaxis [193, 194]

Low risk: Not recommended (included most solid tumor patients).

High Risk: Consider fluoroquinolones prophylaxis (levofloxacin is preferred).

TABLE 6.10. MASCC scoring index for evaluation of febrile neutropenia [196].

Characteristic	Score
Illness extent (choose 1 item below)	
No symptoms	5
Mild symptoms	5
Moderate symptoms	3
No hypotension (SBP ≥90 mmHg without pressors)	5
No chronic obstructive pulmonary disease	4
Solid tumors (if have hematologic malignancy—no previous fungal infection)	4
No dehydration	3
Outpatient at onset of fever	3
Age <60 yo (does not apply for patients ≤16 yo)	2

Therapeutic Options [193, 194]

Common antibiotic and antifungal treatments are outline in Tables 6.11 and 6.12.

Low Risk Patients

- Patients can be managed in home, ambulatory clinic, or hospital.
- Both IV and/or oral antibiotics are reasonable.
- Close monitoring before and after antibiotics administration, especially within the first 72 h, is required.
- Anti-pseudomonas antibiotics should be used the first line.
- If oral antibiotics are chosen, ciprofloxacin plus amoxicillin/clavulanate are the first line therapy.

High Risk Patients

- Patients should be managed in the hospital setting.
- IV antibiotics is required.
- Monotherapy with anti-pseudomonas antibiotics can be used as the first line for uncomplicated patients.
- Details of drug dose and spectrum (see Tables 6.11 and 6.12).
- Add site-specific evaluation and therapy when indicated.

TABLE 6.11. Common antibiotics used for FN [2, 194].

Drug name	Dose	Adverse effects	Comments	Dose adjustment due to renal dysfunction
Gram-positive active antibiotics				
Vancomycin	15 mg/kg IV Q12h; c.diff: 125 mg PO Q6h	Rash, red man syndrome	Not effective for vancomycin-resistant enterococcus (VRE)	Yes
Linezolid	600 mg IV/PO BID	Thrombocytopenia, Serotonin syndrome (rare), peripheral neuropathy (long-term use)	Effective for MRSE and VRE Cautious for when used during immunosuppressive chemotherapy	No
Daptomycin	6 mg/kg IV daily	Myositis and rhabdomyolysis	Check CK prior to start treatment and once a week thereafter Not effective for pneumonia due to inactivation by pulmonary surfactant Effective for MRSA and VRE	Yes
Dalfopristin/ quinopristin	7.5 mg/kg IV Q8h	Myalgia, arthralgia	Effective for VRE, but not effective for *Enterococcus faecalis* Less common use due to its side effects Central line access required	No
Ceftaroline	600 mg IV Q12h	Uncommon	Has both gram-positive and negative activity including MRSA Not effective for *Enterococcus faecalis* Seroconversion of Coombs' test	Yes
Gram-negative active antibiotics (including pseudomonas)				
Pipercillin/ tazobactam	4.5 g IV Q6h	Allergy	Empiric drug choice for FN Active for most gram-positive, negative and anaerobe organisms Not recommended for meningitis False positive for galactomannan test	Yes

Cefepime	2 g IV Q8h	Uncommon	Empiric drug choice for FN Active for most gram-positive, negative organisms Not effective for anaerobes and Enterococcus spp. Recommended for suspected/proven CNS infection	Yes
Imipenem/ cilastatin sodium	500 mg IV Q6h	Nausea/vomiting; seizure	Empiric drug choice for FN Active for most gram-positive, negative and anaerobe organisms Preferred for ESBL or serious Enterobacter infections May lower seizure threshold for CNS tumor/infection or renal insufficiency	Yes
Meropenem	1 g IV Q8h (2 g IV Q8h for meningitis)	Uncommon, seizure	Empiric drug choice for FN Active for most gram-positive, negative and anaerobe organisms Preferred for ESBL or serious Enterobacter infections May lower seizure threshold for CNS tumor/infection or renal insufficiency	Yes
Ceftazidine	2 g IV Q8h	Uncommon	Not effective for anaerobes and Enterococcus spp. Less common use for FN due to increasing resistance at some centers	Yes
Other antibiotics				
Ciprofloxacin	500–750 mg PO BID or 400 mg IV Q8h	QTc prolongation	Minimal gram-positive coverage Not effective for anaerobes Oral combination with amoxicillin/clavulanate or clindamycin for low risk patients	Yes
Levofloxacin	500–750 mg PO/ IV daily	QTc prolongation	More gram-positive coverage in addition to gram-negative organisms Not effective for anaerobes Drug of choice of prophylaxis for selective high risk patients	Yes
Aminoglycoside	Varies with different agents	Renal toxicity, ototoxicity	Effective mainly for gram-negative organisms Synergistic effect when used with beta lactams for *S. aureus* and Enterobacter spp. Reserve for severe infections Pharmacokinetic monitoring is required	Yes

TABLE 6.12. Common antifungals used for FN [2, 194].

Drug name	Dose	Adverse effects	Comments	Dose adjustment due to renal dysfunction
Fluconazole	400 mg IV/PO daily	Minimal	Effective for many Candida spp Variable activity against *Candida glabrata*, but not effective for *Candida krusei* Not effective for molds	Yes
Voriconazole	6 mg/kg IV Q12h × 2, then 4 mg/kg IV Q12h; or 200 mg po bid	QTc prolongation; drug interactions with CYP3A4 substrates	Effective for Candida and Aspergillus species Not effective for Zycomycetes Primary therapy for invasive aspergillosis Use with caution with IV form in patients with renal dysfunction	No
Posaconazole	Prophylaxis: 200 mg PO TID Treatment: 200 mg PO QID followed by 400 mg PO BID	QTc prolongation drug interactions with CYP3A4 substrates	Effective for Candida and Aspergillus and some Zycomycetes spp Administer with a full meal or liquid nutritional supplements PPIs can decrease absorption of posaconazole Use with caution with IV form in patients with renal dysfunction	No
Amphotericin B deoxycolate	0.5–1.5 mg/kg IV Q24h	Infusion reaction, renal toxicity, electrolyte wasting	Effective for Candida and Aspergillus and some Zycomycetes spp Prehydration Premedication with acetaminophen, antihistamine, and meperidine	Yes

Liposomal amphotericin B	3–10 mg/kg IV Q24h	Less infusion reactions and nephrotoxicity, electrolyte wasting than plain amphotericin B	Effective for Candida and Aspergillus and some Zycomycetes spp Prehydration Premedication with acetaminophen, antihistamine, and meperidine	Yes
Amphotericin B lipid complex	5 mg/kg IV Q24h	Less infusion reactions and nephrotoxicity, electrolyte wasting than plain amphotericin B	Effective for Candida and Aspergillus and some Zycomycetes spp Prehydration Premedication with acetaminophen, antihistamine, and meperidine	Yes
Amphotericin B colloidal dispersion	5 mg/kg IV Q24h	Substantial infusion reactions, nephrotoxicity, electrolyte wasting	Effective for Candida and Aspergillus and some Zycomycetes spp. Prehydration Premedication with acetaminophen, antihistamine, and meperidine	Yes
Caspofungin	70 mg IV once followed by 50 mg IV Q24h	AST/ALT elevation (less common)	Effective for Candida and Aspergillus spp only Not effective for Zycomycetes Primary therapy for invasive Candida infection Salvage therapy for aspergillosis	No, but does adjustment is required for liver dysfunction
Micafungin	Treatment: 100 mg IV Q24h Prophylaxis: 50 mg IV Q24	Uncommon	Effective for Candida and Aspergillus spp only Not effective for Zycomycetes Primary therapy for invasive Candida infection	No
Anidulafungin	200 mg IV once followed by 100 mg IV Q24h	Uncommon	Effective for Candida and Aspergillus spp. only Not effective for Zycomycetes Primary therapy for invasive Candida infection	No

Clinically Unstable Patients

- Empiric treatment: broad spectrum β-lactam (meropenem, imipenem/cilastatin, pipercillin/tazobactam plus an aminoglycoside and vancomycin).
- Strongly consider adding fluconazole and echinocandin antifungal if patient not on antifungal prophylaxis.
- Consider additional stress dose of hydrocortisone, especially for patients with septic shock.

Indications for Antibiotics with Gram-Positive Coverage

- Clinically apparent, serious, catheter-related infection.
- Blood culture positive for gram-positive bacteria prior to final identification and susceptibility test.
- Known colonization with penicillin/cephalosporin-resistant pneumococci, methicillin-resistant *Staphylococcus aureus*, vancomycin-resistant enterococus.
- Severe mucositis.
- Hypotension or septic shock without identified pathogen (clinically unstable).
- Soft tissue or skin infection.

Follow-Up [193]

- Changes of empiric antibiotics should be based on clinical and microbiology data.
- If infection is identified, then change antibiotics to appropriate coverage for the site and the drug susceptibility of the pathogen.
- If vancomycin or other gram-positive coverage antibiotics are part of the initial empiric therapy, it can be discontinued after 2 days without evidence of infection.
- After initial empiric standard regimen, antibiotics for hemodynamically unstable patients should be expanded to

include coverage for persistent gram-negative, gram-positive, anaerobic bacteria and antifungals.

- Empiric antifungals can be considered for patients with persistent fever over 4–7 days of broad spectrum antimicrobials and with no identified source of fever.

Treatment Duration [194]

- For fever of unknown origin, initial antibiotic therapy should continue until ANC ≥0.5 × 109/L and increasing.
- For documented infection, continue antibiotics at least to ANC ≥0.5 × 109/L; however, a full course of therapy can also be based on the infection site and pathogen. Can consult with institutional infectious disease specialist.
- Skin/soft tissue: 7–14 days.
- Bloodstream infection (uncomplicated).
  - Gram-positive: 7–14 days.
  - Gram-negative: 10–14 days.
  - *S. aureus*: at least 2 weeks after first negative blood culture, treatment course can be prolonged with the involvement of endovascular structure.
  - Yeast: at least 2 weeks after the first negative blood culture.
- Sinusitis/bacterial pneumonia: 10–21 days.
- Invasive fungal infection:
  - Candida: at least 2 weeks after the first negative blood culture.
  - Mold: (e.g., Aspergillus): at least 12 weeks.
- Viral infection.
  - HSV/VZV: 7–10 days.
  - Influenza: at least 5 days, maybe prolonged until symptom resolution in immunocompromised patients.

Extravasation

Background [197]

Extravasation causes 0.5–6 % of adverse events associated with chemotherapy administration. Based on the characteristics and potential tissue damage, chemotherapy agents can be classified as irritant, vesicant and nonirritant, non-vesicant. However, it is often controversial regarding which drugs are vesicants or irritants. Because of limited clinical trial data, treatment for extravasation may vary from institution to institution.

Definitions [198]

- Irritant: An agent which may cause a local inflammatory reaction, but without tissue necrosis.
- Vesicant: An agent which may cause severe tissue necrosis.

Table 6.13 compares and contrasts irritants and vesicants.

Risk Factors [197]

- Vein physiology—fragile, small, sclerotic veins, blood flow, and vessel size.
- Pharmacologic—duration and amount of chemotherapy exposure, drug administration sequence (see Table 6.13).
- Physiologic—superior vena cava syndrome, peripheral neuropathy, lymphedema, phlebitis.

TABLE 6.13. Comparison of irritant and vesicant.

	Irritant	Vesicant
Physiology	Local inflammatory reaction	Tissue injury and/or necrosis
Duration of injury	Short-term	Longer, or permanent
Symptoms	Burning, tender, erythema	Burning, itching, blistering, pain
Blood return	Intact	No

- Radiologic—previous local irradiation.
- Mechanical—needle insertion technique, injection site, multiple venipuncture attempts.

Prevention [197–200]

- Use of central venous catheter if possible.
- Careful administration with frequent checking of blood return.
- IV sites should be started from as distant from hand, dorsum of the foot, or any joints as possible.
- Do not administer chemotherapy distal from a recent venipuncture site.
- Consider using hot compress to dilate veins before administration.
- Educate patients to report any pain, tingling, burning symptoms.
- Monitor IV sites frequently during infusion.

Clinical Management [199, 200]

General Management Protocol (see Table 6.14)

- Stop infusion.
- Aspirate any drugs via intravenous cannula.
- Do not flush the line.
- Instill antidotes if available.
- Remove the catheter.
- Cold or warm packs as recommended.
- Consider taking a picture of the site with extravasation and mark the border.
- Monitor the site for 24 h, at 1 and 2 weeks and as necessary for redness, swelling, pain, ulceration and necrosis.
- Early surgery for severe and large amount of extravasation when necessary.

TABLE 6.14. Classification of chemotherapy agents and management of extravasation.

Chemotherapy agent	Irritant or vesicant classification	Suggested extravasation management protocol
Bevacizumab	Non-vesicant/nonirritant	
Bleomycin sulfate	Non-vesicant/nonirritant (drug can be administered intramuscularly or subcutaneously)	
Carboplatin	Irritant at greater than 10 mg/mL	Cold protocol + DMSO
Cisplatin	Vesicant at high doses	Extravasation of more than 20 mL of 0.5 mg/mL concentration. If less than this, no treatment. If more, see sodium thiosulfate
Cyclophosphamide	Non-vesicant/nonirritant	
Dacarbazine	Irritant	Warm protocol
Docetaxel	Irritant potential vesicant	Cold protocol + DMSO
Doxorubicin	Vesicant	Cold protocol + DMSO OR cold protocol + dexrazoxane extravasations of less than 1–2 mL often heal spontaneously. If greater than 3 mL, ulceration often results.
Doxorubicin liposome	Irritant	Cold protocol
Epirubicin	Vesicant	Cold protocol + DMSO OR Cold protocol + dexrazoxane
Etoposide	Irritant	Warm protocol. Treatment with hyaluronidase is needed only if large amount of concentrated solution extravasates, e.g., amounts one half or more of the planned total dose of etoposide

Fluorouracil	Irritant	Cold protocol
Gemcitabine hydrochloride	Non-vesicant/nonirritant	
Ifosfamide	Non-vesicant/nonirritant	
Irinotecan	Irritant	Cold protocol
Leuprolide acetate	Non-vesicant/nonirritant	Intramuscular use only
Melphalan	Irritant	No specific recommendation
Methotrexate sodium	Non-vesicant/nonirritant	
Mitomycin	Vesicant	Cold protocol + DMSO protect extravasation from sunlight
Oxaliplatin	Irritant vesicant properties have been reported	Extravasation of moderate to high doses led to inflammation but not necrosis. Sodium thiosulfate, OR High-dose dexamethasone 8 mg BID × 10 days may be considered. avoid cold protocol
Paclitaxel	Irritant, potential vesicant	Cold protocol
Paclitaxel protein-bound	Irritant, potential vesicant	Cold protocol
Pemetrexed disodium	Non-vesicant/nonirritant	
Topotecan hydrochloride	Irritant	Cold protocol
Vinca alkaloids (vincristine, vinorelbine, vinblastine)	Vesicant	Hyaluronidase and warm protocol

Cold Protocol

- Immediately after medical treatment is completed, apply ice pack to the affected area for 15–20 min at least 4 times per day for the first 24–48 h by any of the following means:
  - Cool wash cloth.
  - Instant cool/ice pack.
- Elevate limb at all times and exercise at least every 4–6 h to reduce immobility.

Warm Protocol

- Immediately after medical treatment is completed apply warmth to the affected area for 15–20 min at least 4 times per day for the first 24–48 h by any of the following means:
  - Heating pad (K pad) on moderate setting.
  - Instant warm pack.
- Elevate and extend limb to promote circulation at all times and exercise at least every 4–6 h to reduce immobility.

Antidotes [197, 199–202]

- Sodium Thiosulfate.
  - Mix 0.4 mL of 25 % sodium thiosulfate with 2.1 mL Sterile Water for Injection (resulting in 1/6 molar solution).
  - Inject 2 mL of the sodium thiosulfate solution subQ into the extravasation site using a 25-gauge or smaller needle.
  - Follow cold protocol.
- Hyaluronidase.
  - Inject 1 mL (200 units) as five separate injections in a clockwise manner, each containing 0.2 mL of hyaluronidase, subQ around the extravasation site.
  - Change needle with each injection.

- Hyaluronidase must not be given IV; death has resulted.
- Follow warm protocol.
- DO NOT APPLY ICE.
- Dimethylsulfoxide (DMSO).
- For anthracycline extravasation management:
  - Consider for cases that may be difficult to delineate between a local infusion reaction (phlebitis, irritation) versus a small volume extravasation.
  - When opposite arm/extremity/area other than affected area is not available for IV access.
    - Begin DMSO immediately after the nurse has aspirated any residual extravasate and removed the IV device.
- Conflicting literature exists as to the benefit of this adjuvant therapy.
- Dimethylsulfoxide 99 %: Using cotton ball or small gauze pad, invert DMSO bottle to wet cotton ball or small gauze then apply topically every 6 h for 14 days or every 8 h for 7 days, leave uncovered.

- Dexrazoxane (Totect™).
  - As an alternative treatment of anthracycline extravasations.
  - Consider systemic treatment when:
    - Centrally placed venous catheter extravasations may result in extensive underlying soft tissue involvement, Large volume extravasations (when ulceration and necrosis is likely to occur),
    - Significant amount of time (>1 h) has elapsed between discovery of the extravasation and initiation of extravasation management.
    - Therapy must be initiated within 6 h of extravasation.
- Cold protocol should be held 15 min prior to infusion through 15 min after infusion.
- Recommended dose:

- Days 1 and 2: 1,000 mg/m^2 (2,000 mg max dose) IV.
- Day 3: 500 mg/m^2 (1,000 mg max dose).
- Reduce dose by 50 % for patients with a creatinine clearance less than 40 mL/min.
- Dilute in 1,000 mL 0.9 % NaCl and infuse over 1–2 h in opposite extremity/area than the one affected by the extravasation.
- On days 2 and 3, premedicate with prochlorperazine 10 mg PO or dexamethasone 12 mg PO.

Background [203]

Hypersensitivity reactions (HSRs) are most commonly seen in gynecologic oncology patients receiving platinums (carboplatin, cisplatin, and oxaliplatin) and taxanes (paclitaxel and docetaxel); however, they were reported in other agents such as liposomal doxorubicin. HSRs are often unpredictable and symptoms vary dramatically. This article focuses on carboplatin/cisplatin and paclitaxel/docetaxel HSRs and their clinical management.

Incidence [1–5, 204]

- Carboplatin: 1–6 % overall, however, incidence is up to 44 %.
- Cisplatin: 5–20 %.
- Paclitaxel and docetaxel: 10 % without premedication and 2 % with premedication.

Mechanism [203–205]

- Platinums: true allergic reactions and most acute HSR if IgE mediated activation of basophils and mast cells. Types of HSRs are outlined in Table 6.15.
- Taxanes: generally an infusion-related, but not Ig-E mediated. Often attributed to Cremophor (paclitaxel) and

TABLE 6.15. Type of hypersensitivity reaction of platinums and their characteristics.

Type of hypersensitivity reactions	Antigen	Mediated by	Mechanism	Involved in platinum hypersensitivity	Symptoms related
I	Soluble antigen	IgE	Mast cell and basophil degranulation	Carboplatin, cisplatin, oxaliplatin (most)	Early onset symptoms: itching, chest pain, rash, anaphylactic reactions
II	Cell- or matrix associated antigen	IgG, IgM	Phagocyte and NK-cell activation	Oxaliplatin	Hemolysis, thrombocytopenia
III	Soluble antigen	IgG	Immune complex, phagocyte and NK-cell activation, complement fixation	Oxaliplatin	Chronic urticaria, joint pain, proteinuria
IV	Soluble or cell-associated antigen	T-cell	Macrophage and eosinophil activation, cytotoxicity	Carboplatin, cisplatin	Delayed reactions, hours or even days after infusion

Tween 80 (docetaxel). It is the direct activation of basophils and mast cells.

Clinical Presentation and Grading [179, 203]

Severity grading of HSR is outlined in Table 6.16.

Platinum Hypersensitivity

- Often occurs following re-exposure, after the completion of the initial treatment (>6 doses).
- Symptoms can occur anytime during the infusion, or after completion of the infusion.
- Commonly HSR symptoms are more severe.
- Half of HSR are still mild but anaphylaxis can occur.

Taxane Hypersensitivity

- Often occurs during the first and second cycle of paclitaxel/docetaxel.
- Typically occurs with the first a few minutes.
- Symptoms are often milder, but anaphylaxis can still occur.

Prevention [195, 203, 204]

- Preparation for the possible HSR.
  - Obtain all necessary treatment/monitoring equipment including blood pressure monitor, IV antihistamines, IV emergent steroids (e.g., hydrocortisone), IV epinephrine, and oxygen.
- Premedication 30 min before chemotherapy (most taxanes).
  - H1 antagonist (diphenhydramine 50 mg IV).
  - H2 antagonist (ranitidine 50 mg IV or famotidine 20 mg IV).
  - Steroid (dexamethasone 20 mg IV).

TABLE 6.16. Grading of HSR.

	Grade				
	1	2	3	4	5
Hypersensitivity (allergic reaction)	Transient flushing or rash, drug fever <38.0 °C, intervention not indicated	Intervention or infusion interruption indicated; responds promptly to symptomatic treatment (e.g., antihistamines, NSAIDS, narcotics); prophylactic medications indicated for ≤24 h	Prolonged (e.g., not rapidly responsive to symptomatic medication and/or brief interruption of infusion); recurrence of symptoms following initial improvement; hospitalization indicated for clinical sequelae (e.g., renal impairment, pulmonary infiltrates)	Life-threatening consequences; urgent intervention indicated	Death
Acute infusion reactions (cytokine release syndrome)	Mild reaction; infusion interruption not indicated; intervention not indicated	Therapy or infusion interruption indicated but responds promptly to symptomatic treatment (e.g., antihistamines, NSAIDS, narcotics, IV fluids); prophylactic medications indicated for ≤24 h	Prolonged (e.g., not rapidly responsive to symptomatic medication and/or brief interruption of infusion); recurrence of symptoms following initial improvement; hospitalization indicated for clinical sequelae (e.g., renal impairment, pulmonary infiltrates)	Life-threatening consequences; pressor or ventilator support indicated	Death

TABLE 6.17. 12-Step rapid desensitization protocol for chemotherapy agents.

Step	Solution	Rate (mL/h)	Time (in minutes)	Volume infused per step (mL)
1	100-fold dilution of final target concentration	2.0	15	0.50
2		5.0	15	1.25
3		10.0	15	2.50
4		20.0	15	5.00
5	Tenfold dilution of final target concentration	5.0	15	1.25
6		10.0	15	2.50
7		20.0	15	5.00
8		40.0	15	10.00
9	Concentration was calculated by subtracting the cumulative dose administered in steps 1–8 from the total target dose	10.0	15	2.50
10		20.0	15	5.00
11		40.0	15	10.00
12		75.0	Prolonged to complete target dose	232.50

Desensitization [203, 206]

- Gradual reintroduction of small amounts of drug antigen titrating to the full dose, on prolonged infusion and premedication.
- Various desensitization protocols have been published.
- No single protocol is preferred.
- Desensitization typically takes a much longer time, but recent rapid desensitization protocols have been tested with success. Table 6.17 describes desensitization protocol from the largest study to date.
- Consider substitute with a different platinum or taxane drug.
- Cisplatin for patients with a history of severe carboplatin HSR.
- Docetaxel or nanoalbumin paclitaxel for patients with a history of severe paclitaxel HSR.
- Monitor patients closely for any signs/symptoms of breakthrough reactions during desensitization.

References

1. Taxol [Package Insert] Princeton, NJ: Bristol-Meyer Squibb Company; 2011.
2. Lexicomp Online. Wolters Kluwer Health. Hudson, OH; 2014. http://online.lexi.com. Accessed 11 Jan 2014.
3. Taxotere [Package Insert] Bridgewater, NJ: Sanofi-Aventis; 2013.
4. Platinol [Package Insert] Princeton, NJ: Bristol-Meyer Squibb Company; 2010.
5. Paraplatin [Package Insert] Princeton, NJ: Bristol-Meyer Squibb Company; 2010.
6. Eloxatin [Package Insert] Bridgewater, NJ: Sanofi-Aventis; 2013.
7. Camptosar [Package Insert] New York, NY: Pfizer; 2012.
8. Hycamtin [Package Insert] Research Triangle Park, NC: Glaxo Smith Kline; 2010.
9. Doxil [Package Insert] Horsham, PA: Janssen Products; 2013.
10. Doxorubicin [Package Insert] Bedford, OH: Bedford Laboratories; 2012.
11. Ellence [Package Insert] New York, NY: Pfizer Inc.; 2013.
12. Gemzar [Package Insert] Indianapolis, IN: Eli Lilly and Company; 2013.
13. Navelbine [Package Insert] Parsippany, NJ: Pierre Fabre Pharmaceuticals Inc.; 2007.
14. Vinblastine [Package Insert] Bedford, OH: Bedford Laboratories; 2012.
15. Vincristine [Package Insert] Lake Forest, IL: Hospira, Inc.; 2013.
16. Methotrexate Injection [Package Insert] Lake Forest, IL: Hospira, Inc.; 2011.
17. Cosmogen [Package Insert] Deerfield, IL: Ovation Pharmaceuticals, Inc.; 2008.
18. Cytoxan [Package Insert] Princeton, NJ: Bristol-Myers Squibb Company; 2005.
19. Hexalen [Package Insert] Woodcliff Lake, NJ: Eisai Inc.; 2009.
20. Xeloda [Package Insert] South San Francisco, CA: Genentech, Inc.; 2013.
21. Fluorouracil [Package Insert] Irvine, CA: Gensia Sicor Pharmaceuticals, Inc.; 1999.
22. Ifex [Package Insert] Princeton, NJ: Bristol Myers Squibb Company; 2007.

23. Alkeran Injection [Package Insert] Rockville, MD: ApoPharma USA Inc.; 2011.
24. Alimta [Package Insert] Indianapolis, IN: Eli Lilly and Company; 2013.
25. Dacarbazine [Package Insert] Bedford, OH: Bedford Laboratories; 2007.
26. Temodar [Package Insert] Whitehouse Station, NJ: Merck & Co., Inc.; 2013.
27. Votrient [Package Insert] Research Triangle Park, NC: GlaxoSmithKline; 2013.
28. Etoposide Injection [Package Insert] Bedford, OH: Bedford Laboratories; 2012.
29. Etoposide Capsule [Package Insert] Morgantown, WV: Mylan Pharmaceuticals Inc.; 2013.
30. Bleomycin [Package Insert] Lake Forest, IL: Hospira, Inc.; 2012.
31. Rose PG, Bundy BN, Watkins EB, Thigpen JT, Deppe G, Maiman MA, et al. Concurrent cisplatin-based radiotherapy and chemotherapy for locally advanced cervical cancer. N Engl J Med. 1999;340(15):1144–53.
32. Rose PG, Ali S, Watkins E, Thigpen JT, Deppe G, Clarke-Pearson DL, et al. Long-term follow-up of a randomized trial comparing concurrent single agent cisplatin, cisplatin-based combination chemotherapy, or hydroxyurea during pelvic irradiation for locally advanced cervical cancer: a Gynecologic Oncology Group Study. J Clin Oncol. 2007;25(19):2804–10.
33. Keys HM, Bundy BN, Stehman FB, Muderspach LI, Chafe WE, Suggs 3rd CL, et al. Cisplatin, radiation, and adjuvant hysterectomy compared with radiation and adjuvant hysterectomy for bulky stage IB cervical carcinoma. N Engl J Med. 1999; 340(15):1154–61.
34. Lanciano R, Calkins A, Bundy BN, Parham G, Lucci 3rd JA, Moore DH, et al. Randomized comparison of weekly cisplatin or protracted venous infusion of fluorouracil in combination with pelvic radiation in advanced cervix cancer: a gynecologic oncology group study. J Clin Oncol. 2005;23(33):8289–95.
35. Peters 3rd WA, Liu PY, Barrett 2nd RJ, Stock RJ, Monk BJ, Berek JS, et al. Concurrent chemotherapy and pelvic radiation therapy compared with pelvic radiation therapy alone as adjuvant therapy after radical surgery in high-risk early-stage cancer of the cervix. J Clin Oncol. 2000;18(8):1606–13.

36. Moore DH, Blessing JA, McQuellon RP, Thaler HT, Cella D, Benda J, et al. Phase III study of cisplatin with or without paclitaxel in stage IVB, recurrent, or persistent squamous cell carcinoma of the cervix: a gynecologic oncology group study. J Clin Oncol. 2004;22(15):3113–9.
37. Monk BJ, Sill MW, McMeekin DS, Cohn DE, Ramondetta LM, Boardman CH, et al. Phase III trial of four cisplatin-containing doublet combinations in stage IVB, recurrent, or persistent cervical carcinoma: a Gynecologic Oncology Group study. J Clin Oncol. 2009;27(28):4649–55.
38. Kitagawa R, Katsumata N, Shibata T. A randomized, phase III trial of paclitaxel plus carboplatin (TC) versus paclitaxel plus cisplatin (TP) in stage IVb, persistent or recurrent cervical cancer: Japan Clinical Oncology Group study (JCOG0505). J Clin Oncol. 2012;30.
39. Long 3rd HJ, Bundy BN, Grendys Jr EC, Benda JA, McMeekin DS, Sorosky J, et al. Randomized phase III trial of cisplatin with or without topotecan in carcinoma of the uterine cervix: a Gynecologic Oncology Group Study. J Clin Oncol. 2005; 23(21):4626–33.
40. Tewari KSS, Long M, Ramondetta HJ, Landrum LM, Oaknin A, Reid TJ, Leitao MM, Michael HE, Monk BJ. Incorporation of bevacizumab in the treatment of recurrent and metastatic cervical cancer: a phase III randomized trial of the Gynecologic Oncology Group. J Clin Oncol. 2013;31 Suppl 18:3. Abstract.
41. Weiss GR, Green S, Hannigan EV, Boutselis JG, Surwit EA, Wallace DL, et al. A phase II trial of carboplatin for recurrent or metastatic squamous carcinoma of the uterine cervix: a Southwest Oncology Group study. Gynecol Oncol. 1990;39(3): 332–6.
42. Kudelka AP, Winn R, Edwards CL, Downey G, Greenberg H, Dakhil SR, et al. An update of a phase II study of paclitaxel in advanced or recurrent squamous cell cancer of the cervix. Anticancer Drugs. 1997;8(7):657–61.
43. Monk BJ, Sill MW, Burger RA, Gray HJ, Buekers TE, Roman LD. Phase II trial of bevacizumab in the treatment of persistent or recurrent squamous cell carcinoma of the cervix: a gynecologic oncology group study. J Clin Oncol. 2009;27(7):1069–74.
44. Garcia AA, Blessing JA, Vaccarello L, Roman LD. Phase II clinical trial of docetaxel in refractory squamous cell carcinoma of the cervix: a Gynecologic Oncology Group Study. Am J Clin Oncol. 2007;30(4):428–31.

45. Look KY, Blessing JA, Gallup DG, Lentz SS. A phase II trial of 5-fluorouracil and high-dose leucovorin in patients with recurrent squamous cell carcinoma of the cervix: a Gynecologic Oncology Group study. Am J Clin Oncol. 1996;19(5):439–41.
46. Schilder RJ, Blessing J, Cohn DE. Evaluation of gemcitabine in previously treated patients with non-squamous cell carcinoma of the cervix: a phase II study of the Gynecologic Oncology Group. Gynecol Oncol. 2005;96(1):103–7.
47. Coleman RE, Harper PG, Gallagher C, Osborne R, Rankin EM, Silverstone AC, et al. A phase II study of ifosfamide in advanced and relapsed carcinoma of the cervix. Cancer Chemother Pharmacol. 1986;18(3):280–3.
48. Sutton GP, Blessing JA, McGuire WP, Patton T, Look KY. Phase II trial of ifosfamide and mesna in patients with advanced or recurrent squamous carcinoma of the cervix who had never received chemotherapy: a Gynecologic Oncology Group study. Am J Obstet Gynecol. 1993;168(3 Pt 1):805–7.
49. Verschraegen CF, Levy T, Kudelka AP, Llerena E, Ende K, Freedman RS, et al. Phase II study of irinotecan in prior chemotherapy-treated squamous cell carcinoma of the cervix. J Clin Oncol. 1997;15(2):625–31.
50. Wagenaar HC, Pecorelli S, Mangioni C, van der Burg ME, Rotmensz N, Anastasopoulou A, et al. Phase II study of mitomycin-C and cisplatin in disseminated, squamous cell carcinoma of the uterine cervix. A European Organization for Research and Treatment of Cancer (EORTC) Gynecological Cancer Group study. Eur J Cancer. 2001;37(13):1624–8.
51. Muderspach LI, Blessing JA, Levenback C, Moore Jr JL. A phase II study of topotecan in patients with squamous cell carcinoma of the cervix: a gynecologic oncology group study. Gynecol Oncol. 2001;81(2):213–5.
52. Bookman MA, Blessing JA, Hanjani P, Herzog TJ, Andersen WA. Topotecan in squamous cell carcinoma of the cervix: a phase II study of the Gynecologic Oncology Group. Gynecol Oncol. 2000;77(3):446–9.
53. Thigpen JT, Brady MF, Alvarez RD, Adelson MD, Homesley HD, Manetta A, et al. Oral medroxyprogesterone acetate in the treatment of advanced or recurrent endometrial carcinoma: a dose-response study by the Gynecologic Oncology Group. J Clin Oncol. 1999;17(6):1736–44.
54. Thigpen T, Brady MF, Homesley HD, Soper JT, Bell J. Tamoxifen in the treatment of advanced or recurrent endometrial carci-

noma: a Gynecologic Oncology Group study. J Clin Oncol. 2001;19(2):364–7.

55. Pinelli DM, Fiorica JV, Roberts WS, Hoffman MS, Nicosia SV, Cavanagh D. Chemotherapy plus sequential hormonal therapy for advanced and recurrent endometrial carcinoma: a phase II study. Gynecol Oncol. 1996;60(3):462–7.
56. Lentz SS, Brady MF, Major FJ, Reid GC, Soper JT. High-dose megestrol acetate in advanced or recurrent endometrial carcinoma: a Gynecologic Oncology Group Study. J Clin Oncol. 1996;14(2):357–61.
57. Fiorica JV, Brunetto VL, Hanjani P, Lentz SS, Mannel R, Andersen W. Phase II trial of alternating courses of megestrol acetate and tamoxifen in advanced endometrial carcinoma: a Gynecologic Oncology Group study. Gynecol Oncol. 2004;92(1):10–4.
58. Ma BB, Oza A, Eisenhauer E, Stanimir G, Carey M, Chapman W, et al. The activity of letrozole in patients with advanced or recurrent endometrial cancer and correlation with biological markers – a study of the National Cancer Institute of Canada Clinical Trials Group. Int J Gynecol Cancer. 2004;14(4):650–8.
59. Rose PG, Brunetto VL, VanLe L, Bell J, Walker JL, Lee RB. A phase II trial of anastrozole in advanced recurrent or persistent endometrial carcinoma: a Gynecologic Oncology Group study. Gynecol Oncol. 2000;78(2):212–6.
60. Randall ME, Filiaci VL, Muss H, Spirtos NM, Mannel RS, Fowler J, et al. Randomized phase III trial of whole-abdominal irradiation versus doxorubicin and cisplatin chemotherapy in advanced endometrial carcinoma: a Gynecologic Oncology Group Study. J Clin Oncol. 2006;24(1):36–44.
61. Thigpen JT, Brady MF, Homesley HD, Malfetano J, DuBeshter B, Burger RA, et al. Phase III trial of doxorubicin with or without cisplatin in advanced endometrial carcinoma: a gynecologic oncology group study. J Clin Oncol. 2004;22(19):3902–8.
62. Homesley HD, Filiaci V, Gibbons SK, Long HJ, Cella D, Spirtos NM, et al. A randomized phase III trial in advanced endometrial carcinoma of surgery and volume directed radiation followed by cisplatin and doxorubicin with or without paclitaxel: a Gynecologic Oncology Group study. Gynecol Oncol. 2009; 112(3):543–52.
63. Sorbe B, Andersson H, Boman K, Rosenberg P, Kalling M. Treatment of primary advanced and recurrent endometrial carcinoma with a combination of carboplatin and paclitaxel-long-term follow-up. Int J Gynecol Cancer. 2008;18(4):803–8.

64. Pectasides D, Xiros N, Papaxoinis G, Pectasides E, Sykiotis C, Koumarianou A, et al. Carboplatin and paclitaxel in advanced or metastatic endometrial cancer. Gynecol Oncol. 2008; 109(2):250–4.
65. Nomura H, Aoki D, Takahashi F, Katsumata N, Watanabe Y, Konishi I, et al. Randomized phase II study comparing docetaxel plus cisplatin, docetaxel plus carboplatin, and paclitaxel plus carboplatin in patients with advanced or recurrent endometrial carcinoma: a Japanese Gynecologic Oncology Group study (JGOG2041). Ann Oncol. 2011;22(3):636–42.
66. Secord AA, Havrilesky LJ, Carney ME, Soper JT, Clarke-Pearson DL, Rodriguez GC, et al. Weekly low-dose paclitaxel and carboplatin in the treatment of advanced or recurrent cervical and endometrial cancer. Int J Clin Oncol. 2007;12(1): 31–6.
67. Scribner Jr DR, Puls LE, Gold MA. A phase II evaluation of docetaxel and carboplatin followed by tumor volume directed pelvic plus or minus paraaortic irradiation for stage III endometrial cancer. Gynecol Oncol. 2012;125(2):388–93.
68. Geller MA, Ivy JJ, Ghebre R, Downs Jr LS, Judson PL, Carson LF, et al. A phase II trial of carboplatin and docetaxel followed by radiotherapy given in a "Sandwich" method for stage III, IV, and recurrent endometrial cancer. Gynecol Oncol. 2011; 121(1):112–7.
69. Deppe G, Cohen CJ, Bruckner HW. Treatment of advanced endometrial adenocarcinoma with cis-dichlorodiammine platinum (II) after intensive prior therapy. Gynecol Oncol. 1980;10(1):51–4.
70. Seski JC, Edwards CL, Herson J, Rutledge FN. Cisplatin chemotherapy for disseminated endometrial cancer. Obstet Gynecol. 1982;59(2):225–8.
71. Burke TW, Munkarah A, Kavanagh JJ, Morris M, Levenback C, Tornos C, et al. Treatment of advanced or recurrent endometrial carcinoma with single-agent carboplatin. Gynecol Oncol. 1993;51(3):397–400.
72. Green 3rd JB, Green S, Alberts DS, O'Toole R, Surwit EA, Noltimier JW. Carboplatin therapy in advanced endometrial cancer. Obstet Gynecol. 1990;75(4):696–700.
73. Thigpen JT, Buchsbaum HJ, Mangan C, Blessing JA. Phase II trial of adriamycin in the treatment of advanced or recurrent endometrial carcinoma: a Gynecologic Oncology Group study. Cancer Treat Rep. 1979;63(1):21–7.

74. Muggia FM, Blessing JA, Sorosky J, Reid GC. Phase II trial of the pegylated liposomal doxorubicin in previously treated metastatic endometrial cancer: a Gynecologic Oncology Group study. J Clin Oncol. 2002;20(9):2360–4.
75. Ball HG, Blessing JA, Lentz SS, Mutch DG. A phase II trial of paclitaxel in patients with advanced or recurrent adenocarcinoma of the endometrium: a Gynecologic Oncology Group study. Gynecol Oncol. 1996;62(2):278–81.
76. Lincoln S, Blessing JA, Lee RB, Rocereto TF. Activity of paclitaxel as second-line chemotherapy in endometrial carcinoma: a Gynecologic Oncology Group study. Gynecol Oncol. 2003; 88(3):277–81.
77. Garcia AA, Blessing JA, Nolte S, Mannel RS. A phase II evaluation of weekly docetaxel in the treatment of recurrent or persistent endometrial carcinoma: a study by the Gynecologic Oncology Group. Gynecol Oncol. 2008;111(1):22–6.
78. Aghajanian C, Sill MW, Darcy KM, Greer B, McMeekin DS, Rose PG, et al. Phase II trial of bevacizumab in recurrent or persistent endometrial cancer: a Gynecologic Oncology Group study. J Clin Oncol. 2011;29(16):2259–65.
79. Sutton G, Brunetto VL, Kilgore L, Soper JT, McGehee R, Olt G, et al. A phase III trial of ifosfamide with or without cisplatin in carcinosarcoma of the uterus: a Gynecologic Oncology Group study. Gynecol Oncol. 2000;79(2):147–53.
80. Sutton G, Kauderer J, Carson LF, Lentz SS, Whitney CW, Gallion H. Adjuvant ifosfamide and cisplatin in patients with completely resected stage I or II carcinosarcomas (mixed mesodermal tumors) of the uterus: a Gynecologic Oncology Group study. Gynecol Oncol. 2005;96(3):630–4.
81. Homesley HD, Filiaci V, Markman M, Bitterman P, Eaton L, Kilgore LC, et al. Phase III trial of ifosfamide with or without paclitaxel in advanced uterine carcinosarcoma: a Gynecologic Oncology Group study. J Clin Oncol. 2007;25(5):526–31.
82. Pink D, Lindner T, Mrozek A, Kretzschmar A, Thuss-Patience PC, Dorken B, et al. Harm or benefit of hormonal treatment in metastatic low-grade endometrial stromal sarcoma: single center experience with 10 cases and review of the literature. Gynecol Oncol. 2006;101(3):464–9.
83. Chu MC, Mor G, Lim C, Zheng W, Parkash V, Schwartz PE. Low-grade endometrial stromal sarcoma: hormonal aspects. Gynecol Oncol. 2003;90(1):170–6.
84. Cheng X, Yang G, Schmeler KM, Coleman RL, Tu X, Liu J, et al. Recurrence patterns and prognosis of endometrial stromal sar-

coma and the potential of tyrosine kinase-inhibiting therapy. Gynecol Oncol. 2011;121(2):323–7.

85. O'Cearbhaill R, Zhou Q, Iasonos A, Soslow RA, Leitao MM, Aghajanian C, et al. Treatment of advanced uterine leiomyosarcoma with aromatase inhibitors. Gynecol Oncol. 2010;116(3):424–9.
86. Hensley ML, Maki R, Venkatraman E, Geller G, Lovegren M, Aghajanian C, et al. Gemcitabine and docetaxel in patients with unresectable leiomyosarcoma: results of a phase II trial. J Clin Oncol. 2002;20(12):2824–31.
87. Hensley ML, Blessing JA, Degeest K, Abulafia O, Rose PG, Homesley HD. Fixed-dose rate gemcitabine plus docetaxel as second-line therapy for metastatic uterine leiomyosarcoma: a Gynecologic Oncology Group phase II study. Gynecol Oncol. 2008;109(3):323–8.
88. Hensley ML, Blessing JA, Mannel R, Rose PG. Fixed-dose rate gemcitabine plus docetaxel as first-line therapy for metastatic uterine leiomyosarcoma: a Gynecologic Oncology Group phase II trial. Gynecol Oncol. 2008;109(3):329–34.
89. Hensley ML, Ishill N, Soslow R, Larkin J, Abu-Rustum N, Sabbatini P, et al. Adjuvant gemcitabine plus docetaxel for completely resected stages I-IV high grade uterine leiomyosarcoma: results of a prospective study. Gynecol Oncol. 2009;112(3):563–7.
90. Sutton G, Blessing JA, Malfetano JH. Ifosfamide and doxorubicin in the treatment of advanced leiomyosarcomas of the uterus: a Gynecologic Oncology Group study. Gynecol Oncol. 1996;62(2):226–9.
91. Le Cesne A, Judson I, Crowther D, Rodenhuis S, Keizer HJ, Van Hoesel Q, et al. Randomized phase III study comparing conventional-dose doxorubicin plus ifosfamide versus high-dose doxorubicin plus ifosfamide plus recombinant human granulocyte-macrophage colony-stimulating factor in advanced soft tissue sarcomas: a trial of the European Organization for Research and Treatment of Cancer/Soft Tissue and Bone Sarcoma Group. J Clin Oncol. 2000;18(14):2676–84.
92. Omura GA, Major FJ, Blessing JA, Sedlacek TV, Thigpen JT, Creasman WT, et al. A randomized study of adriamycin with and without dimethyl triazenoimidazole carboxamide in advanced uterine sarcomas. Cancer. 1983;52(4):626–32.
93. Losa R, Fra J, Lopez-Pousa A, Sierra M, Goitia A, Una E, et al. Phase II study with the combination of gemcitabine and DTIC in patients with advanced soft tissue sarcomas. Cancer Chemother Pharmacol. 2007;59(2):251–9.

94. Garcia-Del-Muro X, Lopez-Pousa A, Maurel J, Martin J, Martinez-Trufero J, Casado A, et al. Randomized phase II study comparing gemcitabine plus dacarbazine versus dacarbazine alone in patients with previously treated soft tissue sarcoma: a Spanish Group for Research on Sarcomas study. J Clin Oncol. 2011;29(18):2528–33.
95. Dileo P, Morgan JA, Zahrieh D, Desai J, Salesi JM, Harmon DC, et al. Gemcitabine and vinorelbine combination chemotherapy for patients with advanced soft tissue sarcomas: results of a phase II trial. Cancer. 2007;109(9):1863–9.
96. Petrioli R, Coratti A, Correale P, D'Aniello C, Grimaldi L, Tanzini G, et al. Adjuvant epirubicin with or without Ifosfamide for adult soft-tissue sarcoma. Am J Clin Oncol. 2002;25(5): 468–73.
97. Look KY, Sandler A, Blessing JA, Lucci 3rd JA, Rose PG. Phase II trial of gemcitabine as second-line chemotherapy of uterine leiomyosarcoma: a Gynecologic Oncology Group (GOG) Study. Gynecol Oncol. 2004;92(2):644–7.
98. Sutton GP, Blessing JA, Barrett RJ, McGehee R. Phase II trial of ifosfamide and mesna in leiomyosarcoma of the uterus: a Gynecologic Oncology Group study. Am J Obstet Gynecol. 1992;166(2):556–9.
99. Sutton G, Blessing J, Hanjani P, Kramer P. Phase II evaluation of liposomal doxorubicin (Doxil) in recurrent or advanced leiomyosarcoma of the uterus: a Gynecologic Oncology Group study. Gynecol Oncol. 2005;96(3):749–52.
100. Sutton G, Blessing JA, Ball H. Phase II trial of paclitaxel in leiomyosarcoma of the uterus: a gynecologic oncology group study. Gynecol Oncol. 1999;74(3):346–9.
101. Gallup DG, Blessing JA, Andersen W, Morgan MA. Evaluation of paclitaxel in previously treated leiomyosarcoma of the uterus: a gynecologic oncology group study. Gynecol Oncol. 2003;89(1):48–51.
102. Anderson S, Aghajanian C. Temozolomide in uterine leiomyosarcomas. Gynecol Oncol. 2005;98(1):99–103.
103. Nasti G, Errante D, Talamini R, Rizzardini G, Fasan M, Landonio G, et al. Vinorelbine is an effective and safe drug for AIDS-related Kaposi's sarcoma: results of a phase II study. J Clin Oncol. 2000;18(7):1550–7.
104. van der Graaf WT, Blay JY, Chawla SP, Kim DW, Bui-Nguyen B, Casali PG, et al. Pazopanib for metastatic soft-tissue sarcoma

(PALETTE): a randomized, double-blind, placebo-controlled phase 3 trial. Lancet. 2012;379(9829):1879–86.
105. Ozols RF, Bundy BN, Greer BE, Fowler JM, Clarke-Pearson D, Burger RA, et al. Phase III trial of carboplatin and paclitaxel compared with cisplatin and paclitaxel in patients with optimally resected stage III ovarian cancer: a Gynecologic Oncology Group study. J Clin Oncol. 2003;21(17):3194–200.
106. Vasey PA, Atkinson R, Coleman R, Crawford M, Cruickshank M, Eggleton P, et al. Docetaxel-carboplatin as first line chemotherapy for epithelial ovarian cancer. Br J Cancer. 2001;84(2): 170–8.
107. McGuire WP, Hoskins WJ, Brady MF, Kucera PR, Partridge EE, Look KY, et al. Cyclophosphamide and cisplatin compared with paclitaxel and cisplatin in patients with stage III and stage IV ovarian cancer. N Engl J Med. 1996;334(1):1–6.
108. Armstrong DK, Bundy B, Wenzel L, Huang HQ, Baergen R, Lele S, et al. Intraperitoneal cisplatin and paclitaxel in ovarian cancer. N Engl J Med. 2006;354(1):34–43.
109. Katsumata N, Yasuda M, Takahashi F, Isonishi S, Jobo T, Aoki D, et al. Dose-dense paclitaxel once a week in combination with carboplatin every 3 weeks for advanced ovarian cancer: a phase 3, open-label, randomized controlled trial. Lancet. 2009; 374(9698):1331–8.
110. Burger RA, Brady MF, Bookman MA, Fleming GF, Monk BJ, Huang H, et al. Incorporation of bevacizumab in the primary treatment of ovarian cancer. N Engl J Med. 2011;365(26):2473–83.
111. Perren TJ, Swart AM, Pfisterer J, Ledermann JA, Pujade-Lauraine E, Kristensen G, et al. A phase 3 trial of bevacizumab in ovarian cancer. N Engl J Med. 2011;365(26):2484–96.
112. Parmar MK, Ledermann JA, Colombo N, du Bois A, Delaloye JF, Kristensen GB, et al. Paclitaxel plus platinum-based chemotherapy versus conventional platinum-based chemotherapy in women with relapsed ovarian cancer: the ICON4/ AGO-OVAR-2.2 trial. Lancet. 2003;361(9375):2099–106.
113. Gronlund B, Hogdall C, Hansen HH, Engelholm SA. Results of reinduction therapy with paclitaxel and carboplatin in recurrent epithelial ovarian cancer. Gynecol Oncol. 2001;83(1): 128–34.
114. Pfisterer J, Plante M, Vergote I, du Bois A, Hirte H, Lacave AJ, et al. Gemcitabine plus carboplatin compared with carboplatin in patients with platinum-sensitive recurrent ovarian cancer: an

intergroup trial of the AGO-OVAR, the NCIC CTG, and the EORTC GCG. J Clin Oncol. 2006;24(29):4699–707.
115. Aghajanian C, Blank SV, Goff BA, Judson PL, Teneriello MG, Husain A, et al. OCEANS: a randomized, double-blind, placebo-controlled phase III trial of chemotherapy with or without bevacizumab in patients with platinum-sensitive recurrent epithelial ovarian, primary peritoneal, or fallopian tube cancer. J Clin Oncol. 2012;30(17):2039–45.
116. Nagourney RA, Brewer CA, Radecki S, Kidder WA, Sommers BL, Evans SS, et al. Phase II trial of gemcitabine plus cisplatin repeating doublet therapy in previously treated, relapsed ovarian cancer patients. Gynecol Oncol. 2003;88(1):35–9.
117. Rose PG, Mossbruger K, Fusco N, Smrekar M, Eaton S, Rodriguez M. Gemcitabine reverses cisplatin resistance: demonstration of activity in platinum- and multidrug-resistant ovarian and peritoneal carcinoma. Gynecol Oncol. 2003;88(1): 17–21.
118. Strauss HG, Henze A, Teichmann A, Karbe I, Baumgart A, Thomssen C, et al. Phase II trial of docetaxel and carboplatin in recurrent platinum-sensitive ovarian, peritoneal and tubal cancer. Gynecol Oncol. 2007;104(3):612–6.
119. Kushner DM, Connor JP, Sanchez F, Volk M, Schink JC, Bailey HH, et al. Weekly docetaxel and carboplatin for recurrent ovarian and peritoneal cancer: a phase II trial. Gynecol Oncol. 2007;105(2):358–64.
120. Wagner U, Marth C, Largillier R, Kaern J, Brown C, Heywood M, et al. Final overall survival results of phase III GCIG CALYPSO trial of pegylated liposomal doxorubicin and carboplatin vs paclitaxel and carboplatin in platinum-sensitive ovarian cancer patients. Br J Cancer. 2012;107(4):588–91.
121. Alberts DS, Liu PY, Wilczynski SP, Clouser MC, Lopez AM, Michelin DP, et al. Randomized trial of pegylated liposomal doxorubicin (PLD) plus carboplatin versus carboplatin in platinum-sensitive (PS) patients with recurrent epithelial ovarian or peritoneal carcinoma after failure of initial platinum-based chemotherapy (Southwest Oncology Group Protocol S0200). Gynecol Oncol. 2008;108(1):90–4.
122. Burger RA, Sill MW, Monk BJ, Greer BE, Sorosky JI. Phase II trial of bevacizumab in persistent or recurrent epithelial ovarian cancer or primary peritoneal cancer: a Gynecologic Oncology Group study. J Clin Oncol. 2007;25(33):5165–71.

123. Kaye SB, Piccart M, Aapro M, Francis P, Kavanagh J. Phase II trials of docetaxel (Taxotere) in advanced ovarian cancer – an updated overview. Eur J Cancer. 1997;33(13):2167–70.
124. Rose PG, Blessing JA, Ball HG, Hoffman J, Warshal D, DeGeest K, et al. A phase II study of docetaxel in paclitaxel-resistant ovarian and peritoneal carcinoma: a Gynecologic Oncology Group study. Gynecol Oncol. 2003;88(2):130–5.
125. Markman M, Blessing J, Rubin SC, Connor J, Hanjani P, Waggoner S. Phase II trial of weekly paclitaxel (80 mg/m^2) in platinum and paclitaxel-resistant ovarian and primary peritoneal cancers: a Gynecologic Oncology Group study. Gynecol Oncol. 2006;101(3):436–40.
126. Markman M, Webster K, Zanotti K, Kulp B, Peterson G, Belinson J. Phase 2 trial of single-agent gemcitabine in platinum-paclitaxel refractory ovarian cancer. Gynecol Oncol. 2003;90(3): 593–6.
127. D'Agostino G, Amant F, Berteloot P, Scambia G, Vergote I. Phase II study of gemcitabine in recurrent platinum-and paclitaxel-resistant ovarian cancer. Gynecol Oncol. 2003;88(3):266–9.
128. Mutch DG, Orlando M, Goss T, Teneriello MG, Gordon AN, McMeekin SD, et al. Randomized phase III trial of gemcitabine compared with pegylated liposomal doxorubicin in patients with platinum-resistant ovarian cancer. J Clin Oncol. 2007;25(19):2811–8.
129. Rose PG, Blessing JA, Mayer AR, Homesley HD. Prolonged oral etoposide as second-line therapy for platinum-resistant and platinum-sensitive ovarian carcinoma: a Gynecologic Oncology Group study. J Clin Oncol. 1998;16(2):405–10.
130. Vergote I, Himmelmann A, Frankendal B, Scheistroen M, Vlachos K, Trope C. Hexamethylmelamine as second-line therapy in platin-resistant ovarian cancer. Gynecol Oncol. 1992;47(3):282–6.
131. Monk BJ, Choi DC, Pugmire G, Burger RA. Activity of bevacizumab (rhuMAB VEGF) in advanced refractory epithelial ovarian cancer. Gynecol Oncol. 2005;96(3):902–5.
132. Cannistra SA, Matulonis UA, Penson RT, Hambleton J, Dupont J, Mackey H, et al. Phase II study of bevacizumab in patients with platinum-resistant ovarian cancer or peritoneal serous cancer. J Clin Oncol. 2007;25(33):5180–6.

133. Teneriello MG, Tseng PC, Crozier M, Encarnacion C, Hancock K, Messing MJ, et al. Phase II evaluation of nanoparticle albumin-bound paclitaxel in platinum-sensitive patients with recurrent ovarian, peritoneal, or fallopian tube cancer. J Clin Oncol. 2009;27(9):1426–31.
134. Fracasso PM, Blessing JA, Morgan MA, Sood AK, Hoffman JS. Phase II study of oxaliplatin in platinum-resistant and refractory ovarian cancer: a gynecologic group study. J Clin Oncol. 2003;21(15):2856–9.
135. Gordon AN, Fleagle JT, Guthrie D, Parkin DE, Gore ME, Lacave AJ. Recurrent epithelial ovarian carcinoma: a randomized phase III study of pegylated liposomal doxorubicin versus topotecan. J Clin Oncol. 2001;19(14):3312–22.
136. Muggia FM, Hainsworth JD, Jeffers S, Miller P, Groshen S, Tan M, et al. Phase II study of liposomal doxorubicin in refractory ovarian cancer: antitumor activity and toxicity modification by liposomal encapsulation. J Clin Oncol. 1997;15(3):987–93.
137. Ferrandina G, Ludovisi M, Lorusso D, Pignata S, Breda E, Savarese A, et al. Phase III trial of gemcitabine compared with pegylated liposomal doxorubicin in progressive or recurrent ovarian cancer. J Clin Oncol. 2008;26(6):890–6.
138. ten Bokkel Huinink W, Gore M, Carmichael J, Gordon A, Malfetano J, Hudson I, et al. Topotecan versus paclitaxel for the treatment of recurrent epithelial ovarian cancer. J Clin Oncol. 1997;15(6):2183–93.
139. McGuire WP, Blessing JA, Bookman MA, Lentz SS, Dunton CJ. Topotecan has substantial antitumor activity as first-line salvage therapy in platinum-sensitive epithelial ovarian carcinoma: a Gynecologic Oncology Group study. J Clin Oncol. 2000;18(5):1062–7.
140. Sehouli J, Stengel D, Harter P, Kurzeder C, Belau A, Bogenrieder T, et al. Topotecan weekly versus conventional 5-day schedule in patients with platinum-resistant ovarian cancer: a randomized multicenter phase II trial of the North-Eastern German Society of Gynecological Oncology Ovarian Cancer Study Group. J Clin Oncol. 2011;29(2):242–8.
141. Burger RA, DiSaia PJ, Roberts JA, O'Rourke M, Gershenson DM, Homesley HD, et al. Phase II trial of vinorelbine in recurrent and progressive epithelial ovarian cancer. Gynecol Oncol. 1999;72(2):148–53.

142. Miller DS, Blessing JA, Krasner CN, Mannel RS, Hanjani P, Pearl ML, et al. Phase II evaluation of pemetrexed in the treatment of recurrent or persistent platinum-resistant ovarian or primary peritoneal carcinoma: a study of the Gynecologic Oncology Group. J Clin Oncol. 2009;27(16):2686–91.
143. Markman M, Hakes T, Reichman B, Lewis Jr JL, Rubin S, Jones W, et al. Ifosfamide and mesna in previously treated advanced epithelial ovarian cancer: activity in platinum-resistant disease. J Clin Oncol. 1992;10(2):243–8.
144. Wolf JK, Bodurka DC, Verschraegen C, Sun CC, Branham D, Jenkins AD, et al. A phase II trial of oral capecitabine in patients with platinum – and taxane – refractory ovarian, fallopian tube, or peritoneal cancer. Gynecol Oncol. 2006;102(3): 468–74.
145. Bodurka DC, Levenback C, Wolf JK, Gano J, Wharton JT, Kavanagh JJ, et al. Phase II trial of irinotecan in patients with metastatic epithelial ovarian cancer or peritoneal cancer. J Clin Oncol. 2003;21(2):291–7.
146. Markman M, Iseminger KA, Hatch KD, Creasman WT, Barnes W, Dubeshter B. Tamoxifen in platinum-refractory ovarian cancer: a Gynecologic Oncology Group Ancillary Report. Gynecol Oncol. 1996;62(1):4–6.
147. del Carmen MG, Fuller AF, Matulonis U, Horick NK, Goodman A, Duska LR, et al. Phase II trial of anastrozole in women with asymptomatic mullerian cancer. Gynecol Oncol. 2003;91(3): 596–602.
148. Papadimitriou CA, Markaki S, Siapkaras J, Vlachos G, Efstathiou E, Grimani I, et al. Hormonal therapy with letrozole for relapsed epithelial ovarian cancer. Long-term results of a phase II study. Oncology. 2004;66(2):112–7.
149. Bowman A, Gabra H, Langdon SP, Lessells A, Stewart M, Young A, et al. CA125 response is associated with estrogen receptor expression in a phase II trial of letrozole in ovarian cancer: identification of an endocrine-sensitive subgroup. Clin Cancer Res. 2002;8(7):2233–9.
150. Ramirez PT, Schmeler KM, Milam MR, Slomovitz BM, Smith JA, Kavanagh JJ, et al. Efficacy of letrozole in the treatment of recurrent platinum- and taxane-resistant high-grade cancer of the ovary or peritoneum. Gynecol Oncol. 2008;110(1):56–9.
151. Marinaccio M, D'Addario V, Serrati A, Pinto V, Cagnazzo G. Leuprolide acetate as a salvage-therapy in relapsed epithelial ovarian cancer. Eur J Gynaecol Oncol. 1996;17(4):286–8.

152. Veenhof CH, van der Burg ME, Nooy M, Aalders JG, Pecorelli S, Oliveira CF, et al. Phase II study of high-dose megestrol acetate in patients with advanced ovarian carcinoma. Eur J Cancer. 1994;30A(5):697–8.
153. Wilailak S, Linasmita V, Srisupundit S. Phase II study of high-dose megestrol acetate in platinum-refractory epithelial ovarian cancer. Anticancer Drugs. 2001;12(9):719–24.
154. Hesketh PJ. Chemotherapy-induced nausea and vomiting. N Engl J Med. 2008;358(23):2482–94. doi:10.1056/NEJMra0706547.
155. Hesketh PJ, Grunberg SM, Gralla RJ, Warr DG, Roila F, de Wit R, et al. The oral neurokinin-1 antagonist Aprepitant for the prevention of chemotherapy-induced nausea and vomiting: a multinational, randomized, double-blind, placebo-controlled trial in patients receiving high-dose cisplatin-the Aprepitant Protocol 052 Study Group. J Clin Oncol. 2003;21(22):4112–9.
156. Wiser W, Berger A. Practical management of chemotherapy-induced nausea and vomiting. Oncology (Williston Park). 2005;19(5):637–45.
157. Hawkins R, Grunberg S. Chemotherapy-induced nausea and vomiting: challenges and opportunities for improved patient outcomes. Clin J Oncol Nurs. 2009;13(1):54–64. doi:10.1188/09.CJON.54-64.
158. Wilhelm SM, Dehoorne-Smith ML, Kale-Pradhan PB. Prevention of postoperative nausea and vomiting. Ann Pharmacother. 2007;41(1):68–78.
159. Richardson JL, Marks G, Levine A. The influence of symptoms of disease and side effects of treatment on compliance with cancer therapy. J Clin Oncol. 1988;6(11):1746–52.
160. Roila F, Herrstedt J, Aapro M, Gralla RJ, Einhorn LH, Ballatori E, et al. Guideline update for MASCC and ESMO in the prevention of chemotherapy- and radiotherapy-induced nausea and vomiting: results of the Perugia consensus conference. Ann Oncol. 2010;21 suppl 5:v232–43. doi:10.1093/annonc/mdq194.
161. National Comprehensive Cancer Network. Antiemesis. Version 1.2014. Accessed 11 Jan 2014. http://www.nccn.org/professionals/physician_gls/pdf/antiemesis.pdf.
162. Marty M, Pouillart P, Scholl S, Droz JP, Azab M, Brion N, et al. Comparison of 5-hydroxytryptamine3 (serotonin) antagonist ondansetron (GR 38032F) with high-dose metoclopramide in the control of cisplatin-induced emesis. N Engl J Med. 1990;322(12):816–21. doi:10.1056/NEJM199003223221205.

163. Boccia RV, Gordan LN, Clark G, Howell JD, Grunberg SM, Sancuso Study Group. Efficacy and tolerability of transdermal granisetron for the control of chemotherapy-induced nausea and vomiting associated with moderately and highly emetogenic multi-day chemotherapy: a randomized, double-blind, phase III study. Support Care Cancer. 2011;19(10):1609–17.
164. Zofran [Package Insert]. Research Triangle Park, NC: GlaxoSmithKline; 2011.
165. Basch E, Prestrud AA, Hesketh PJ, Kris MG, Feyer PC, Somerfield MR, et al. Antiemetics: American Society of Clinical Oncology clinical practice guideline update. J Clin Oncol. 2011;29(31):4189–98. doi:10.1200/JCO.2010.34.4614.
166. Anzamet [Package Insert]. Bridgewater, NJ: Sanofi-Aventis; 2011.
167. Emend [Package Insert]. Whitehouse Station, NJ: Merck Sharp & Dohme Corp; 2010.
168. Navari RM, Gray SE, Kerr AC. Olanzapine versus Aprepitant for the prevention of chemotherapy-induced nausea and vomiting: a randomized phase III trial. J Support Oncol. 2011;9(5): 188–95. doi:10.1016/j.suponc.2011.05.002.
169. Jordan K, Kinitz I, Voigt W, Behlendrof T, Wolf HH, Schmoll HJ. Safety and efficacy of a triple antiemetic combination with the NK-1 antagonist Aprepitant in highly and moderately emetogenic multiple-day chemotherapy. Eur J Cancer. 2009;45(7):1184–7.
170. Einhorn LH, Brames MJ, Dreicer R, Nichols CR, Cullen Jr MT, Bubalo J. Palonosetron plus dexamethasone for prevention of chemotherapy-induced nausea and vomiting in patients receiving multiple-day cisplatin chemotherapy for germ cell cancer. Support Care Cancer. 2007;15(11):1293–300.
171. Shaw C, Taylor L. Treatment-related diarrhea in patients with cancer. Clin J Oncol Nurs. 2012;16(4):413–7. doi:10.1188/12.CJON.413-417.
172. Wadler S, Benson AB, Engelking C, Catalano R, Field M, Kornblau SM, et al. Recommended guidelines for the treatment of chemotherapy-induced diarrhea. J Clin Oncol. 1998;16:3169.
173. Benson AB, Ajani JA, Catalano RB, Engelking C, Kornblau SM, Martenson JA, et al. Recommended guidelines for the treatment of chemotherapy-induced diarrhea. J Clin Oncol. 2004;22(14):2918–26. doi:10.1200/JCO.2004.04.132.
174. Gupta E, Lestingi TM, Mick R, Ramirez J, Vokes EE, Ratain MJ. Metabolic fate of Irinotecan in humans: correlation of glucuronidation with diarrhea. Cancer Res. 1994;54(14):3723–5.

175. Diasio RB, Beavers TL, Carpenter JT. Familial deficiency of dihydropyrimidine dehydrogenase. Biochemical basis for familial pyrimidinemia and severe 5-fluorouracil-induced toxicity. J Clin Invest. 1988;81(1):47–51.
176. Harris BE, Carpenter JT, Diasio RB. Severe 5-fluorouracil toxicity secondary to dihydropyrimidine dehydrogenase deficiency. A potentially more common pharmacogenetic syndrome. Cancer. 1991;68(3):499–501.
177. Pullarkat ST, Stoehlmacher J, Ghader V, Xiong YP, Ingles SA, Sherrod A, et al. Thymidylate synthase gene polymorphism determines response and toxicity of 5-FU chemotherapy. Pharmacogenomics J. 2001;1(1):65.
178. Xu JM, Wang Y, Ge FJ, Lin L, Liu ZY, Sharma MR. Severe irinotecan-induced toxicity in a patient with UGT1A1 28 and UGT1A1 6 polymorphisms. World J Gastroenterol. 2013;19(24):2899–903. doi:10.3748/wjg.v19.i24.3899.
179. Common Terminology Criteria for Adverse Events Version 4.03. http://evs.nci.nih.gov/ftp1/CTCAE/CTCAE_4.03_2010–06–14_QuickReference_5x7.pdf. Accessed 4 Jan 2014.
180. Abigerges D, Armand JP, Chabot GG, Da Costa L, Fadel E, Cote C, et al. Irinotecan (CPT-11) high-dose escalation using intensive high-dose loperamide to control diarrhea. J Natl Cancer Inst. 1994;86(6):446. doi:10.1093/jnci/86.6.446.
181. Stavraka C, Ford A, Ghaem-Maghami S, Crook T, Agarwal R, Gabra H, et al. Gynecol Oncol. 2012;125(1):59–64. doi:10.1016/j.ygyno.2011.12.421.
182. Argyriou AA, Bruna J, Marmiroli P, Cavaletti G. Chemotherapy-induced peripheral neurotoxicity (CIPN): an update. Crit Rev Oncol Hematol. 2012;82(1):51–77.
183. Stubblefield MD, Burstein HJ, Burton AW, Custodio CM, Deng GE, Ho M, et al. NCCN task force report: management of neuropathy in cancer. J Natl Compr Canc Netw. 2009;7:S-1–26.
184. Beijers AJ, Jongen JL, Vreugdenhil G. Chemotherapy-induced neurotoxocity: the value of neuroprotective strategies. Neth J Med. 2012;70(1):18–25.
185. Grisold W, Cavaletti G, Windebank AJ. Peripheral neuropathies from chemotherapeutics and targeted agents: diagnosis, treatment, and prevention. Neuro Oncol. 2012;14 Suppl 4:iv45–54. doi:10.1093/neuonc/nos203.
186. Chamberlain MC. Neurotoxicity of cancer treatment. Curr Oncol Rep. 2010;16:60–7. doi:10.1007/s11912-009-0072-9.

187. Piccolo J, Kolesar JM. Prevention and treatment of chemotherapy-induced peripheral neuropathy. Am J Health Syst Pharm. 2014;71(1):19–25. doi:10.2146/ajhp130126.
188. Weber B, Largillier R, Ray-Coquard I, Yazbek G, Meunier J, Alexandre J, et al. A potentially neuroprotective role for erythropoietin with paclitaxel treatment in ovarian cancer patients: a prospective phase II GINECO trial. Support Care Cancer. 2013;21(7):1947–54.
189. Loprinzi CL, Qin R, Dakhill SR, Fehrenbacher L, Flynn KA, Atherton P, et al. Phase III randomized, placebo-controlled, double-blind study of intravenous calcium and magnesium to prevent oxaliplatin-induced sensory neurotoxicity (N08CB/Alliance). J Clin Oncol. 2013. doi:10.1200/JCO.2013.52.0536.
190. Hensley ML, Hagerty KL, Kewalramani T, Green DM, Meropol NJ, Wasserman TH, et al. American Society of Clinical Oncology 2008 clinical practice guideline update: use of chemotherapy and radiation therapy protectants. J Clin Oncol. 2009;27(1):127–45. doi:10.1200/JCO.2008.17.2627.
191. Dale DC, McCarter GC, Crawford J, Lyman GH. Myelotoxicity and dose intensity of chemotherapy: reporting practices from randomized clinical trials. J Natl Compr Canc Netw. 2003; 1(3):440–54.
192. Kuderer NM, Dale DC, Crawford J, Cosler LE, Lyman GH. Mortality, morbidity, and cost associated with febrile neutropenia in adult cancer patients. Cancer. 2006;106(10):2258–66.
193. Freifeld AG, Bow EJ, Sepkowitz KA, Boeckh MJ, Ito JI, Mullen CA, et al. Clinical practice guideline for the use of antimicrobial agents in neutropenic patients with cancer: 2010 Update by the Infectious Diseases Society of America. Clin Infect Dis. 2011; 52(4):427–31.
194. National Comprehensive Cancer Network. Prevention and treatment of cancer-related infection. Version 1.2013. Accessed 25 Dec 2013. http://www.nccn.org/professionals/physician_gls/pdf/infections.pdf.
195. Green MR. Symptom management. In: ASHP and ACCP Inc. 2013 Oncology Pharmacy Preparatory Review Course, 2013 ed. Lenex, KS: American College of Clinical Pharmacy, 2013: 1072–1079.
196. Klastersky J, Paesmans M, Rubenstein EB, Boyer M, Elting L, Feld R, et al. The Multinational Association for Supportive Care in Cancer risk index: a multinational scoring system for

identifying low-risk febrile neutropenic cancer patients. J Clin Oncol. 2000;18(16):3038–51.

197. Goolsby TV, Lombardo FA. Extravasation of chemotherapeutic agents: prevention and treatment. Semin Oncol. 2006;33(1):139–43.
198. Chu E, DeVita Jr VT, Copur MS, et al., editors. Physician's cancer chemotherapy drug manual. Sudbury: Jones and Bartlett; 2008.
199. Perry MC. The chemotherapy source book. 4th ed. Philadelphia: Lippincott Williams & Wilkins; 2008.
200. Schulmeister L. Extravasation management: clinical update. Semin Oncol Nurs. 2011;27(1):82–90.
201. Bertelli G, Gozza A, Forno GB, Vidili MG, Silvestro S, Venturini M, et al. Topical dimethylsulfoxide for the prevention of soft tissue injury after extravasation of vesicant cytotoxic drugs: a prospective clinical study. J Clin Oncol. 1995;13(11):2851–5.
202. Mouridsen HT, Langer SW, Buter J, Eidtmann H, Rosti G, de Wit M, et al. Treatment of anthracycline extravasation with Savene (dexrazoxane): results from two prospective clinical multicentre studies. Ann Oncol. 2007;18(3):546–50.
203. National Comprehensive Cancer Network. Epithelial ovarian cancer. Version 2.2013. Accessed 20 July 2013. http://www.nccn.org/professionals/physician_gls/pdf/ovarian.pdf.
204. Makrilia N, Syrigou E, Kaklamanos I, Manolopoulos L, Saif MW. Hypersensitivity reactions associated with platinum antineoplastic agents: a systematic review. Met Based Drugs. 2010;2010. pii:207084.
205. Castells M, Sancho-Serra Mdel C, Simarro M. Hypersensitivity to antineoplastic agents: mechanisms and treatment with rapid desensitization. Cancer Immunol Immunother. 2012;61(9):1575–84.
206. Castells MC, Tennant NM, Sloane DE, Hsu FI, Barrett NA, Hong DI, et al. Hypersensitivity reactions to chemotherapy: outcomes and safety of rapid desensitization in 413 cases. J Allergy Clin Immunol. 2008;122(3):574–80.

Section 3
Radiation Therapy

Chapter 7 Radiation Therapy in Gynecologic Cancer

Susan G.R. McDuff and Catheryn M. Yashar

Biology of Radiation Therapy

Definitions

- Roentgen = R = unit of exposure: The amount of X-rays or gamma radiation that will produce 1 cm^3 of air at 0 °C.
- 1 Gray = 1 J/kg = 100 cGray = 100 rads.
- Curie (Ci) unit of activity = 3.7×10^{10} disintegrations/s.

Compton Effect

- Principle employed in therapeutic radiation (high energy levels).
  - Incident photon comes into contact with an outer orbiting electron and some of its energy is given to the electron in the form of kinetic energy.
    This fast electron then breaks out of its orbit and can ionize other atoms of the absorber.
    - Breaking vital chemical bonds, initiating chain of events that translate into radiation changes.

S.G.R. McDuff, M.D., Ph.D. • C.M. Yashar, M.D. (✉)
Department of Radiation Medicine and Applied Sciences,
University of California San Diego Health System,
3855 Health Sciences Drive #0843, La Jolla, CA 92093-0843, USA
e-mail: susan.mcduff@gmail.com; cyashar@ucsd.edu

R.N. Eskander and R.E. Bristow (eds.), *Gynecologic Oncology: A Pocketbook*, DOI 10.1007/978-1-4939-1976-5_7,

Photoelectric Effect

- Principle employed at lower energies (commonly diagnostic radiology).
  - Incident photon smashes into a bound electron in the shell of an atom of the absorbing material and all the energy is transferred.
  - An inner orbiting electron is released from orbit after absorbing energy, and the vacancy is filled by and outer electron dropping in to take its place.
  - A new photon of characteristic radiation is produced.

Radiobiology

- How does radiation kill cancer?
  - DNA damage is the primary mechanism by which radiation kills cancer cells [1, 2].
  - Radiation damages DNA by creating:
    - Single- or double-strand DNA breaks.
    - Base damage.
    - Abnormal cross-links between DNA strands.
    - Abnormal cross-links between proteins and DNA.
  - Radiation can damage DNA directly or create free radicals which themselves induce DNA damage.
  - Radiation can also injure cell membranes, which may induce cell death via apoptosis.

Radiosensitivity

- The goal of radiation therapy is to selectively eliminate neoplastic cells while sparing normal tissues [2].
- *Radiosensitivity* refers to how susceptible a cell is to the effects of radiation.
  - Radiosensitivity is characterized by the extent, rapidity, and duration of response [2].
  - Radiosensitivity is determined by how quickly a given cell can repair DNA damage.

- Malignant cells are preferentially destroyed by radiation due to differential DNA repair capabilities.
- Following low doses of radiation (e.g., 1–2 Gy), tumor cells and normal cells sustain sublethal damage to their DNA.
  - Normal cells can repair sublethal damage relatively quickly compared to tumor cells and that is why radiation is typically administered in a fractionated schedule (low doses every day). This schedule gives normal cells a chance for repair while malignant cells accrue mutations.
  - Hypofractionation schedules allow for radiation delivery in relatively larger doses, less than once daily.
- Tumors differ in their radiosensitivity.
  - Some tumors regress with relatively low doses of radiation while others require far greater doses.

Importance of Oxygen

- The more oxygen present, the more sensitive a cell will be to radiation.

  If oxygen is present, oxygen molecules may attach themselves to damaged DNA, thereby "fixing" the damage.
  - Hypoxic cells are more resistant to injury caused by radiation than non-hypoxic cells.
    - Tirapazamine is an experimental drug that causes DNA damage only in the setting of hypoxia, and may be beneficial in targeting hypoxic regions of the tumor that are less sensitive to radiation.
      - Initial investigations have failed to find a survival benefit associated with tirapazamine in cervical cancer [3].
    - GOG 219 investigated the impact of tirapazamine on PFS and OS in patients with 1B2-4A cervical cancer limited to the pelvis.

- No difference in 3-year PFS or OS between tirapazamine and control arms.
- Increased toxicity with tirapazamine.

Importance of Cycling

- Cycling cells are more susceptible to radiation than non-cycling cells.
- A higher proportion of mitotic cells means that more of the tumor will be susceptible to radiation.
  - Cell position within the cell cycle is also important.
    - Cells in late G2 and mitosis phase are the most sensitive.
    - Paclitaxel is a chemotherapeutic agent that arrests cells in mitosis and thus makes arrested cells more susceptible to radiation damage.

Radiocurability

- *Radiocurability* refers to the ability of a patient to be cured [2].
  - Radiocurability depends on the sensitivity of the tumor, the tolerance of surrounding tissues, and the disease burden.
    - For example, squamous cell carcinoma of the cervix is a relatively radioresistant tumor (requiring doses >70 Gy to obtain a cure); however, it is highly curable because it is accessible to high-dose irradiation as normal surrounding tissues (i.e., the cervix and vagina) can themselves sustain relatively high doses of radiation without undue toxicity.

Therapeutic Ratio

- The *Therapeutic Ratio* is the ratio that quantifies the amount of radiation that induces tumor cell death with the amount that causes normal tissue toxicity.

– Calculated by the toxic dose divided by the therapeutic dose, and the goal of much research in radiation therapy is to maximize the therapeutic ratio, such that the dose required to produce a therapeutic effect is much lower than the dose required to produce a toxic effect.

Radiation Sensitizers

- Radiosensitizers are agents, like paclitaxel, that increase the toxicity of radiation.
- Examples:
  - Chemotherapeutic agents:
    - Cisplatin (inhibits the ability of cells to repair DNA damage), 5-fluorouracil, adriamycin, and gemcitabine.
  - Hypoxic cell sensitizers: improve the response of hypoxic cells to radiation.
    - Misonidazole.
- *Radiation protectors* (radioprotectors) are agents that decrease the toxicity of radiation on normal tissues.
  - Endogenous sulfhydryl compounds and amifostine are examples of radioprotectors.

Inverse Square Law

- The dose of radiation at a given point is inversely proportional to the square of the distance from the source of the radiation ($I = 1/d^2$) [2].
  - The inverse square law explains why the bladder and rectum can be relatively spared from receiving high doses of radiation when radiation is placed directly in the vagina (brachytherapy).
  - The dose rate at 2 cm from the source is one-fourth that at 1 cm.

  - The inverse square law dictates why it is important to stand at the door of the room of a brachytherapy patient in order to minimize exposure.

Introduction to Medical Radiation

Overview of Radiation Delivery Modalities: Two Main Types

External Beam Radiation Therapy (EBRT)

- Radiation in the form of electrons, photons, or protons is delivered to body tissues from sources at a distance from the body (e.g., linear accelerators, Figs. 7.1 and 7.2).
  - No radioactive sources within the body.
  - Radiation is delivered without machinery touching the patient directly.
- Specialized forms of external beam radiation therapy.
  - Stereotactic radiotherapy.
    - Uses a standard linear accelerator to deliver high-dose to precise locations in the body.
  - Stereotactic radiosurgery (SRS) delivers radiation to precise locations in the brain.
  - Stereotactic body radiotherapy (SBRT) delivers radiation to precise locations in the body.
  - Proton therapy.
    - Uses a beam of protons to deliver radiation to malignant tissue.
    - Main benefit: improves radiation localization and minimizes exit dose (which can minimize total dose to normal tissues, especially when tumor and normal tissues are juxtaposed).

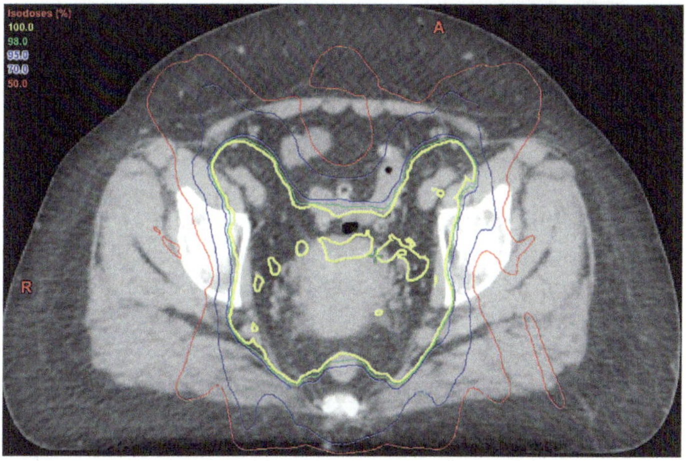

FIG. 7.1. Axial CT view of an image-guided IMRT plan for cervical cancer. Image courtesy of C. Yashar.

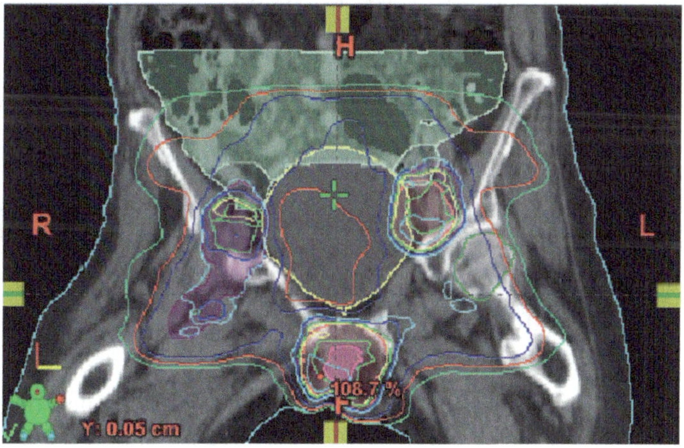

FIG. 7.2. Coronal CT view of an image-guided IMRT plan for vulvar cancer. Image courtesy of C. Yashar.

- Cyber Knife.
  - Radiation is delivered from a robotic arm and targets radiation at any body part from any direction using fiducial markers as guidance
- Gamma Knife.
  - Utilizes cobalt and aims gamma radiation to precise locations in the brain for the treatment of brain tumors with the intent of delivering an ablative dose of radiation in one treatment session.

Local Irradiation (Brachytherapy)

- Radiation emitted from natural isotopes (e.g., iridium, cesium) is predominantly used for interstitial radiation therapy, intracavitary radiation therapy, or brachytherapy [2].
- What is brachytherapy?
  - Radiation is delivered to tissues from sources that are placed inside the body close to the tumor.
  - Intracavitary brachytherapy:
    - Radioactive source is placed directly in a body cavity (e.g., the vagina, Figs. 7.3, 7.4, and 7.5).
  - Interstitial radiation therapy:
    - Radioactive source is placed directly in the tumor bed or body tissue (e.g., the prostate) that isn't a natural cavity.
  - Typically delivered at either a low-dose-rate (LDR) or high-dose-rate (HDR) system.
    - *LDR systems* require hospital admission such that the patient may stay in a shielded room and are less frequently used in the modern era of radiation oncology.
      - LDR systems deliver dose at a rate of around 50–120 cGy/h.

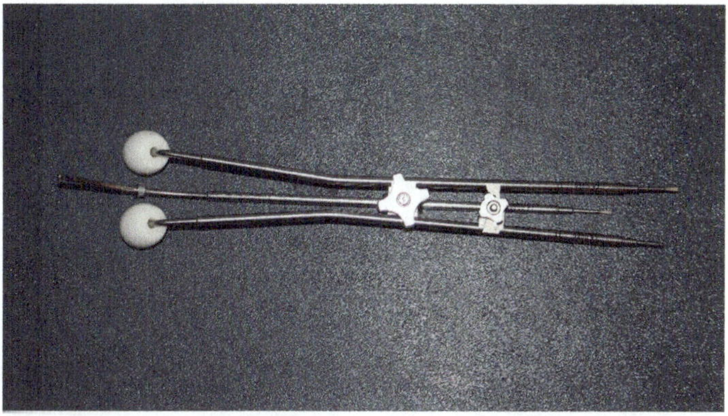

FIG. 7.3. Applicator used for treating cancer of the cervix, endometrium, and vagina. Image courtesy of C. Yashar.

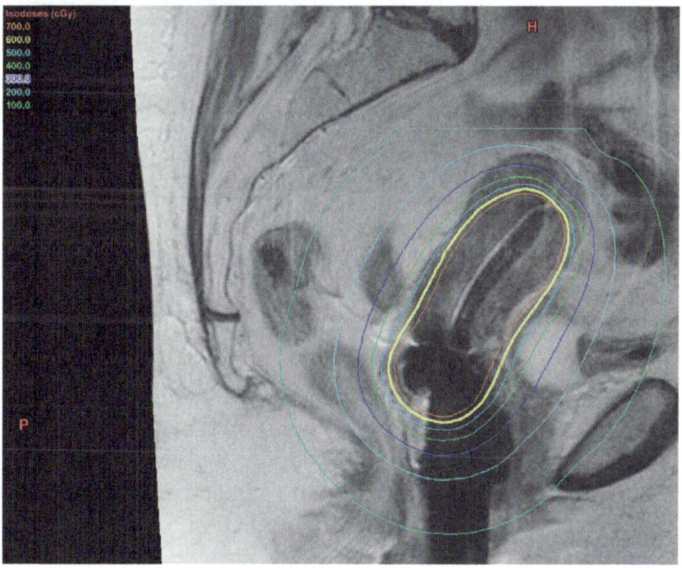

FIG. 7.4. Sagittal MRI display with brachytherapy equipment in place. *Colored lines* represent distribution of dose around the applicator, with dose decreasing as a function of the inverse square law. Image courtesy of C. Yashar.

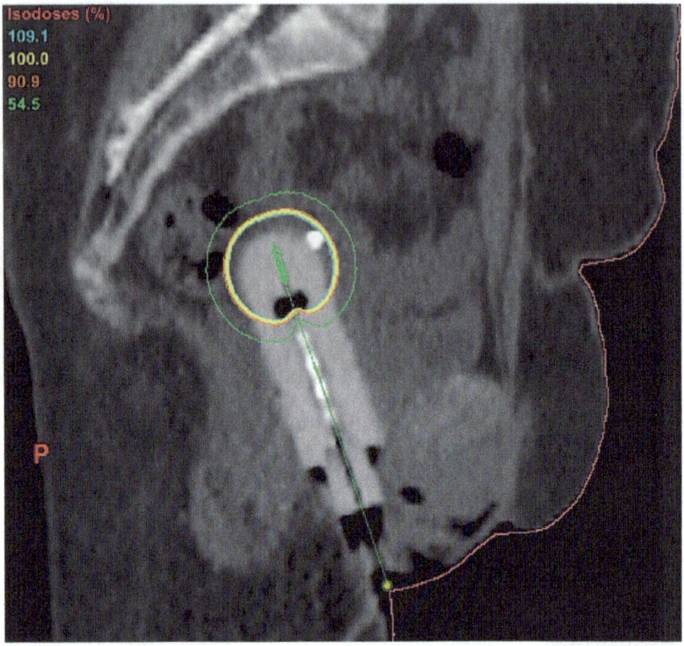

FIG. 7.5. Vaginal cuff brachytherapy. Image courtesy of C. Yashar.

- *HDR systems* are more frequently employed and deliver doses at 100 cGy/min.
- HDR systems are typically employed on an outpatient basis.
- Applicators that can be loaded with radioactive materials (primarily iridium) are used to administer intracavitary radiation.
- Needles that can contain radioactive materials are used to deliver interstitial radiation.
  - Permanent radioactive seeds can be placed in the body. These seeds remain even after decay of the source (Table 7.1) [4, 5].

TABLE 7.1. Radiation dose and organ tolerance [4, 5].

Organ	Tolerance dose (cGy)
Bone marrow	2,000
Spinal cord	5,000
Femoral head	5,000
Stomach	4,500
Bowel	5,000
Rectum	5,000
Ureter	7,500–8,000
Bladder	6,500
Ovary	600–1,000
Uterus	10,000–20,000
Cervix	9,000
Vagina	9,000–10,000
Vulva	2,000–3,000

Radiation Field Margins (for 3D CT-Based Planning) [6]

- Postoperative therapy of cervical cancer and endometrial cancer.
  - Clinical Target Volume (CTV) Definition—identifies target that may contain microscopic spread of disease.
    - Common, external, and internal iliac lymph node regions, and the upper 3.0 cm of vagina and paravaginal soft tissue lateral to the vagina.
      - For patients with cervical cancer (or endometrial cancer with cervical stromal invasion), the CTV should include the presacral lymph node region.
    - Superior border of CTV: begin 7 mm below the L4-L5 interspace (although there is consideration with 2D planning of covering all the common nodes which may join to form the aorta/inferior vena cava more cephalad than the conventional 2D border of L4/L5).
    - Inferior border of CTV: extend to 3.0 cm below the upper extent of the vagina (defined by the vaginal marker) or to 1.0 cm above the inferior extent of the obturator foramen, whichever is lower.
    - Uniform 3D planning target volume expansion: 7 mm.

ı Field Margins (for Bony Anatomy-
ınning)

- Pelvic radiation Stage 1B–4A cervical cancer and endometrial cancer.
  - Superior border: L4-L5 (with 3D therapy, transition to confluence of the common iliac arteries and veins may be practiced, ~L3).
  - Lateral border 1.5 cm beyond lateral margin of bony pelvis.
  - Inferior border mid-point of obturator foramen (allows coverage of upper vagina) or 4 cm below vagina marker, whichever is lower.
  - Posterior border: coverage of at least S3 and with more advanced disease the sacral hollow.
  - Anterior border: Just anterior to symphysis pubis.

Para-aortic Radiation

- Addition of para-aortic radiation to pelvic treatment requires that superior border be moved to body of L1 vertebra, with lateral borders of para-aortic filed encompassing the vertebral processes.
- Anterior border of para-aortic fields is 2 cm anterior to anterior surface of vertebral bodies.
- Posterior border is 2 cm posterior to anterior surface of vertebral bodies.

Inguinal Radiation

- Anterior field
  - Superior border: line 2 cm superior and parallel to inguinal ligament.
  - Lateral border: vertical line parallel to midline at anterior superior ileac spine.
  - Inferior border: 8 cm inferior and parallel to inguinal ligament and 1 cm below most inferior portion of the vulva.

- Medial border: 2 cm from midline bilaterally.
- (Above leads to a pair of parallelograms).

- Posterior field.
    - Superior border: mid-SI joint.
    - Lateral border: 2 cm lateral to widest portion of true bony pelvis.
    - Inferior border: mid-point of obturator foramen.

Brachytherapy Landmarks [7]

Point A: 2 cm above external OS and 2 cm lateral to midline (refers to uterus). Represents the parametria.

Point B: 3 cm lateral to point A, or 5 cm lateral to midline (should represent the pelvic sidewall).

The remainder of the chapter provides detail regarding specific radiation protocols used to treat the initial presentation of the most common gynecologic malignancies involving the endometrium, cervix, vagina, and vulva, as well as a brief overview of ovarian cancer, primary peritoneal carcinoma, fallopian tube carcinoma. A general overview of palliative treatment options will be provided at the end of the chapter.

Use of Radiation Therapy in the Most Common Gynecologic Malignancies

Endometrial Cancer

- Most common gynecologic malignancy diagnosed in the USA [8].
- Standard of care: up-front surgery (with consideration of lymph node dissection) serves to stage the cancer.
    - Low risk patients are typically not given a nodal dissection at the time of surgery and are often observed following surgery.
    - *Vaginal brachytherapy*: used for more deeply invasive lesions, higher-grade lesions, older patients, or patients

with lymphovascular space invasion as isolated high risk factor.

- *Pelvic and paraaortic irradiation*: reserved for the highest risk Stage I patients with multiple high risk factors, high risk Stage I patients without a nodal dissection, and advanced stage patients.
- See Table 7.2 for a summary of the key research studies and clinical trials that comprise the basis for the above general treatment recommendations [9, 10, 14–17].

Key Research Studies in the Treatment of Early Stage (Stage I–II) Endometrial Carcinoma

- Aalders et al. (1980)
  - Randomized controlled trial designed to study the benefit of additional pelvic external beam radiation therapy (EBRT) following surgery and vaginal brachytherapy in the treatment of Stage I endometrial carcinoma [9].
  - Five hundred and forty patients with Stage I endometrial carcinoma received a total abdominal hysterectomy and bilateral salpingo-oophorectomy (with no pelvic lymph node dissection) followed by postoperative vaginal cuff brachytherapy. Patients were then randomized to no further treatment versus additional treatment with EBRT to the draining pelvic lymphatics.
  - EBRT significantly reduced the risk of local recurrence (1.9 % vaginal and pelvic recurrence rate in EBRT group vs. 6.9 % recurrence rate in the no additional treatment group, $p < 0.01$).
    - EBRT group non-significantly developed more distant metastases than the no additional treatment group (9.9 % vs. 5.4 %, $0.10 > p > 0.05$) [9].
    - There was no overall survival benefit for additional EBRT observed at 9 years (90 % in the control group vs. 87 % in the EBRT group).

TABLE 7.2. Summary of clinical trials guiding the use of radiation therapy in the management of endometrial cancer [9, 10, 14–17].

Study	FIGO stage (eligible patients)	Control group	Comparison group(s)	Overall survival (OS)	Recurrence risk	Toxicity
Aalders et al. [9]	Surgical Stage I (540)	Surgery plus brachytherapy (BT) alone	Surgery and BT plus EBRT	(1) No OS benefit for additional EBRT (90 % in BT-alone group vs. 87 % in BT + EBRT) (2) Subset analysis: OS benefit for BT + EBRT in Stage IC Grade 3 patients (82 % vs. 72 %)	EBRT decreased risk of pelvic recurrence (1.9 % in EBRT group vs. 6.9 % in brachytherapy alone, $p<0.01$)	Complications reported include: rectovaginal fistula, urethral stricture (in BT-alone group) and small-bowel obstruction, bladder necrosis (in the BT + EBRT group)
PORTEC-1, Creutzberg et al. [10]	Stage IB (G2–3) or IC (G1–2) (715), specifically no IC3 patients	Surgery alone	Surgery and postoperative EBRT	No survival benefit for additional EBRT (81 %) versus surgery alone (85 %, ns)	Locoregional failures greater in surgery-alone group (14 %) versus surgery + EBRT (4 %, p<0.001)	Treatment-related complications greater in radiotherapy group (25 %) versus surgery-alone group (6 %, $p<0.001$); mostly grade 1 toxicity

(continued)

TABLE 7.2. (continued)

Study	FIGO stage (eligible patients)	Control group	Comparison group(s)	Overall survival (OS)	Recurrence risk	Toxicity
GOG-99, Keys et al. [14]	Stage IB–II (392)	Surgery alone	Surgery and postoperative EBRT	No overall survival benefit for additional EBRT (92 % in EBRT group vs. 86 % in surgery-alone group, $p=0.5$)	EBRT reduced risk of recurrence (12 % vs. 3 % in surgery-alone group, $p<0.01$); Among HIR subset, 26 % in surgery alone group versus 6 % with additional EBRT	Significantly more hematologic, gastrointestinal, genitourinary, and cutaneous toxicities in EBRT group
PORTEC-2, Nout et al. [15]	Stage I–IIA with high-intermediate risk features (427)	Surgery plus EBRT	Surgery plus vaginal brachytherapy	No difference in survival, 85 % versus 80 % (ns)	No difference in vaginal recurrence, locoregional relapse or isolated pelvic recurrences	Acute grade 1–2 toxicity higher in EBRT group (54 % vs. 13 % in BT group, ss)
JGOG-2033, Susumu et al. [16]	Stage IC–IIIC (385)	Surgery plus EBRT	Surgery plus chemotherapy (cyclophosphamide, doxorubicin, and cisplatin)	(1) Low/intermediate risk patients: no survival difference (2) Survival benefit in high-risk patients for chemotherapy (90 % vs. 74 % for EBRT group, $p=0.006$)	(1) Low/intermediate risk patients: no progression-free survival benefit (PFS) (2) PFS benefit in high-risk patients for chemotherapy (84 % vs. 66 % for EBRT group, $p=0.024$)	No difference in toxicity between groups (1.6 % of EBRT group had grade 3–4 toxicity vs. 4.7 % of chemotherapy group)

Italy, Maggi et al. [17]	High-risk endometrial, Stage IC G3, II G3, and III (345)	Surgery plus EBRT	Surgery plus chemotherapy (cisplatin, doxorubicin, cyclophosphamide)	No overall survival difference (69 % in EBRT group vs. 66 % in chemotherapy group, ns)	No PFS difference (63 % in EBRT group vs. 63 % in chemotherapy group, ns)	EBRT associated with gastrointestinal and genitourinary side effects; Chemotherapy associated with hematologic, nausea, and vomiting

- *Poor prognostic indicators identified*: age >60 years, FIGO Stage IB (previously termed FIGO Stage IC), histologic Grade 3, and lymphovascular invasion [9].
- A subset analysis revealed that only patients with poorly differentiated (grade 3) tumors, infiltrating more than half of the myometrial thickness, benefit from additional external beam radiation therapy (overall survival 82 % in the EBRT group vs. 72 % in the no additional treatment group) [9].

– The Post Operative Radiation Therapy in Endometrial Carcinoma 1 (PORTEC-1) trial.

- Randomized controlled trial designed to address the benefit of postoperative radiation therapy following initial surgery for endometrial carcinoma [10–13].
- Seven hundred and fifteen patients with Stage IB (grade 2–3) or Stage IC (grade 1–2) received a total abdominal hysterectomy and bilateral salpingo-oophorectomy (with no pelvic lymph node dissection). Patients were then randomized to receive EBRT versus no further therapy.
- Significant reduction in local recurrence with EBRT (5.8 % in the EBRT group vs. 15.5 % in the NAT group at 15 years, $p<0.001$), but no overall survival benefit [13].
- EBRT was more likely to be associated with adverse events, with up to 26 % of patients in the EBRT arm experiencing toxicity (mostly grade 1–2) compared to 4 % patients in the control arm [11], with side effects from the radiation therapy seen to persist at 15 years post-treatment [13].
- Given the absence of a survival benefit for EBRT and the relatively high rate of toxicity, EBRT is recommended to only be given to patients determined to be at high risk of recurrence.

  - Risk factors: age >60 years, grade 3 lesions, deep myometrial invasion.

    - Patients with 2 of these 3 high risk features (high intermediate risk, HIR, patients) were seen to have a 20 % risk of locoregional recurrence without radiation therapy, which decreased to 5 % following EBRT [10].
  - Thus, after PORTEC-1, it was felt that there remained an indication for EBRT in HIR patients, but should be avoided in low-intermediate risk patients [13].
- GOG-99 trial
  - Conducted to assess the benefit of postoperative radiation therapy versus no additional treatment following surgery for endometrial carcinoma on recurrence-free interval as the primary outcome [14].
  - In this study, 392 patients with intermediate or high-intermediate risk were randomized following total abdominal hysterectomy with bilateral salpingo-oophorectomy (with select patients receiving pelvic lymph node dissection) to postoperative radiation therapy versus no additional treatment.
  - Significantly lower recurrence rate in the EBRT treated group compared to the group receiving no additional treatment, which was especially pronounced in the high intermediate risk patient subset (6 % in the EBRT group vs. 26 % in the no additional treatment group at 2 years, $p<0.01$) [14].
  - Conclusion: postoperative radiation therapy significantly decreases the risk of recurrence in early stage endometrial carcinoma, but should be limited to patients with high intermediate risk features [14].
- PORTEC-2
  - Because most recurrences for limited-stage endometrial carcinoma following surgery occur in the vaginal cuff, PORTEC-2 was designed to compare the efficacy of vaginal brachytherapy with pelvic EBRT for preventing vaginal recurrence following hysterectomy [15].

  - In this study, 427 intermediate or high-risk endometrial carcinoma patients received total abdominal hysterectomy with bilateral saplingooophorectomy (and no lymph node dissection) and were then randomized to receiving either EBRT or vaginal brachytherapy.
  - At 5 years, vaginal brachytherapy is as effective as EBRT for preventing vaginal recurrence.

- No difference in locoregional-relapse, isolated pelvic recurrence, distant metastases, or overall survival [15].
  - Vaginal brachytherapy was associated with significantly less acute grade 1–2 gastrointestinal toxicity than the EBRT group (13 % vs. 54 %).
  - Conclusion: vaginal brachytherapy should be used in place of EBRT as the standard-of-care adjunctive therapy for patients that fit PORTEC-2 criteria [15].

- *Chemotherapy:* used for patients with more advanced disease, or higher-risk limited stage disease.
- JGOG-2033 trial
  - Conducted to compare postoperative pelvic radiation with chemotherapy for patients with >50 % myometrial invasion (Stage IC–IV) [16].
  - In this trial, 385 patients were randomized following TAH/BSO or radical hysterectomy (with the majority of patients receiving pelvic lymph node dissection) to receive either pelvic radiation therapy (AP/PA field to 45–50 Gy) or 3 courses of cisplatin/doxorubicin/cyclophosphamide.
  - At 5 years, no survival differences between the groups (progression-free or overall) [16].
  - On subset analysis, there was no difference for low or intermediate risk patients.
    - In the high-risk group (defined as patients with Stage IC and age >70 years old, or patients with Stage IC, grade 3 disease, Stage II, or Stage IIIA patients), chemotherapy was associated with an overall survival benefit compared to radiation (89.7 % vs. 73.6 %, $p<0.01$) [16].

- Maggi et al. (2006)
  - Compared EBRT versus combined platinum-based chemotherapy following surgery for high-risk endometrial carcinoma [17].
  - Three hundred and forty-five patients with high-risk endometrial carcinoma (defined as Stage IC, grade 3, Stage IIC, grade III, with >50 % myometrial invasion, and Stage III patients) were randomized to receiving either EBRT (to 45–50 Gy) or 5 cycles of cisplatin/doxorubicin/cyclophosphamide chemotherapy.
  - At 5 years, there were no differences in overall-survival or progression-free survival between the groups [17].
    - The authors noted that there was a trend toward delayed local relapse with radiation therapy, and a trend for delayed progression to distant metastatic disease with chemotherapy, but these trends were not significant [17].

Key Research Studies in the Treatment of Locally Advanced (Stage III–IV) Endometrial Carcinoma

- For patients with higher-stage endometrial carcinoma, surgery, chemotherapy, and radiation therapy are all vital treatment components.
- Hogberg et al. presented the pooled results from two randomized studies (NSGO-EC-9501/EORTC-55991 and MaNGO ILIADE-III) designed to address the benefit of chemotherapy following surgery and radiation therapy for advanced endometrial carcinoma [18].
  - Five hundred and thirty-four patients with high-risk Stage I–III endometrial carcinoma patients received TAH/BSO were randomized to receive radiation therapy alone or sequential radiation therapy and chemotherapy.

  - Additional chemotherapy improves progression-free survival, and there was a trend to improving overall survival [18].

- GOG 184 trial
  - Randomized patients with advanced endometrial carcinoma (Stage III or IV) treated with surgery and tumor-volume directed pelvic irradiation to receive either cisplatin and doxorubicin or cisplatin, doxorubicin, and paclitaxel chemotherapy.
    - No difference in recurrence-free survival between arms.
    - The addition of paclitaxel was associated with increased toxicity [19].

- GOG 122
  - Randomized trial designed to compare whole-abdominal radiation versus chemotherapy in patients with Stage III–IV endometrial carcinoma and no greater than 2 cm of residual disease following hysterectomy [20].
  - Three hundred and ninety-six patients who received a TAH/BSO were then randomized to receive either whole abdominal radiation (AP/PA fields to 30 Gy with 15 Gy boost to lymph nodes) or 8 cycles of doxorubicin and cisplatin chemotherapy.
  - At 5 years, significant improvement in overall survival for the chemotherapy group (55 %) compared to the group receiving abdominal radiation therapy (42 %), however with greater acute toxicity observed in the chemotherapy arm [20].
    - Approximately half of the patients in both arms experienced recurrence; patients in the chemotherapy arm tended to have higher rates of pelvic recurrence, whereas patients in the chemotherapy arm had fewer distant recurrences [20].

- The whole abdominal radiation dose was relatively low with an outdated administration compared to techniques employed today.

- *Sandwich trials*: administered adjuvant radiation therapy "sandwiched" between courses of chemotherapy.
  - Einstein et al. presented the results from a phase II prospective study designed to assess the tolerability of sequential chemotherapy with radiation therapy for advanced endometrial carcinoma [21]. Following surgery, patients were given a sequence of paclitaxel, radiation therapy, and carboplatin.
    - The treatment was well-tolerated, and the authors reported overall survival of 6.3 years for Stage I/II, 3.0 years for stage III/IV [21].
  - Secord et al. [22] presented the results of a multicenter retrospective analysis of patients with Stage III and IV endometrial carcinoma to assess the whether there was benefit for a particular sequencing of chemotherapy and radiation following surgery.
    - "Sandwich" chemotherapy-radiation-chemotherapy (CRC) was associated with improved survival compared to chemotherapy followed by radiation (CR) and radiation followed by chemotherapy (RC) [22].
- Ongoing trials
  - GOG-0249
    - Designed to assess whether vaginal cuff brachytherapy followed by 3 cycles of chemotherapy (paclitaxel and carboplatin) increases recurrence-free survival compared to EBRT in patients with Stage I–IIA endometrial carcinoma with high-intermediate risk factors.

- PORTEC-3
  - Designed to compare EBRT alone versus concurrent cisplatin-EBRT followed by adjuvant chemotherapy (paclitaxel and carboplatin) in high risk stage I–III patients.
- GOG 0258
  - Addresses the benefit for concurrent cisplatin and tumor-volume directed irradiation followed by carboplatin and paclitaxel versus carboplatin and paclitaxel alone for advanced endometrial carcinoma patients.

Cervical Cancer

- The third most common gynecologic malignancy diagnosed in the USA, following endometrial and ovarian cancer.
- Formerly the most common cause of cancer-related mortality in the USA, however mortality from cervical cancer has decreased dramatically as a result of improved access to Papanicolaou smear screening programs [23].
- Worldwide, however, cervical cancer remains the second most common cause of cancer-related mortality.

Treatment of Microinvasive (Stage IA) Cervical Cancer

- The current primary treatment of Stage IA1 cervical cancer with no lymphovascular space invasion is cervical conization.
- For Stage IA2 disease, or IA1 with lymphovascular space invasion, the treatment is modified or radical hysterectomy with consideration for pelvic lymph node dissection.
- In poor surgical candidates, brachytherapy alone (if stage IA1) or external beam radiation therapy with brachytherapy (stage IA2) are reasonable options [24, 25].

Key Research Studies in the Treatment of Early Stage Non-Bulky (Stage IB1 and IIA <4 cm) Cervical Cancer

- Surgery and radiation are equivalent treatment options for early stage, non-bulky cervical cancer because no trial has shown a survival or disease-free survival advantage for either modality [26, 27].
- However, surgery and radiation therapy differ in their side effect profile.
- Landoni et al. (1997)
  - Randomized 343 patients with Stage IB-IIA cervical cancer to receive radical hysterectomy versus EBRT (to 47 Gy) followed by LDR to a median dose of 76 Gy [26].
  - Patients in the surgical arm who were found to have Stage IIB or greater disease were allowed adjuvant RT, and 63 % of patients in the surgery arm received RT.
  - At 5 years, there was no difference in overall (87 % in the surgery group vs. 90 % in the radiation therapy group) or disease-free survival.
  - For patients with adenocarcinoma histology, there was an overall survival advantage for surgery (70 %) compared to radiation therapy (59 %), as well as a disease-free survival benefit.
  - Surgery was associated with a higher risk of grade 2–3 complications (28 %) compared to radiation therapy (12 %), and patients who had surgery with adjuvant radiation therapy experienced the highest rate of complications [26].
- GOG 71/RTOG 8412
  - Addressed whether surgery plus adjuvant radiation therapy confers benefit beyond radiation therapy alone.
  - Two hundred and fifty-six patients with “bulky” Stage IB cervical cancer (defined as exophytic or “barrel” shaped tumors greater than 4 cm) were randomized to

receive either external beam radiation therapy followed by hysterectomy or external beam radiation therapy alone [27]. Both groups received brachytherapy 1–2 weeks following completion of treatment.

  - At 5 years, no difference in overall survival between the groups.
    - But radiation therapy plus hysterectomy had a lower incidence of local relapse (14 %) compared to the radiation therapy alone (27 %).
  - There was also a trend towards a progression-free survival benefit with the addition of hysterectomy (62 % vs. 53 %, $p = 0.09$) [27].

- The presence of certain risk factors in Stage IB cervical cancer patients can assist in determining which patients will benefit most from adjuvant radiation therapy [28].
- Delgado et al. (1990)
  - Prospectively evaluated 645 patients with Stage 1 squamous cell carcinoma of the cervix to determine prognostic factors associated with disease-free interval [29].
    - Disease-free interval is strongly associated with depth of tumor invasion, tumor size, and capillary-lymphatic space (or lymphovascular space) invasion.
    - These criteria are the "Sedlis criteria."
      - Patients need postoperative radiation therapy if they have 2 or more of the following factors: 1) size >4 cm, 2) deep stromal invasion (invasion of carcinoma to greater than 1/3 of the stroma), and 3) lymphovascular space invasion.
        - The GOG-0263 is evaluating the role of radiation therapy with or without chemotherapy in patients with Stage I or II cervical cancer (with greater than 2/3 Sedlis criteria) following surgery.

Treatment of Early Stage Bulky (Stage IB2 and IIA >4 cm) and Locally Advanced (Stage IIB–IVA) Cervical Cancer

- Radiation and chemotherapy are indicated for early stage bulky cervical cancer [30].
- For patients with clinically visible disease (at least Stage IB2), or with bulky disease (>4 cm) that invades beyond the uterus but without parametrial invasion (Stage IIA), concurrent chemotherapy and radiation afford a significant survival benefit when compared to radiation therapy alone, with or without surgery [31–36].
  - The combination of surgery and chemoradiation is more toxic than primary chemoradiation, so if there is suspicion that postoperative adjuvant therapy will be needed (if a patient is felt to have a high risk of parametrial invasion, positive margins, or positive nodes on surgery) consideration of primary chemoradiation should be entertained [36].
- Standard of care chemotherapy: cisplatin-based chemotherapy.
  - Two randomized controlled trials have demonstrated a survival benefit for the addition of weekly cisplatin-based chemotherapy given concurrently with radiation therapy [34, 35], and three randomized controlled trials have demonstrated a survival benefit for the addition of cisplatin and 5-fluorauracil given concurrently with radiation therapy [32, 33, 36].
    - Pearcey et al. was the only randomized controlled trial comparing radiation therapy alone with radiation therapy plus weekly cisplatin that did not show a survival benefit for the addition of cisplatin [37]. Other investigators have also published on carboplatin and paclitaxel [38].
    - Combination therapies (with gemcitabine or biologics such as bevacizumab) are currently under investigation. See Table 7.2 for a summary of these trials.

Key Research Studies (See Table 7.3 for More Detail)

- GOG 123
  - Randomized 369 patients with Stage IB2 cervical carcinoma to receive radiation therapy alone or RT plus weekly cisplatin [35].
  - There was an overall and progression-free survival benefit for the addition of weekly cisplatin [35], preserved for a median follow-up of 8 years [31].
- GOG 120
  - Three-arm randomized controlled trial that assigned patients to receive radiation therapy and weekly cisplatin, radiation therapy plus hydroxyurea, or radiation therapy plus cisplatin, FU, and hydroxyurea [34].
  - Similar overall survival and progression-free survival benefits were seen when the two arms containing cisplatin-based chemotherapy were used compared to radiation therapy plus hydroxyurea alone [34].
  - Comparable survival benefits were seen in the GOG 85 trial ([32]; comparing radiation therapy with hydroxyurea with radiation therapy and cisplatin plus fluorouracil), as well as GOG 109 ([36]; comparing radiation therapy alone with radiation therapy and cisplatin plus fluorouracil).
- RTOG 90-01
  - Addressed the distinction between extended-field radiation therapy (with coverage of the para-aortic lymph nodes) versus radiation therapy plus cisplatin and fluorouracil [33].
  - Survival benefit found for the addition of cisplatin/FU chemotherapy.
- NCI Canada study
  - The only randomized controlled trial that did not show a benefit for the addition of cisplatin-based chemotherapy to radiation therapy in the treatment of cervical cancer [37].

Table 7.3. Summary of clinical trials guiding the use of radiation therapy, chemotherapy, and surgery in the management of cervical cancer [26, 32–37].

Study	FIGO stage (eligible patients)	Control group	Comparison group(s)	Overall survival (OS)	Progression-free survival (PFS)	Toxicity
Keys et al. [35] GOG 123	IB2 (369)	Radiotherapy	Radiotherapy plus weekly cisplatin	Greater OS in cisplatin + RT group 83 % versus RT alone 74 % ($p=0.008$)	Greater PFS in cisplatin + RT group 79 % versus RT alone 63 % ($p<0.001$)	Grade 3 and 4 toxicity greater in radiotherapy plus cisplatin group (21 % vs. 2 %)
Whitney et al. [32] GOG 85/ SWOG 8695 intergroup	IIB-IVA (368)	Radiotherapy plus hydroxyurea (HU)	Radiotherapy plus cisplatin and fluorouracil (FU)	Greater OS in cisplatin/FU group 55 % versus HU group 43 % ($p=0.018$)	Greater PFS in cisplatin/FU 57 % versus HU group 47 % ($p=0.033$)	Leukopenia greater with HU (24 % vs. 4 %)
Morris et al. [33] RTOG 90-01	IB2-IVA (386)	Extended-field radiotherapy (with coverage of para-aortic lymph nodes)	Radiotherapy plus cisplatin and FU	Greater OS in RT + cisplatin group 73 % versus RT-alone group 58 % ($p=0.004$)	Greater PFS in RT + cisplatin/FU group 40 % versus RT alone group 67 % ($p<0.001$)	Higher rate of reversible hematologic side effects in RT + cisplatin/FU group versus RT alone group

(continued)

TABLE 7.3. (continued)

Study	FIGO stage (eligible patients)	Control group	Comparison group(s)	Overall survival (OS)	Progression-free survival (PFS)	Toxicity
Rose et al. [34] GOG 120	IIB-IVA (526)	Radiotherapy plus hydroxyurea	1. Radiotherapy plus weekly cisplatin 2. Radiotherapy plus cisplatin, FU, HU	Cisplatin 75 % versus cisplatin/FU/HU 75 % versus HU 60 % (relative Risk 0.6 for cisplatin groups)	Cisplatin 67 % versus cisplatin/FU/HU 64 % versus HU 47 % (Relative Risk 0.56 for cisplatin groups)	Grade 3 and 4 toxicity more likely in 3-drug group compared to the other groups
Peters et al. 36] GOG 109/ intergroup 0107/ SWOG 8797/ RTOG 9112	IB or IIA (243)	Radiotherapy	Radiotherapy plus cisplatin and FU	Greater OS in the cisplatin/FU group 81 % versus RT alone group 71 % ($p=0.007$)	Greater PFS in the cisplatin/FU group 80 % versus RT alone group 63 % ($p=0.003$)	Greater grade 3 and 4 toxicity in the RT + cisplatin/ FU group
Pearcey et al. [37] NCI Canada	IB-IVA (253)	Radiotherapy	Radiotherapy plus weekly cisplatin	No difference in OS, 62 % in cisplatin + RT versus 58 % in RT alone group ($p>0.05$)	No difference in PFS between groups ($p>0.05$)	Greater decrease in hemoglobin levels in the cisplatin + RT group (30 %) versus RT-alone group (20 %)

Landoni et al. [26]	IB-IIA (343)	Radiotherapy	Surgery (with adjuvant RT delivered for surgical stage pT2b or greater, less than 3 mm safe cervical stroma, cut through or positive nodes)	No difference in OS between groups ($p > 0.05$)	No difference in PFS between groups ($p > 0.05$)	Greater morbidity in surgery group (28 %) versus RT group (12 %), ($p = 0.0004$)
Sedlis et al. [39] GOG 92	IB (277)	Surgery plus adjuvant radiotherapy	Surgery with no further treatment (NFT)	Follow-up too short for survival analysis	Greater PFS in the surgery + RT group 88 % versus surgery alone group 79 % ($p = 0.008$)	Greater grade 3/4 events in surgery + adjuvant RT group (6 %) versus surgery alone (2 %)

- Two hundred and fifty-three patients were randomized to receive radiation therapy alone or radiation therapy plus weekly cisplatin for patients with Stage IB–IVA cervical cancer [37].
- No difference in overall survival or progression-free survival.
- Hypotheses why their study did not show a benefit of cisplatin when five other trials showed a benefit:
  - The GOG 120 [34] and the GOG 85 [32] trials differed from the NCI Canada study because they did not have an RT-alone arm.
  - GOG 85 [32] and GOG 109 [36] trials paired cisplatin with fluorouracil instead of cisplatin alone.
  - The RTOG 90-01 trial [33] had an RT-only arm; however, the radiation therapy delivered was extended-field and modified to cover the para-aortics.
  - In the GOG 85 and GOG 120 trials, the median duration of radiation treatment was 62 and 64 days, respectively, whereas the treatment duration was 51 days in the NCI Canada study.
  - The addition of fluorouracil may have contributed to the survival benefit seen in GOG 85 and RTOG 90-01.
- The GOG 123 [35] trial was the most similar to the NCI Canada study in that the comparison arms were the same in both studies (radiation therapy alone vs. radiation therapy and weekly cisplatin); however, the GOG 123 trial showed that there was a survival advantage to weekly cisplatin whereas the NCIC study failed to find a benefit.
  - In the GOG 123 (Keys et al.) study, patients were limited to bulky stage IB2 cervical cancer, whereas the NCI Canada study included patients with stage IB–IVA. Moreover, all patients in the GOG 123 trial received an adjuvant extrafascial hysterectomy following either preoperative radiation therapy alone or preoperative radiation therapy with cisplatin.

- Current NCCN guidelines recommend treatment with external beam radiation therapy with concurrent cisplatin-based chemotherapy in addition to brachytherapy for treatment of this subset of patients.

Vulvar Cancer

- Carcinoma of the vulva is a rare gynecologic malignancy, comprising less than 3 % of gynecologic cancers [40].
- In women greater than 50 years of age, vulvar cancer is often associated with non-neoplastic epithelial disorders (e.g., chronic inflammation or lichen sclerosis), and does not generally present with cervical neoplasia or condylomas [40].
- In women younger than 50 years, vulvar cancer is often associated with the human papillomavirus (HPV), and generally presents with precursor lesions and condylomata [40].
- The majority of vulvar cancers are diagnosed in the early stages, although older women tend to present with more advanced disease [40].

Treatment of Limited-Stage (Stage I) Vulvar Cancer

- For resectable Stage I vulvar carcinoma, surgery is the primary treatment.
- Radical vulvectomy with bilateral dissection of inguinal groin nodes was the standard of care, but in modern practice, radical local excision is performed with inguinal lymph node dissection based on depth of invasion [40].
- The risk of recurrence is directly related to surgical margins, with >1 cm margin typically associated with the least risk of local recurrence [41].
- Predictors of recurrence following surgery include:
  - Depth of invasion, tumor thickness, infiltrative growth, lymphovascular invasion, increasing keratin, and greater than 10 mitoses on histology [41].

- Adjuvant radiation can be used in the setting of close or positive margins, positive lymph nodes, high-grade lesions and those lesions with lymphovascular space invasion.
- Faul et al. reported results from a retrospective review of 62 patients with either close (<8 mm) or positive margins following surgery [42].
  - Half of the patients received radiation therapy covering the vulva, bilateral groins and lower pelvis, while the other half of patients were observed.
  - The use of postoperative radiation therapy lowered the rate of locoregional recurrence (69 % of the observed group recurred compared to 33 % in the radiation therapy group) [42].

Treatment of Advanced-Stage (Stage II–IV) Vulvar Cancer

- For unresectable, Stage II–IV vulvar carcinoma, the primary treatment is radiation therapy with interstitial or intracavitary brachytherapy [43].
- Chemotherapy can also be used for more advanced cases; commonly used agents include fluorouracil, cisplatin and carboplatin.
- GOG 101
  - Designed to determine the feasibility of preoperative chemoradiation in patients with advanced vulvar cancer [44].
  - Seventy-three patients with clinical Stage III–IV squamous cell carcinoma received a split course (i.e., with a planned treatment break) of concurrent chemotherapy (cisplatin and 5-fluorouracil) and radiation therapy followed by surgical excision of the residual tumor plus bilateral inguinal lymph node dissection.
  - Following chemoradiation, 47 % patients had no visible vulvar cancer, and only 3 % were found to have residual unresectable disease [44].

- Conclusion: preoperative chemoradiation therapy may decrease the need for total pelvic exenteration in patients with advanced stage vulvar cancer [44].

- GOG 205
  - Designed to improve upon the GOG 101 protocol for utilizing concurrent chemoradiation as the primary treatment of locally advanced vulvar carcinoma [45].
    - The GOG 205 protocol specified weekly cisplatin with radiation therapy (adopting the standard of care for squamous cell carcinoma of the cervix), eliminated the planned treatment break utilized in GOG 101, and delivered a higher total dose to the primary tumor [45].
  - Fifty-eight patients with locally advanced (T3 or T4 tumors not amenable to surgical resection with radical vulvectomy) were given this higher dose of radiation therapy (57.6 Gy) with weekly cisplatin, followed by surgical resection of any residual tumor (or biopsy to confirm no residual tumor) [45].
  - Sixty-four percent of patients achieved a complete clinical response, which was noted to be an improvement from the 47 % cited in the GOG 101 study.
  - Conclusion: based on GOG 101 and GOG 205, primary chemoradiation should be considered as initial treatment for vulvar cancer that would otherwise require pelvic exenteration or partial removal of the closely involved structures (i.e., urethra, vagina, anus, bladder, rectum).

Vaginal Cancer

- Primary vaginal neoplasms are rare, comprising less than 2 % of gynecologic malignancies [46]. If any part of the lesion touches the cervix it is classified as a cervical carcinoma.
- Vaginal squamous cell carcinoma has many of the same risk factors as cervical cancer, and there is a strong

association between the development of vaginal cancer with persistent HPV infection [46].

 – Other risk factors include: infection with HSV or trichomonas, an increasing number of sexual partners, long-term pessary use, smoking, immunosuppression, prior pelvic radiation, and maternal use of diethylstilbestrol.

- Generally, vaginal cancer is preceded by a precursor vaginal intraepithelial neoplasia lesion [46].
- A higher proportion of late-stage disease is seen in Black, Asian Pacific Islander, Hispanic and older women, and a lower 5-year survival rate is seen in these groups [46].
  - Squamous cell carcinoma is the most common histology; however, adenocarcinoma and non-epithelial tumors (e.g., melanoma, sarcoma) are possible and carry a worse prognosis than squamous cell histology.
- Surgery is the standard of care for vaginal carcinoma in situ, and primary radiation therapy (consists of EBRT with a brachytherapy boost) is the standard of care for localized vaginal cancer [47].
  - Brachytherapy can be considered alone for more limited lesions (<2 cm, <0.5 cm thick). Surgical options are generally considered to result in increased morbidity than radiation.
- Most of the literature is retrospective, and there are no randomized controlled trials comparing surgery with radiation therapy.

Retrospective Studies

- Number of retrospective studies have documented outcomes of vaginal cancer treated with primary radiation therapy [48–53].
  - Frank et al. reported outcomes from a retrospective series of 193 patients with Stage I–IV vaginal carcinoma treated with EBRT (40–45 Gy) followed by brachytherapy

(to deliver total of 75–80 Gy) [48]. Disease specific survival was 85 % for Stage I patients, 78 % for Stage II, and 58 % for Stage III–IV patients.

    - Most common type of failure was locoregional.
    - Conclusion: primary radiation therapy can provide excellent outcomes for patients with vaginal carcinoma [48].

  - Mock et al. documented outcomes for using HDR brachytherapy alone or in conjunction with EBRT to treat primary vaginal carcinoma, and report that HDR brachytherapy is effective and tolerable [51].
  - Kucera et al. conducted a retrospective series to compare HDR to conventional LDR brachytherapy and found no difference in overall survival with HDR compared to LDR brachytherapy [54].

- Primary radiation therapy is an effective treatment for patients with vaginal carcinoma, especially patients with Stage I disease [53].
- For patients with tumors beyond Stage I, brachytherapy is necessary to enhance locoregional control, and the use of systemic chemotherapy may improve survival in patients with more advanced disease or distant metastases [53].
- Concurrent chemotherapy and radiation therapy can be given in the initial treatment of locally advanced vaginal cancer [55–58].

  - Commonly used agents include 5-fluorouracil, cisplatin, mitomycin.
  - Samant et al. published results from a Canadian retrospective series that included 12 patients with Stage II–IVA vaginal cancer treated with concurrent weekly cisplatin plus radiation therapy (EBRT plus brachytherapy) [56].

    - The overall survival rate after 5 years was 66 %, with 75 % progression-free survival and 92 % locoregional control [56].

- Dalrymple et al. (2004)
  - Fourteen patients with Stage I–III vaginal carcinoma were treated with primary chemoradiation therapy [57]. Patients received either 5-fluorouracil (5-FU), 5-FU/cisplatin, or mitomycin, and the authors reported 65 % survival after a median follow-up of 8 years [57].
- Thus, primary chemoradiation can be effective for the treatment of vaginal cancer and should be considered especially for more advanced cases.

Ovarian Cancer, Primary Peritoneal, and Fallopian Tube Carcinoma

Ovarian Cancer

- For the majority of ovarian cancer histologies (epithelial, sex-cord stromal, and germ cell) the standard of care is a total abdominal hysterectomy with bilateral salpingo-oophorectomy with staging as the initial treatment.
- For epithelial ovarian cancer, current NCCN guidelines suggest that patients with Stage IA–IB Grade 1 disease be observed, and patients with Stage IA–IB Grade 2 or greater disease receive chemotherapy with a taxane/carboplatin.
- Whole abdomen radiation therapy is no longer recommended in the initial treatment of ovarian cancer, but radiation therapy plays an important role in palliative care.

Primary Peritoneal Carcinoma

- Extra-ovarian primary peritoneal carcinoma is similar to serous ovarian carcinoma in terms of clinical presentation, appearance on histology, and response to chemotherapy [59].
- Primary peritoneal carcinoma accounts for nearly 10 % of cases where the presumed diagnosis is ovarian cancer and

it can arise following bilateral oophorectomy that is performed for reasons of prophylaxis or for removal of benign tumors [59, 60].

  - The histology in most cases is serous, although non-serous tumors can be seen [59, 60].

- Debulking surgery and multi-agent cisplatin-based chemotherapy are the standard treatments [60], and radiation therapy can be employed for palliative indications.

Fallopian Tube Carcinoma

- Primary fallopian tube carcinoma is an extremely aggressive but very rare neoplasm, accounting for less than 2 % of gynecologic malignancies [61].
- Primary fallopian tube carcinoma is treated similarly to epithelial ovarian cancer, with surgery and chemotherapy as cornerstones of treatment [61].
- Klein et al. reported the results of a multicenter retrospective study examining outcomes following postoperative adjuvant radiation or chemotherapy for 95 patients with Stage I–II primary fallopian tube carcinoma [62].
  - The authors reported no difference in overall survival between adjuvant radiation therapy versus chemotherapy [62].
- Radiation therapy can also be used in the palliative setting for cases of advanced primary fallopian tube carcinoma.

Palliative Radiation

- Palliative radiotherapy can be employed to ameliorate pain and bleeding that may arise in the advanced stages of a gynecologic malignancy.
- A variety of regimens have been employed in the palliative setting, ranging from treatments in a single dose, daily treatments or twice-daily fractionation schemes.

- RTOG 7905
    - Phase II study of 48 patients designed to document treatment outcomes with palliative radiotherapy and misonidazole for advanced pelvic malignancy [63].
    - Patients received a single dose of 10 Gy repeated at 4 week intervals for a total of 3 fractions. Approximately 68 % of patients exhibited some response, but there was a high rate of complications (49 % crude late complications rate) [63].
- RTOG 8502
    - Prospective longitudinal study designed to improve upon the palliative fractionation scheme employed in RTOG 7905.
    - Women with advanced gynecologic malignancies received palliative radiation therapy to 44 Gy in 3.7 Gy fractions delivered BID for 2 consecutive days followed by a break before the next set of 4 treatments [64].
    - 6.9 % patients had late grade 3+ complications at 18 months, which represents a significant decrease from the 49 % seen in RTOG 7905, and no one receiving less than 30 Gy had late toxicity [64].

References

1. Sarkaria, JN, Bristow RG. "Overview of cancer molecular radiobiology." In *Radiation Oncology Advances*, pp. 115–131. Springer US, 2008.
2. Yashar CM. "Basic Principle in Gynecologic Radiotherapy." *Clinical Gynecology Oncology 7ed. Philadelphia: Mosby* 94 2007.
3. Disilvestro PA, Ali S, Craighead PS, Lucci JA, Lee Y-C, Cohn DE, et al. Phase III randomized trial of weekly cisplatin and irradiation versus cisplatin and tirapazamine and irradiation in stages IB2, IIA, IIB, IIIB, and IVA cervical carcinoma limited to the pelvis: a Gynecologic Oncology Group study. J Clin Oncol. 2014; 32: no. 5, 458–464.

4. Tewari KS, DiSaia PJ. Radiation therapy for gynecologic cancer. J Obstet Gynaecol Res. 2002;28:123–40.
5. Marks LB, Yorke ED, Jackson A, Ten Haken RK, Constine LS, Eisbruch A, et al. Use of normal tissue complication probability models in the clinic. Int J Radiat Oncol Biol Phys. 2010;76: S10–9.
6. Small W, Mell LK, Anderson P, Creutzberg C, De Los Santos J, Gaffney D, et al. Consensus guidelines for delineation of clinical target volume for intensity-modulated pelvic radiotherapy in postoperative treatment of endometrial and cervical cancer. Int J Radiat Oncol Biol Phys. 2008;71:428–34.
7. Viswanathan AN, Thomadsen B. American Brachytherapy Society consensus guidelines for locally advanced carcinoma of the cervix. Part I: general principles. Brachytherapy. 2012;11: 33–46.
8. Jemal A, Bray F, Center MM, Ferlay J, Ward E, Forman D. Global cancer statistics. CA Cancer J Clin. 2011;61:69–90.
9. Aalders J, Abeler V, Kolstad P, Onsrud M. Postoperative external irradiation and prognostic parameters in stage I endometrial carcinoma: clinical and histopathologic study of 540 patients. Obstet Gynecol. 1980;56:419–27.
10. Creutzberg CL, van Putten WL, Koper PC, Lybeert ML, Jobsen JJ, Wárlám-Rodenhuis CC, et al. Surgery and postoperative radiotherapy versus surgery alone for patients with stage-1 endometrial carcinoma: multicentre randomised trial. PORTEC Study Group. Post operative radiation therapy in endometrial carcinoma. Lancet. 2000;355:1404–11.
11. Creutzberg CL, van Putten WL, Koper PC, Lybeert ML, Jobsen JJ, Wárlám-Rodenhuis CC, et al. The morbidity of treatment for patients with Stage I endometrial cancer: results from a randomized trial. Int J Radiat Oncol Biol Phys. 2001;51:1246–55.
12. Scholten AN, van Putten WLJ, Beerman H, Smit VTHBM, Koper PCM, Lybeert MLM, et al. Postoperative radiotherapy for stage 1 endometrial carcinoma: long-term outcome of the randomized PORTEC trial with central pathology review. Int J Radiat Oncol Biol Phys. 2005;63:834–8.
13. Nout RA, van de Poll-Franse LV, Lybeert MLM, Wárlám-Rodenhuis CC, Jobsen JJ, Mens JWM, et al. Long-term outcome and quality of life of patients with endometrial carcinoma treated with or without pelvic radiotherapy in the post operative radiation therapy in endometrial carcinoma 1 (PORTEC-1) trial. J Clin Oncol. 2011;29:1692–700.

14. Keys HM, Roberts JA, Brunetto VL, Zaino RJ, Spirtos NM, Bloss JD, et al. A phase III trial of surgery with or without adjunctive external pelvic radiation therapy in intermediate risk endometrial adenocarcinoma: a Gynecologic Oncology Group study. Gynecol Oncol. 2004;92:744–51.
15. Nout RA, Smit VTHBM, Putter H, Jürgenliemk-Schulz IM, Jobsen JJ, Lutgens LCHW, et al. Vaginal brachytherapy versus pelvic external beam radiotherapy for patients with endometrial cancer of high-intermediate risk (PORTEC-2): an open-label, non-inferiority, randomised trial. Lancet. 2010;375:816–23.
16. Susumu N, Sagae S, Udagawa Y, Niwa K, Kuramoto H, Satoh S, et al. Randomized phase III trial of pelvic radiotherapy versus cisplatin-based combined chemotherapy in patients with intermediate- and high-risk endometrial cancer: a Japanese Gynecologic Oncology Group study. Gynecol Oncol. 2008;108:226–33.
17. Maggi R, Lissoni A, Spina F, Melpignano M, Zola P, Favalli G, et al. Adjuvant chemotherapy vs radiotherapy in high-risk endometrial carcinoma: results of a randomised trial. Br J Cancer. 2006;95:266–71.
18. Hogberg T, Signorelli M, de Oliveira CF, Fossati R, Lissoni AA, Sorbe B, et al. Sequential adjuvant chemotherapy and radiotherapy in endometrial cancer-results from two randomised studies. Eur J Cancer. 2010;46:2422–31.
19. Homesley HD, Filiaci V, Gibbons SK, Long HJ, Cella D, Spirtos NM, et al. A randomized phase III trial in advanced endometrial carcinoma of surgery and volume directed radiation followed by cisplatin and doxorubicin with or without paclitaxel: a Gynecologic Oncology Group study. Gynecol Oncol. 2009;112:543–52.
20. Randall ME, Filiaci VL, Muss H, Spirtos NM, Mannel RS, Fowler J, et al. Randomized phase III trial of whole-abdominal irradiation versus doxorubicin and cisplatin chemotherapy in advanced endometrial carcinoma: a Gynecologic Oncology Group study. J Clin Oncol. 2006;24:36–44.
21. Einstein MH, Frimer M, Kuo DY-S, Reimers LL, Mehta K, Mutyala S, et al. Phase II trial of adjuvant pelvic radiation "sandwiched" between combination paclitaxel and carboplatin in women with uterine papillary serous carcinoma. Gynecol Oncol. 2012;124:21–5.
22. Secord AA, Havrilesky LJ, O'Malley DM, Bae-Jump V, Fleming ND, Broadwater G, et al. A multicenter evaluation of sequential

multimodality therapy and clinical outcome for the treatment of advanced endometrial cancer. Gynecol Oncol. 2009;114:442–7.

23. Franco EL, Duarte-Franco E, Ferenczy A. Cervical cancer: epidemiology, prevention and the role of human papillomavirus infection. CMAJ. 2001;164:1017–25.
24. Grigsby PW, Perez CA. Radiotherapy alone for medically inoperable carcinoma of the cervix: stage IA and carcinoma in situ. Int J Radiat Oncol Biol Phys. 1991;21:375–8.
25. Kolstad P. Follow-up study of 232 patients with stage Ia1 and 411 patients with stage Ia2 squamous cell carcinoma of the cervix (microinvasive carcinoma). Gynecol Oncol. 1989;33:265–72.
26. Landoni F, Maneo A, Colombo A, Placa F, Milani R, Perego P, et al. Randomised study of radical surgery versus radiotherapy for stage Ib-IIa cervical cancer. Lancet. 1997;350:535–40.
27. Keys HM, Bundy BN, Stehman FB, Okagaki T, Gallup DG, Burnett AF, et al. Radiation therapy with and without extrafascial hysterectomy for bulky stage IB cervical carcinoma: a randomized trial of the Gynecologic Oncology Group. Gynecol Oncol. 2003;89:343–53.
28. Wolfson AH, Varia MA, Moore D, Rao GG, Gaffney DK, Erickson-Wittmann BA, et al. ACR Appropriateness Criteria® role of adjuvant therapy in the management of early stage cervical cancer. Gynecol Oncol. 2012;125:256–62.
29. Delgado G, Bundy B, Zaino R, Sevin BU, Creasman WT, Major F. Prospective surgical-pathological study of disease-free interval in patients with stage IB squamous cell carcinoma of the cervix: a Gynecologic Oncology Group study. Gynecol Oncol. 1990;38:352–7.
30. Gaffney DK, Erickson-Wittmann BA, Jhingran A, Mayr NA, Puthawala AA, Moore D, et al. ACR Appropriateness Criteria® on advanced cervical cancer expert panel on radiation oncology-gynecology. Int J Radiat Oncol Biol Phys. 2011;81:609–14.
31. Stehman FB, Ali S, Keys HM, Muderspach LI, Chafe WE, Gallup DG, et al. Radiation therapy with or without weekly cisplatin for bulky stage 1B cervical carcinoma: follow-up of a Gynecologic Oncology Group trial. Am J Obstet Gynecol. 2007;197:503.e1–6.
32. Whitney CW, Sause W, Bundy BN, Malfetano JH, Hannigan EV, Fowler WC, et al. Randomized comparison of fluorouracil plus cisplatin versus hydroxyurea as an adjunct to radiation therapy in stage IIB-IVA carcinoma of the cervix with negative para-aortic lymph nodes: a Gynecologic Oncology Group and Southwest Oncology Group study. J Clin Oncol. 1999;17:1339–48.

33. Morris M, Eifel PJ, Lu J, Grigsby PW, Levenback C, Stevens RE, et al. Pelvic radiation with concurrent chemotherapy compared with pelvic and para-aortic radiation for high-risk cervical cancer. N Engl J Med. 1999;340:1137–43.
34. Rose PG, Bundy BN, Watkins EB, Thigpen JT, Deppe G, Maiman MA, et al. Concurrent cisplatin-based radiotherapy and chemotherapy for locally advanced cervical cancer. N Engl J Med. 1999;340:1144–53.
35. Keys HM, Bundy BN, Stehman FB, Muderspach LI, Chafe WE, Suggs 3rd CL, et al. Cisplatin, radiation, and adjuvant hysterectomy compared with radiation and adjuvant hysterectomy for bulky stage IB cervical carcinoma. N Engl J Med. 1999;340: 1154–61.
36. Peters WA, Liu PY, Barrett RJ, Stock RJ, Monk BJ, Berek JS, et al. Concurrent chemotherapy and pelvic radiation therapy compared with pelvic radiation therapy alone as adjuvant therapy after radical surgery in high-risk early-stage cancer of the cervix. J Clin Oncol. 2000;18:1606–13.
37. Pearcey R, Brundage M, Drouin P, Jeffrey J, Johnston D, Lukka H, et al. Phase III trial comparing radical radiotherapy with and without cisplatin chemotherapy in patients with advanced squamous cell cancer of the cervix. J Clin Oncol. 2002;20:966–72.
38. Mabuchi S, Takahashi R, Isohashi F, Yokoi T, Ito K, Tsutui T, et al. A phase I study of concurrent weekly carboplatin and paclitaxel combined with intensity-modulated pelvic radiotherapy as an adjuvant treatment for early-stage cervical cancer patients with positive pelvic lymph nodes. Int J Gynecol Cancer. 2013;23:1279–86.
39. Sedlis A, Bundy BN, Rotman MZ, Lentz SS, Muderspach LI, Zaino RJ. A randomized trial of pelvic radiation therapy versus no further therapy in selected patients with stage IB carcinoma of the cervix after radical hysterectomy and pelvic lymphadenectomy: a Gynecologic Oncology Group study. Gynecol Oncol. 1999;73:177–83.
40. Stroup AM, Harlan LC, Trimble EL. Demographic, clinical, and treatment trends among women diagnosed with vulvar cancer in the United States. Gynecol Oncol. 2008;108:577–83.
41. Heaps JM, Fu YS, Montz FJ, Hacker NF, Berek JS. Surgical-pathologic variables predictive of local recurrence in squamous cell carcinoma of the vulva. Gynecol Oncol. 1990;38:309–14.

42. Faul CM, Mirmow D, Huang Q, Gerszten K, Day R, Jones MW. Adjuvant radiation for vulvar carcinoma: improved local control. Int J Radiat Oncol Biol Phys. 1997;38:381–9.
43. Kidd E, Moore D, Varia MA, Gaffney DK, Elshaikh MA, Erickson B, et al. ACR Appropriateness Criteria® management of locoregionally advanced squamous cell carcinoma of the vulva. Am J Clin Oncol. 2013;36:415–22.
44. Moore DH, Thomas GM, Montana GS, Saxer A, Gallup DG, Olt G. Preoperative chemoradiation for advanced vulvar cancer: a phase II study of the Gynecologic Oncology Group. Int J Radiat Oncol Biol Phys. 1998;42:79–85.
45. Moore DH, Ali S, Koh W-J, Michael H, Barnes MN, McCourt CK, et al. A phase II trial of radiation therapy and weekly cisplatin chemotherapy for the treatment of locally-advanced squamous cell carcinoma of the vulva: a gynecologic oncology group study. Gynecol Oncol. 2012;124:529–33.
46. Wu X, Matanoski G, Chen VW, Saraiya M, Coughlin SS, King JB, et al. Descriptive epidemiology of vaginal cancer incidence and survival by race, ethnicity, and age in the United States. Cancer. 2008;113:2873–82.
47. Creasman WT, Phillips JL, Menck HR. The National Cancer Data Base report on cancer of the vagina. Cancer. 1998;83:1033–40.
48. Frank SJ, Jhingran A, Levenback C, Eifel PJ. Definitive radiation therapy for squamous cell carcinoma of the vagina. Int J Radiat Oncol Biol Phys. 2005;62:138–47.
49. Sinha B, Stehman F, Schilder J, Clark L, Cardenes H. Indiana University experience in the management of vaginal cancer. Int J Gynecol Cancer. 2009;19:686–93.
50. Hegemann S, Schäfer U, Lellé R, Willich N, Micke O. Long-term results of radiotherapy in primary carcinoma of the vagina. Strahlenther Onkol. 2009;185:184–9.
51. Mock U, Kucera H, Fellner C, Knocke TH, Pötter R. High-dose-rate (HDR) brachytherapy with or without external beam radiotherapy in the treatment of primary vaginal carcinoma: long-term results and side effects. Int J Radiat Oncol Biol Phys. 2003;56:950–7.
52. Stock RG, Mychalczak B, Armstrong JG, Curtin JP, Harrison LB. The importance of brachytherapy technique in the management of primary carcinoma of the vagina. Int J Radiat Oncol Biol Phys. 1992;24:747–53.
53. Perez CA, Grigsby PW, Garipagaoglu M, Mutch DG, Lockett MA. Factors affecting long-term outcome of irradiation in carcinoma of the vagina. Int J Radiat Oncol Biol Phys. 1999;44:37–45.

54. Kucera H, Mock U, Knocke TH, Kucera E, Pötter R. Radiotherapy alone for invasive vaginal cancer: outcome with intracavitary high dose rate brachytherapy versus conventional low dose rate brachytherapy. Acta Obstet Gynecol Scand. 2001;80:355–60.
55. Nashiro T, Yagi C, Hirakawa M, Inamine M, Nagai Y, Sakumoto K, et al. Concurrent chemoradiation for locally advanced squamous cell carcinoma of the vagina: case series and literature review. Int J Clin Oncol. 2008;13:335–9.
56. Samant R, Lau B, E C, Le T, Tam E. Primary vaginal cancer treated with concurrent chemoradiation using Cis-platinum. Int J Radiat Oncol Biol Phys. 2007;69:746–50.
57. Dalrymple JL, Russell AH, Lee SW, Scudder SA, Leiserowitz GS, Kinney WK, et al. Chemoradiation for primary invasive squamous carcinoma of the vagina. Int J Gynecol Cancer. 2004; 14:110–7.
58. Kirkbride P, Fyles A, Rawlings GA, Manchul L, Levin W, Murphy KJ, et al. Carcinoma of the vagina–experience at the Princess Margaret Hospital (1974–1989). Gynecol Oncol. 1995; 56:435–43.
59. Eltabbakh GH, Piver MS. Extraovarian primary peritoneal carcinoma. Oncology (Williston Park). 1998;12:813–9. discussion 820, 825–6.
60. Bhuyan P, Mahapatra S, Mahapatra S, Sethy S, Parida P, Satpathy S. Extraovarian primary peritoneal papillary serous carcinoma. Arch Gynecol Obstet. 2010;281:561–4.
61. Kalampokas E, Kalampokas T, Tourountous I. Primary fallopian tube carcinoma. Eur J Obstet Gynecol Reprod Biol. 2013;169:155–61.
62. Klein M, Rosen A, Lahousen M, Graf A-H, Rainer A. The relevance of adjuvant therapy in primary carcinoma of the fallopian tube, stages I and II: irradiation vs. chemotherapy. Int J Radiat Oncol. 2000;48:1427–31.
63. Spanos WJ, Wasserman T, Meoz R, Sala J, Kong J, Stetz J. Palliation of advanced pelvic malignant disease with large fraction pelvic radiation and misonidazole: final report of RTOG phase I/II study. Int J Radiat Oncol Biol Phys. 1987;13:1479–82.
64. Spanos WJ, Clery M, Perez CA, Grigsby PW, Doggett RL, Poulter CA, et al. Late effect of multiple daily fraction palliation schedule for advanced pelvic malignancies (RTOG 8502). Int J Radiat Oncol Biol Phys. 1994;29:961–7.

Section 4
Critical Care

Chapter 8
Critical Care

Alexandre Buckley and Ana I. Tergas

Mechanical Ventilation

- Mechanical ventilation (MV) is indicated in the case of respiratory failure and can partially or fully replace spontaneous breathing. The basic mechanism of MV is as follows:
  - Performed through a positive pressure mechanism.
  - After an inspiratory trigger, oxygen-containing air is forced into the airway expanding the alveoli and increasing the pressure.
  - After a termination signal, expiration follows passively.

A. Buckley, M.D., A.I. Tergas, M.D., M.P.H. (✉)
Division of Gynecologic Oncology, Department of Obstetrics and Gynecology, Columbia University College of Physicians and Surgeons, 161 Fort Washington Avenue, HIP 8-837, New York, NY 10032, USA
e-mail: alb9106@nyp.org; ait2111@cumc.columbia.edu

R.N. Eskander and R.E. Bristow (eds.), *Gynecologic Oncology: A Pocketbook*, DOI 10.1007/978-1-4939-1976-5_8,

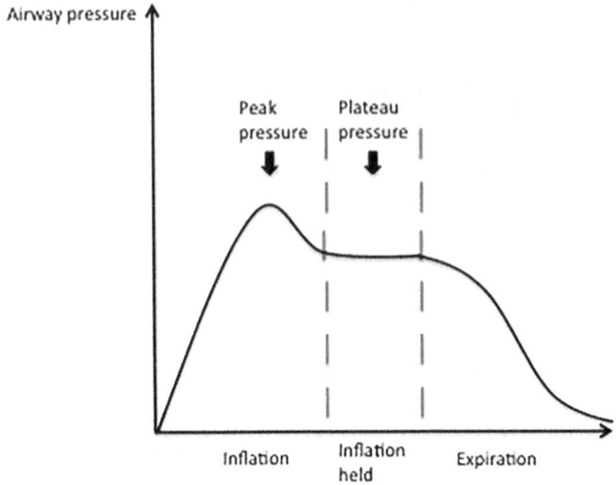

FIG. 8.1. Airway pressure curve at the end of inspiration and held expiration. Initial decrease in peak pressure followed by the plateau pressure.

Lung Mechanics, Monitoring, and Physiology

- Both the upper airway resistance and the lungs elastic recoil (compliance) generate resistance to air flow.
- Peak pressure (Ppeak) occurs at the end of inspiration and is followed by a plateau pressure.
  - The plateau pressure is the pressure in the airway in the hypothetical situation of held inspiration and no expiration.
  - There is an initial decrease in peak pressure followed by the plateau pressure (Fig. 8.1).
- An acute change in upper airway resistance (e.g., endotracheal tube obstruction) would generate an acute increase in Ppeak with unchanged plateau pressure.
- Decreased lung compliance would increase both Ppeak and plateau pressure (e.g., atelectasis, pneumonia, pneumothorax) whereas an endotracheal cuff leak would decrease the Ppeak (Fig. 8.2).

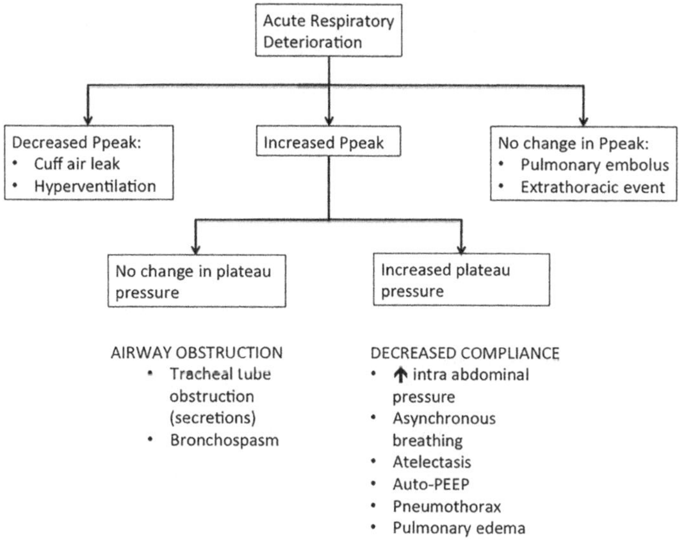

Fig. 8.2. Assessment of acute respiratory deterioration of patients in the ventilator. Decreased lung compliance would increase both Ppeak and plateau pressure (e.g., atelectasis, pneumonia, pneumothorax) whereas an endotracheal cuff leak would decrease the Ppeak.

- Mechanical breaths can be delivered by either pressure-cycled ventilation or volume-cycled ventilation.
  - Advantage of volume cycled ventilation is that a constant volume is assured. However, in noncompliant lungs, intrathoracic pressures can be very high, which can result in lung injury (barotrauma) and have an adverse effect on cardiac output.
  - The increased intrathoracic pressure associated with mechanical ventilation can reduce ventricular filling by impeding venous return and reducing cardiac distensibility. Ventricular output is usually facilitated by the positive intrathoracic pressure. The end result in cardiac output and blood pressure will depend on which of the two effects predominates.

TABLE 8.1. Modes of mechanical ventilation [1].

			Type of breath		
Mode	Breath strategy	Trigger	Mandatory	Assisted	Spontaneous
CMV	Volume or pressure cycled	Ventilator	Yes	No	No
AC	Volume or pressure cycled	Ventilator and patient	Yes	Yes	No
IMV/ SIMV	Volume or pressure cycled	Ventilator and patient	Yes	Yes	Yes
PSV	Pressure-cycled	Patient	No	Yes	No

AC assist control, *CMV* controlled mechanical ventilation, *IMV/SIMV* intermittent mandatory ventilation/synchronized mandatory ventilation, *PSV* pressure support ventilation

Modes of Mechanical Ventilation

- Modes of mechanical ventilation are classified by the type of breath they deliver.
  - The ventilator settings can control, assist, or support the volume or pressure the clinician has determined to be delivered. Each breath is triggered either by the ventilator or the patient (Table 8.1) [1].

Some of the most frequently used modes are assist control (AC), synchronized intermittent mandatory ventilation (SIMV) and pressure support.

- Controlled Mechanical Ventilation (CMV).
  - Minute ventilation is established by the respiratory rate and the tidal volume chosen by the practitioner.
  - The patient does not do any effort to trigger or assist with the respiration.
- Assist Controlled (AC) Mode.
  - Clinician determines the minute ventilation by setting the respiratory rate and tidal volume.
  - The patient can increase the minute ventilation if she triggers a respiration.
  - Each patient-initiated breath receives the set tidal volume that has been established.

TABLE 8.2. The principles of lung-protective ventilation.

1. Prevention of trauma due to excessive volume (tidal volume 4–8 mL/kg of PBW, with predicted plateau volume <30 cm H_2O)
2. Prevention of atelectasis by positive end-expiratory pressure (PEEP) ≥5 cm H_2O and recruitment maneuvers (prolonged inspiration at 30–50 cm H_2O for 30–40 s, a sigh breath with high tidal volume, high pressure during PSV) [3]
3. Adequate ventilation (respiratory rate: 20–35)
4. Prevention of hyperoxia (peripheral oxygen saturation SpO_2 88–95 %)

PBW predicted body weight. PBW females = 45.5 + 0.91 × (height − 152.4); PBW males = 50 + 0.91 × (height − 152.4)

- Synchronized Intermittent Mandatory Ventilation (SIMV).
  - Clinician determines the minute ventilation by setting the respiration rate and tidal volume.
  - Breaths are synchronized with patient's inspiratory effort.
  - SIMV differs from AC in that the patient can also increase the minute ventilation by spontaneous breathing without ventilator assistance.

Initiation of Mechanical Ventilation

Consider the following parameters:

1. Use of invasive or noninvasive mechanical ventilation.
2. Mode of mechanical ventilation.
3. Amount of support to be delivered.
4. Initial ventilator settings.

The selection of the mode is generally based on clinician familiarity and institutional preferences [2]. Recent data suggests that lung-protective mechanical ventilation used for acute respiratory distress syndrome (ARDS) is safe and potentially beneficial in patients who do not have ARDS [3] (Table 8.2). The ideal level of respiratory support allows sufficient rest to the respiratory muscles, without causing atrophy, while attaining adequate ventilation. The AC mode delivers the highest level of support and can be used to initiate mechanical ventilation.

Management of Mechanical Ventilation After Initiation [4]

1. Reduce tidal volume (Vt) by 1 mL/kg every 2 h until Vt=6 mL/kg and measure plateau pressure. Continue reducing Vt until plateau pressure <30 cm H_2O or Vt=4 mL/kg.
2. Monitor arterial blood gas and correct with respiratory rate and Vt settings as necessary.
3. Goals: Vt=6 mL/kg, plateau pressure <30 cm H_2O and pH=7.30–7.45.

Acute Respiratory Distress Syndrome (ARDS)

In 2011, The European Society of Intensive Care Medicine, endorsed by the American Thoracic Society and the Society of Critical Care Medicine, developed the Berlin definition for ARDS. It is described as an acute, diffuse, inflammatory lung injury leading to increased vascular permeability, increased lung weight, and loss of aerated lung tissue. Diffuse alveolar damage leads to increased dead space and decreased lung compliance. The clinical result is hypoxemia and diffuse bilateral radiographic opacities [5] (Table 8.3).

TABLE 8.3. The Berlin definition for ARDS (the ARDS definition task force) [5].

Acute respiratory distress syndrome		
Timing		Within 1 week of a known clinical insult or new worsening respiratory symptoms
Chest imaging		Bilateral opacities-not fully explained by effusions, lobar/lung collapse, or nodules
Origin of edema		Respiratory failure not fully explained by cardiac failure or fluid overload. Need objective assessment (e.g., echocardiography) to exclude hydrostatic edema if no risk factor present
	Mild	200 mmHg < PaO_2/FiO_2 ≤300 mmHg with PEEP or CPAP ≥5 cm H_2O
Oxygenation	Moderate	100 mmHg < PaO_2/FiO_2 ≤200 mmHg with PEEP ≥5 cm H_2O
	Severe	PaO_2/FiO_2 ≤100 mmHg with PEEP ≥5 cm H_2O

Mild, moderate and severe stages of ARDS have 27, 32, and 45 % mortality rate, respectively and a median duration of mechanical ventilation in survivors of 5, 7, and 9 days, respectively

ARDS severity correlates well with mortality and with increased median duration of mechanical ventilation (Table 8.3) [5]. Mild, moderate, and severe ARDS are associated with 27, 32, and 45 % mortality, respectively.

Consensus exists about using mechanical ventilator strategies to decrease ventilator-associated lung injury in ARDS.

Low tidal volume ventilation (*LTVV*) is associated with decreased mortality and more days off the ventilator [6, 7]. Lung-protective ventilation principles should be employed (Table 8.2).

- The Vt should be adjusted based on plateau pressure.
- The plateau pressure should be measured every 4 h or after each change in PEEP or Vt.
- The goal plateau pressure is <30 cm H_2O.
- Oxygenation goal during LTVV is a PaO_2 between 55 and 80 mmHg or a SpO_2 between 88 and 95 %. This is achieved by adjusting PEEP and FiO_2.
- To achieve these goals, *permissive hypercapnia might be necessary*.

The *open lung ventilation* approach uses LTVV combined with increased PEEP.

- LTVV is used in order to avoid overdistension.
- Elevated PEEP is used to avoid cyclic atelectasis. The high PEEP approach has been shown to improve oxygenation, decrease ICU mortality, and only in severe ARDS decrease hospital mortality [8, 9].

Weaning from the Ventilator and Extubation

Assess for safe discontinuation of the ventilator as soon as possible. Prolonged intubation can lead to increased complications (e.g., upper respiratory airway edema, infection) and costs. Balance risks of premature extubation, such as loss of airway, compromise of gas exchange, aspiration and respiratory muscle fatigue [10]. In order to prevent either early or late extubation, weaning trials have been established. Approximately 10–20 % of extubation attempts fail, despite successful weaning trials. Those patients have a higher mortality rate of 20–50 % [11].

TABLE 8.4. Recommendations to wean mechanical ventilation.

Recommendations to wean mechanical ventilation
Initiate weaning trial when:
1. Resolution/improvement of the condition for which intubation is required
2. Cardiovascular stability without the need of vasopressors
3. No continuous sedation
4. Adequate oxygenation (PaO_2/FiO_2 ≥150 mmHg with PEEP ≤5–8 cm H_2O, FiO_2 ≤0.4–0.5) and pH ≥7.25
Perform daily spontaneous breathing trial (SBT) for 30–120 min
Patient succeeds SBT if:
1. Adequate respiration pattern
2. Adequacy of gas exchange
3. Hemodynamic stability
4. Subjective comfort
Before extubation assess airway patency (cuff leak) and patient's capacity to protect the airway (cough reflex)

Criteria for performing a weaning trial (Table 8.4):

1. Resolution/improvement of the condition for which intubation is required.
2. Cardiovascular stability without the need of vasopressors.
3. No continuous sedation.
4. Adequate oxygenation (PaO_2/FiO_2 ≥150 mmHg with PEEP ≤5–8 cm H_2O, FiO_2 ≤0.4–0.5) and pH ≥7.25.

The weaning technique that has been shown to be the most successful is a daily spontaneous breathing trial (SBT) in which the patient is left to breathe through the T-tube for 30–120 min. During the SBT, minimal pressure support can be given to account for the resistance the T-tube generates.

Clinical signs and symptoms to monitor during SBT:

- Frequency and depth of breathing.
- Adequacy of gas exchange (arterial blood gas).
- Hemodynamic stability (blood pressure, heart rate and respiratory rate).
- The patient's subjective comfort level.

Once the patient has passed the SBT, the decision to discontinue the endotracheal tube should follow the assessment of airway patency (cuff leak) and the ability of the patient to protect the airway (cough reflex).

The cuff leak evaluates the volume escaping between the endotracheal tube and the trachea as a predictor of airway obstruction after extubation:

- With the endotracheal tube cuff inflated, the patient is placed in assist-control settings.
- Aspirate the tube and the upper airway (evaluating cough reflex).
- Measure the inspiratory and expiratory tidal volumes (read on the ventilator). These volumes are expected to be similar.
- Next, the tidal inspiratory and expiratory volumes are measured with the cuff deflated. If the difference of these volumes is above 110 cc it should be interpreted as a patent airway and the negative predictive value for stridor after extubation approaches 98 % [12].

Management of Sepsis and Fluid Resuscitation

Sepsis

Sepsis is a complex clinical condition in which an infection induces a systemic inflammatory response. The landmark signs of sepsis are:

- Systemic inflammation.
- Vasodilation.
- Leukocytosis.
- Increased vascular permeability.

Sepsis can lead to multiple organ dysfunction syndrome (MODS), which has a high mortality rate. Adequate and timely treatment of sepsis is key to success of patient's management. Early goal-directed therapy within 6 h of diagnosis decreases in-hospital mortality by more than 15 % [13].

The in-hospital mortality rate for sepsis is reported to be about 16 % [14]. Escherichia coli and MRSA infections are the most common sepsis-associated infections. Complication of device, implant or graft is the most common reason for sepsis-related hospitalization [14].

The progression to MODS from an infectious origin can be thought as a continuum from infection, bacteremia, sepsis, severe sepsis, septic shock to multiple organ dysfunction syndrome [15].

Systemic inflammatory response syndrome (SIRS) is characterized by dysregulated inflammation, which can be associated to noninfectious processes (e.g., pancreatitis, autoimmune disorders, vasculitis, burns). Sepsis and severe sepsis definitions and criteria can be found in Tables 8.5 and 8.6. Septic shock is defined as sepsis-induced hypotension refractory to adequate fluid resuscitation.

Management of Sepsis

- Have a high index of suspicion, as early recognition is crucial to optimize patient outcomes.
- Stabilize the airway.
  - Provide supplemental oxygen along with intubation for mechanical ventilation if necessary.
- Assess perfusion through vital signs (blood pressure, heart rate, core temperature), mental status, urine output, temperature, and lactate level.
- Correct physiologic abnormalities.
- If infection is suspected, collect blood cultures and start broad-spectrum antibiotics.
  - Draw blood cultures prior to starting antibiotics, but do not delay the start of antibiotics for more than 45 min [15]. Delay in antibiotics initiation is a strong predictor of mortality [16].
  - Draw blood cultures from at least two different sites and culture for both aerobic and anaerobic pathogens. Perform other cultures or send other body fluids when clinically relevant (i.e., line sample when vascular access in place).
- Continue broad-spectrum antibiotics until the source of infection is identified.

TABLE 8.5. Diagnostic criteria for sepsis.

Sepsis-presence (probable or documented) of infection together with systemic manifestations of infection

Systemic manifestations of infection

- Fever (>38.3 °C)
- Hypothermia (core temperature <36 °C)
- Heart rate >90 min or more than two SD above the normal value for age
- Tachypnea
- Altered mental status
- Significant edema or positive fluid balance (>20 mL/kg over 24 h)
- Hyperglycemia (plasma glucose >140 mg/dL or 7.7 mmol/L) in the absence of diabetes
- Leukocytosis (WBC count >12,000 μL)
- Leukopenia (WBC count <4,000 μL)
- Normal WBC count with greater than 10 % immature forms
- Plasma C-reactive protein more than two SD above the normal value
- Plasma procalcitonin more than two SD above the normal value

Hemodynamic variables

- Arterial hypotension (SBP <90 mmHg, MAP <70 mmHg, or an SBP decrease >40 mmHg in adults or less than two SD below normal for age)

Organ dysfunction variables

- Arterial hypoxemia ($PaO_2/FiO_2 < 300$)
- Acute oliguria (urine output <0.5 mL/kg/h for at least 2 h despite adequate fluid resuscitation)
- Creatinine increase >0.5 mg/dL or 44.2 μmol/L
- Coagulation abnormalities (INR >1.5 or aPTT >60 s)
- Ileus (absent bowel sounds)
- Thrombocytopenia (platelet count <100,000 μL-1)
- Hyperbilirubinemia (plasma total bilirubin >4 mg/dL or 70 μmol/L)

Tissue perfusion variables

- Hyperlactatemia (>1 mmol/L)
- Decreased capillary refill or mottling

Establishing central venous access allows for fluid resuscitation, medication administration, blood draws and blood transfusions, and hemodynamic monitoring by measuring the central venous pressure (CVP) and the superior vena cava oxygenation saturation ($ScvO_2$).

The Society of Critical Care Medicine and the European Society of Intensive Care Medicine has put forth a "Surviving

TABLE 8.6. Severe sepsis.

Sepsis-induced tissue hypoperfusion or organ dysfunction (any of the following thought to be due to the infection)
• Sepsis-induced hypotension
• Lactate above upper limits laboratory normal
• Urine output <0.5 mL/kg/h for more than 2 h despite adequate fluid resuscitation
• Acute lung injury with PaO_2/FiO_2 <250 in the absence of pneumonia as infection source
• Acute lung injury with PaO_2/FiO_2 <200 in the presence of pneumonia as infection source
• Creatinine >2.0 mg/dL (176.8 μmol/L)
• Bilirubin >2 mg/dL (34.2 μmol/L)
• Platelet count <100,000 μL
• Coagulopathy (international normalized ratio >1.5)

TABLE 8.7. Surviving sepsis campaign care bundle.

Sepsis care bundle
To be completed within 3 h:
1. Measure lactate level
2. Obtain blood cultures prior to administration of antibiotics
3. Administer broad spectrum antibiotics
4. Administer 30 mL/kg crystalloid for hypotension or lactate ≥4 mmol/L
To be completed within 6 h:
1. Apply vasopressors (for hypotension that does not respond to initial fluid resuscitation) to maintain a mean arterial pressure (MAP) ≥65 mmHg
2. In the event of persistent arterial hypotension despite adequate volume resuscitation (septic shock) or initial lactate ≥4 mmol/L (36 mg/dL):
(a) Measure central venous pressure (CVP)
(b) Measure central venous oxygen saturation ($ScvO_2$)
3. Remeasure lactate if initial lactate was elevated

Sepsis Campaign Bundle" protocol that sets time-sensitive guidelines for the management of sepsis (Table 8.7).

During the first 6 h of resuscitation, other guidelines for the treatment of sepsis-induced hyporperfusion include the following additional parameters [15]:

- Central venous pressure (CVP) 8–12 mmHg.
- Urine output ≥0.5 mL/kg/h.

- Superior vena cava oxygenation saturation ($ScvO_2$) or mixed venous oxygen saturation (SvO2) 70 or 65 %, respectively.

Intravenous Fluid Resuscitation

Relative intravascular hypovolemia is typical and may be severe. Unless there is evidence of heart failure, large volumes of fluids are indicated as initial therapy. Crystalloids are the fluid of choice during resuscitation. Albumin can be considered when patients require substantial amounts of crystalloids. Hydroxyethyl starches are not recommended due to potential harm. Generally, the central venous pressure goal is 8–12 mmHg, but if the patient is on a ventilator, aim for 12–15 mmHg. IV fluids should be administered in well-defined and rapidly infused boluses (e.g., 500 mL every 30 min). Early goal-directed therapy for severe sepsis and septic shock typically requires a mean volume of about 5 L in the first 6 h of resuscitation [13].

Before and after each bolus, assess the following:

- Volume status.
- Tissue perfusion.
- Blood pressure.
- Pulmonary edema.

Vasopressors and Inotropes

Vasopressors induce vasoconstriction, whereas inotropes increase cardiac contractility. The mean arterial pressure goal of 65 mmHg or higher can be achieved by fluid resuscitation as first line therapy. If the patient doesn't respond to fluid boluses or fluids are impairing gas exchange due to pulmonary edema, vasopressors should be used as a second line therapy.

The manner in which vasopressors and inotropes are used is largely based on expert opinion and the use of surrogate end points. A Cochrane Database Systematic review shows no superiority of any particular vasopressor; however, dopamine was shown to have an increased risk of arrhythmias [17].

- Repletion of intravascular volume is crucial for vasopressors to be effective. If maximal doses of a first agent are inadequate, then a second drug should be added.
- Vasopressors act on the following adrenergic receptors: Alpha-1, Beta-1, Beta-2 as well as the dopaminergic receptors:
  - Alpha-1 receptors are mainly located in the vascular walls and they cause vasoconstriction.
  - Beta-1 receptors are located in the heart and they induce a positive inotropic and chronotropic effect.
  - Beta-2 receptors are located in blood vessels and induce vasodilation.
  - Dopamine receptors are located in the renal, splanchnic, coronary and cerebral vasculature. Their activation leads to vasodilation, although a subtype of dopamine receptors cause vasoconstriction by induction of norepinephrine release.
- The main agents used are Norepinephrine (levophed), phenylephrine, dopamine and dobutamine (Table 8.8).
- Vasoactive drugs should be administered through a central venous access. A peripheral access can be used temporarily until central venous access is obtained.

The choice of the agent in septic shock can be made in the basis of whether the patient has hyperdynamic septic shock (low systemic vascular resistance and high cardiac output) or hypodynamic septic shock (low vascular resistance with low cardiac output).

- In hyperdynamic septic shock, a prominent alpha-1 vasoconstrictor effect can be achieved with norepinephrine or phenylephrine.
- In hypodynamic septic shock, both beta-1 and alpha-1 inotropic and vasoconstriction effect can be obtained with norepinephrine. Norepinephrine is the usual first drug of choice for septic shock.

Table 8.8. Vasoactive medications.

Drug	Receptor activity				Clinical effect	IV starting dose	Contraindications/caution
	alpha-1	beta-1	beta-2	Dopamine		mcg/min (titrate)	
Norepinephrine	Strong effect	Moderate effect	No effect	No effect	Increased SVR, stable/increased CO	8–12	Hypersensitivity, severe hypovolemia, DVT (except for lifesaving procedures), concomitan
Epinephrine	Strong effect	Strong effect	Moderate effect	No effect	Increased cardiac output, decreased SVR (low dose) or increased SVR (higher dose)	1	Hypersensitivity, CAD, glaucoma
Phenylephrine	Strong effect					100–180	Hypersensitivity, uncontrolled/ severe HTN, ventricular tachycardia, glaucoma
Dopamine dose (mcg/kg/min)							
0.5–2	No effect	Mild effect	No effect	Moderate effect	Increased CO	NA	Hypersensitivity, idiopathic hypertrophic subaortic stenosis
5–10		Moderate effect	No effect	Moderate effect	Mild increase of CO and SVR	NA	
10–20	Moderate effect	Moderate effect	No effect	Moderate effect	Moderate increase of SVR	NA	

- *Dobutamine should be avoided in septic shock* as it leads to vasodilation, worsening hypotension. It is used predominantly in cases of cardiogenic shock.

Central Venous Access Placement and Interpretation

Central venous access is a common procedure among hospitalized patients, especially in the intensive care unit. Central venous access is also needed in patients requiring recurrent venous access for plasmapheresis, hemodialysis, drug administration such as chemotherapy, and other indications (Table 8.9).

When placing central venous catheters, avoid:

- Areas of increased risk of infection,
- Anatomically distorted areas, or
- Sites potentially needed for chronic access (hemodialysis).

Device Selection

The two major types:

- Tunneled catheters (permanent).
- Non-tunneled catheters

Table 8.9. Indications for central venous access

• Administration of medications otherwise vesicant through peripheral venous access (vasopressors, chemotherapy, others)
• Hemodynamic monitoring
• Plasmapheresis, apheresis, hemodialysis
• Poor peripheral venous access
• Cardiac pacing
• Inferior vena cava filter placement
• Thrombolytic therapy
• Stenting

Catheter choice depends on the indication for CVA, and the risks and benefits must be carefully considered. Specific elements to consider are:

- The number of lumens the catheter allows.
- The bore of the lumen.
- Risk of infection. Tunneled central venous catheters have a lower rate of infection compared to non-tunneled catheters [18].
- Risk of thrombosis. Catheters with fewer lumens, and therefore smaller diameters, are preferred to reduce the risk of thrombosis [19].

Site Selection

- The site selection is based upon access needs and the operator's expertise.
- Commonly used veins are the jugular veins, subclavian vein, and femoral vein.
- The puncture site should not be contaminated or potentially become contaminated.
- Avoid sites with distorted anatomy.
- If a patient has unilateral lung disease, it is generally recommended to attempt central venous access on the side of the disease to avoid injury to the normal lung from complications such as pneumothorax.

Catheter Infection

A summary of the guidelines recommendations to prevent catheter-related infections is found in Table 8.10 [20].

In a patient with fever and a central venous catheter:

- Obtain blood cultures from peripheral blood and from the catheter.
- Growth of *Staphylococcus aureus*, coagulase negative Staphylococcus or Candida should raise the suspicion for a catheter related blood stream infection.

TABLE 8.10. CVC recommendations to prevent catheter-related infection.

CVC recommendations to prevent catheter-related infection
• Educate, train and periodically assess knowledge and adherence to guidelines of all personnel involved in insertion and care of catheters
• *Selection of catheters and sites*
– Weigh risks and benefits of placing a CVC at a recommended site to reduce infectious complications against mechanical complications (pneumothorax, subclavian vein laceration)
– Avoid femoral vein
– Use subclavian site rather than jugular or femoral site to minimize infection risk for nontunneled catheters
– Avoid subclavian site for hemodialysis patients
– Use ultrasound guidance
– Use minimum number of ports or lumens
– Promptly remove non essential catheters
– If aseptic technique not ensured, replace catheter as soon as possible (within 48 h)
• *Aseptic technique*
– Hand hygiene and aseptic technique
– Use maximal sterile barrier precautions
– Prepare and clean skin with antiseptic
– Use sterile gauze or sterile, transparent, semipermeable dressing to cover the catheter site
– Replace gauze every 2 days or transparent dressing every 7 days for short term CVC sites
• *Replacement of CVCs, PICCs and hemodialysis catheters*
– Do not routinely replace CVC, PICC, hemodialysis catheters, or pulmonary artery catheters to prevent catheter-related infections
– Do not replace CVC or PICC on the basis of fever alone
– Do not use guidewire exchanges routinely for non-tunneled catheters to prevent infection
– Do not use guidewire exchanges to replace a non-tunneled catheter suspected of infection
– Use a guidewire exchange to replace a malfunctioning non-tunneled catheter if no evidence of infection is present

- Empiric treatment should include Vancomycin to cover S. aureus and additional gram-negative coverage (i.e., Zosyn) in critically ill patients and suspected sepsis.

If the catheter is the origin of infection, it should be removed in the following situations:

- Severe sepsis.
- Suppurative thrombophlebitis.
- Endocarditis.

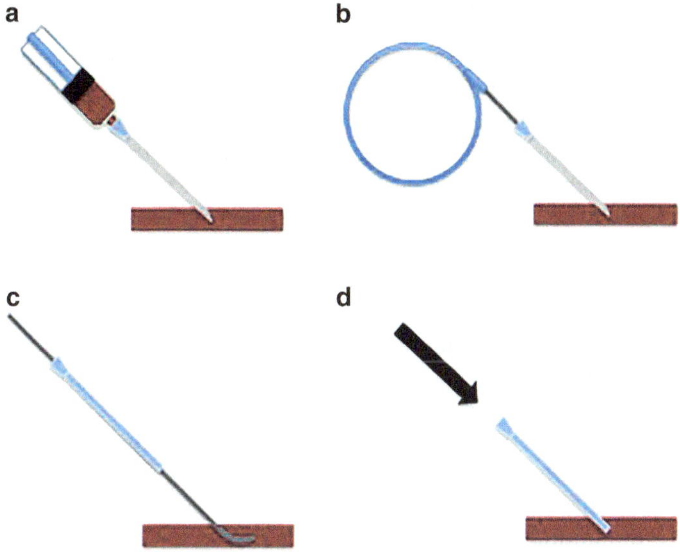

FIG. 8.3. Seldinger technique. Using the modified Seldinger technique to place the catheter. (**a**) Under ultrasound guidance, access the targeted blood vessel with a syringe. (**b**) Remove the syringe and thread the wire through the needle. (**c**) Remove the needle and pass the catheter. (**d**) Remove the wire and secure the catheter.

- Metastatic complications such as pulmonary embolism, peripheral embolism in the setting of arterial catheters.
- A blood stream infection that persists 72 h after appropriate antibiotic therapy.
- Infection due to *S. aureus*, fungi, or mycobacteria.
- Tunnel or pocket infections [21].

Central Venous Access Device Placement

In preparation for placement, gather all the necessary equipment, select the most appropriate puncture site, position the patient flat or in slight Trendelenberg, and prepare the field in an aseptic manner. Once everything is prepared and a surgical time-out has been performed, place the catheter using the modified Seldinger technique, as demonstrated in Fig. 8.3. Analgesia and sedation can be used for patient's comfort.

Pulmonary Artery Catheter Insertion

- Is introduced through the sheath with the curve oriented in such a way that it facilitates the passage through the cardiac chambers.
- When advancing the catheter the balloon at the tip should be completely inflated (1.5 mL) to avoid vessel, endocardium or cardiac valves injuries (The balloon should be deflated when withdrawn).
- Continuous hemodynamic monitoring should be performed during the procedure. Monitor the waveforms by location of the pulmonary artery catheter tip.
- The final position of the catheter in the pulmonary artery is such that the pulmonary capillary wedge pressure (PCWP) is obtained whenever 75–100 % of the balloon is insufflated.
- Confirm correct position (no more than 3–5 cm away from the midline) with chest X-ray.
- Secure the catheter to the skin and record the length of catheter in the patient's chart.

Interpretation of Pulmonary Artery Catheter (Swan–Ganz Catheter) Waveforms

Swan–Ganz catheter allows the measurement of pressures and sampling of blood from the right cardiac chambers and the pulmonary artery [22]. The left atrial pressure can be approximated by measuring the pulmonary capillary wedge pressure (PCWP). These functions allow the diagnosis and management of various clinical conditions, as described in Table 8.11.

Pressure Waveforms and Interpretation

The catheter must be recalibrated prior to use by opening the system to the air to establish atmospheric pressure as zero and level the air-fluid reference of the catheter with the heart.

TABLE 8.11. Clinical use of Swan–Ganz catheter.

Diagnosis
- Etiology of shock
- Hypovolemic
- Cardiogenic
- Sepsis
- Pulmonary embolism

Pulmonary edema (cardiogenic versus non-cardiogenic)
Pulmonary hypertension
Pericardial tamponade
Therapy
- Pharmacologic therapy
- Fluid management
- Sepsis
- Myocardial infarction
- Heart failure

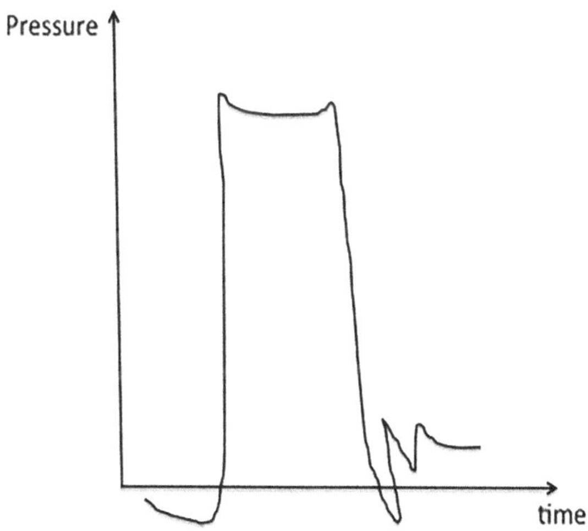

FIG. 8.4. Adequate pulmonary artery catheter dynamic response. Quickly open and close the valve in the continuous flush device. A square wave should appear, followed by ringing and return to baseline.

Following calibration, the dynamic response must be assessed. Quickly open and close the valve in the continuous flush device. A square wave should appear, followed by ringing and return to baseline (Fig. 8.4).

Right Atrium Pressure Waveform

As seen in Fig. 8.5, the "*a*" component of the wave reflects the atrial systole, the "*c*" component reflects the closure of the tricuspid valve, the "*v*" reflects the ventricular systole and the "*y*" reflects the decreasing in pressure after opening of the tricuspid valve.

Conditions that can elevate the normal right atrial pressure (0–7 mmHg):

- Right ventricular infarction.
- Pulmonary hypertension.
- Cardiac tamponade.
- Constrictive pericarditis.
- Volume overload.
- Atrial fibrillation and flutter.
- Others.

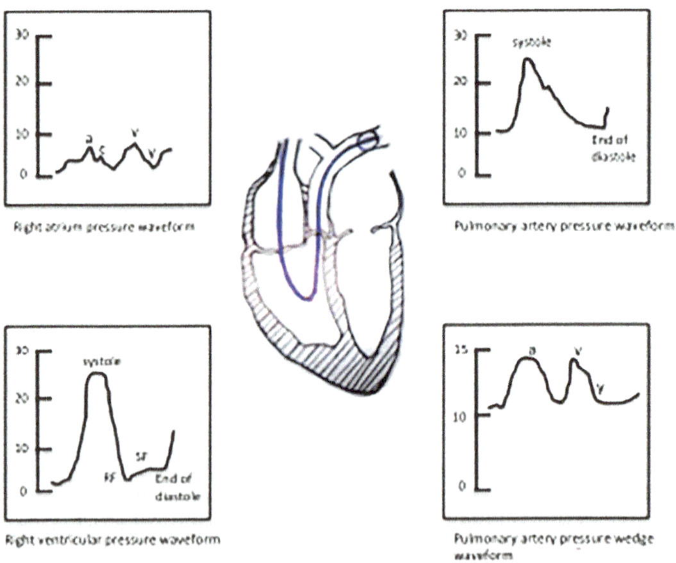

FIG. 8.5 Cardiac pressure waveforms as read by pulmonary artery catheter. The "*a*" component of the wave reflects the atrial systole, the "*c*" component reflects the closure of the tricuspid valve, the "*v*" reflects the ventricular systole and the "*y*" reflects the decreasing in pressure after

Right Ventricular (RV) Pressure Waveform

Figure 8.5 shows the shape and components of the waveform. Ventricular systole is represented by rapid peak followed by a slow elevation on the pressure that represents the ventricular diastole.

- The normal right ventricular systolic pressure ranges from 15 to 25 mmHg.
- The normal end-diastolic pressure ranges from 3 to 12 mmHg.
- Elevated RV systolic pressure can be seen with pulmonary embolism, pulmonary hypertension, pulmonic stenosis.
- RV end-diastolic pressure is seen with ventricular infarction, cardiac constriction and tamponade, RV failure.

Pulmonary Artery Waveform (Measured During Insertion of the Catheter)

The waveform has an upstroke, representing the systole, and a downstroke with a dicrotic notch representing the diastole and the closure of the pulmonic valve (Fig. 8.5).

- Normal systolic pulmonary pressure ranges from 15 to 25 mmHg.
- Normal diastolic pulmonary pressure ranges from 8 to 15 mmHg.

Elevations in PA pressure are seen in:

- Left heart failure.
- Pulmonary embolism.
- Primary lung disease.
- Mitral valve disease.
- Others.

Pulmonary Artery Wedge Pressure (PAWP) Waveform

The waveform is similar to the right atrium waveform. The PAWP estimates the left ventricular end-diastolic pressure (LVEDP) and therefore is affected by respiration. The PAWP should be measured at the end of inspiration.

- Normal values vary from 6 to 15 mmHg.
- Elevation of the "*a*" wave can be seen with increased resistance to left ventricular filling in conditions such as:
- Left ventricular volume overload.
- Mitral stenosis.
- Left ventricular systolic dysfunction or diastolic dysfunction.
- Elevation of the "*v*" wave may represent mitral regurgitation or an acute left atrium volume overload.

Some situations might have discordant PAWP and left ventricular end-diastolic pressure. The PAWP might be higher than the LVEDP in conditions affecting the anatomic structures before the mitral valve (e.g., mitral valve stenosis or regurgitation, pulmonary embolus and others). In the other hand, the PAWP might be lower than the LVEDP in conditions affecting anatomic structures after the mitral valve (decreased left ventricule compliance, aortic valve regurgitation).

Acid–Base Disorders

The acid–base balance is maintained by the kidneys and the lungs. Each one of these organs controls different buffer systems. The kidneys excrete acids mainly by combining hydrogen to two different buffer systems that involve phosphate and ammonia. The lungs manage the acid–base balance through elimination of carbon dioxide.

When assessing the acid–base balance in a patient, the bicarbonate–carbon dioxide buffer system is used:

$$CO_2 + H_2O \leftrightarrow HCO_3^- + H^+$$

The pH is calculated using the Henderson-Hasselbach equation:

$$pH = 6.10 + \log\left(\left[HCO_3^-\right] + \left[0.03 \times pCO_2\right]\right)$$

Table 8.12. Arterial sample values.

Normal arterial sample values
pH = 7.4 ± 0.04
HCO_3 24 ± 3 mEq/L
PCO_2 40 ± 4 mmHg

Table 8.13. Definitions of acid–base disorders.

Acid–base disorders definitions
Acidemia: arterial pH below the normal range (7.36)
Alkalemia: arterial pH above the normal range (7.44)
Acidosis: process that tends to lower the pH
Alkalosis: process that tends to increase the pH
Metabolic acidosis: acidosis by reduction of HCO_3
Metabolic alkalosis: alkalosis by elevation of HCO_3
Respiratory acidosis: acidosis by elevation of PCO_2
Respiratory alkalosis: alkalosis by reduction of PCO_2
Simple acid–base disorder:Presence of one metabolic or respiratory disorder with its appropriate respiratory or metabolic compensation process
Mixed acid–base disorder: Simultaneous presence of more than one acid–base disorder

Under simple acid–base disorders, either the lungs or the kidneys respond by compensating the imbalance. The respiratory response is rapid and commences within 30 min of an aberration in pH balance. Complete respiratory compensation is usually achieved within 12–24 h. The renal system response is somewhat delayed relative to the respiratory response and commences in 6–12 h. Complete renal compensation is usually achieved in 3–5 days.

The acid–base disorders not only affect the pH and buffer systems but also electrolytes like sodium and potassium, therefore, these are part of the variables to be assessed. Normal values for pH, bicarbonate and partial pressure of CO_2 vary depending on the sample origin (Table 8.12). Peripheral venous blood samples have a pH range 0.02–0.04 lower than the arterial sample, the HCO_3 1–2 mEq/L higher and the PCO_2 3–8 mmHg higher than the arterial sample. Definitions of acid–base disorders are listed in Table 8.13.

Metabolic Acidosis

- During metabolic acidosis, serum HCO_3 decreases and respiratory compensation (increased minute ventilation) will cause PCO_2 to decrease.
- For each 1 mEq/L reduction in serum HCO_3, the PCO_2 decreases by 1.2 mmHg.
- An inability to compensate metabolic acidosis can be seen in respiratory or neurologic disease.
- Respiratory compensation in severe metabolic acidosis (HCO_3<6 mEq/L) is typically limited to a PCO_2 of 8–12 mmHg.
- Pharmacologic intervention might be necessary to correct acidosis at PCO_2 values higher than 8–12 mmHg.
- Calculate the anion gap to determine the cause of metabolic acidosis.
- Anion gap = $([Na^+]+[K^+])-([Cl^-]+[HCO_3^-])$.
- Normal range is 3–11 mEq/L.
- A high anion gap indicates an excess of anions such as lactate, ketoacids, PO_4^{3-}, and SO_4^{2-}.
- The patient should be evaluated for conditions that lead to an excess of these anions (Table 8.14).

TABLE 8.14. Conditions causing elevated and normal anion gap.

High anion gap
Lactic acidosis
Ketoacidosis
Renal failure (decreased acid excretion and HCO_3 reabsorption)
Methanol
Uremia
Aspirin
Other toxins
Normal anion gap (or hyperchloremic acidosis/loss of HCO_3 is compensated by Cl reabsorption)
Diarrhea
Renal tubular acidosis
Ammonium chloride, acetazolamide ingestion
Total parenteral nutrition
Addison's disease
Ureterenterostomy

Metabolic Alkalosis

During metabolic acidosis HCO_3 increases and usual respiratory compensation will cause PCO_2 to go in the same direction. For each 1 mEq/L increase in serum HCO_3, the PCO_2 raises by 0.7 mmHg.

Main Causes of Metabolic Alkalosis

- Gastric loss of H^+ and loss of chloride that stimulates reabsorption of HCO_3 by the kidneys (e.g., vomiting, nasogastric suctioning).
- Renal loss of H^+: Thiazide and loop diuretics like furosemide cause sodium and chloride loss by the kidneys with compensatory HCO_3 reabsorption to maintain electrical neutrality.
- Volume depletion generates sodium and HCO_3 reabsorption by the kidneys as well as activation of the renin–aldosterone system promoting H^+ secretion by the distal tubules.
- Hypokalemia stimulates H^+ transmembrane shift into the cells and H^+ secretion by the distal tubules.
- Chronic CO_2 retention.
- Administration of organic anions as lactate, acetate and citrate.

Metabolic alkalosis can cause neurologic manifestations, compensatory hypoventilation (to increase PCO_2), and decreased systemic oxygenation.

Respiratory Acidosis

The acute response to respiratory acid–base disorders is initiated within minutes by the blood, extracellular fluid and cell buffering but this response is modest. A more significant response is generated by the kidneys that starts within a few hours but takes 3–5 days to be completed.

In acute respiratory acidosis, the compensatory response increases the HCO_3 by 1 mEq/L for each 10 mmHg increase of serum PCO_2.

Respiratory Alkalosis

The compensatory response to acute respiratory alkalosis causes the serum HCO_3 to fall 2 mEq/L for every 10 mmHg decline in the PCO_2.

Mixed Acid–Base Disorders

Mixed acid–base disorders are characterized by more than one primary disorder. The expected compensatory effect is typically insufficient and intervention is required.

Management of Acid–Base Disorders

Management of acid–base disorders is cause-specific. However, severe life threatening situations grant specific interventions to correct the pH and electrolyte imbalance.

Metabolic Acidosis

Severe acidosis has major adverse physiologic consequences listed in Table 8.15. In certain organic acidosis treatment of the

TABLE 8.15. Adverse effects of severe acidosis

Cardiovascular
Impairment of cardiac contractility and reduction of cardiac output
Arteriolar dilation and venoconstriction
Increased pulmonary vascular resistance
Decreased renal and hepatic blood flow
Decreased threshold to arrhythmias
Attenuation to catecholamines responsiveness
Respiratory
Hyperventilation
Respiratory muscle fatigue
Dyspnea
Metabolic
Insulin resistance
Inhibition of anaerobic glycolysis
Hyperkalemia
Increased protein catabolism
Cerebral
Decreased mental status and coma

underlying cause can revert the metabolic disorder within hours. By contrast, in hyperchloremic acidosis where HCO_3 is lost (e.g diarrhea, kidneys), exogenous alkali might be required.

The goal of treatment is to correct and prevent adverse effects listed in Table 8.15.

- Respiratory compensation has its limits and therapy should be implemented to maintain a pH above 7.2 and a HCO_3 above 8–10 mmol/L.
- The mainstay of alkali therapy is sodium bicarbonate. Administration of sodium bicarbonate entails certain risks and should be given judiciously.
- The load of sodium bicarbonate can be calculated as:
  - ΔHCO_3 desired in mmol × weight in kg × space of distribution.
    - To avoid risks of overtreatment a 50 % space of distribution is proposed to start.

For example, in a patient you want to bring HCO_3 from 4 to 8 mmol/L and weights 70 kg, the HCO_3 to be administrated is:

$$4 \times 70 \times 0.5 = 140\,\text{mmol}$$

The sodium bicarbonate should be administrated in an infusion rather than a bolus. About 30 min should be allowed after infusion to judge clinical effect and further treatment.

Metabolic Alkalosis

The goal of treatment is to reverse the underlying cause of HCO_3 production and/or HCO_3 retention:

- Patients with gastric loss of H^+ can be treated with antacids like H_2 blockers and proton pump inhibitors.
- Discontinue exogenous administration of alkali as lactate and citrate.
- Enhance renal bicarbonate excretion (correct hypovolemia, hypochloremia, hypokalemia).

References

1. Wolters Kluwer Health UpToDate® Modes of Mechanical Ventilation; http://www.uptodate.com/contents/image?imageKey=PULM/77391&topicKey=PULM%2F1640&source=outline_link&search=mechanical+ventilation&utdPopup=true.
2. Esteban A, et al. How is mechanical ventilation employed in the intensive care unit? An international utilization review. Am J Respir Crit Care Med. 2000;161:1450.
3. Kilickaya O, et al. Initial ventilator settings for critically ill patients. Crit Care. 2013;17(2):123.
4. James MM, Beilman GJ. Mechanical ventilation. Surg Clin N Am. 2012;92:1463–74.
5. Ranieri VM, Rubenfeld GD, Thompson BT, Ferguson ND, Caldwell E, Fan E, Camporota L, Slutsky AS. Acute respiratory distress syndrome: the Berlin definition. JAMA 2012; 307(23):2526–33.
6. Ranieri VM, Rubenfeld GD, Thompson BT, Ferguson ND, Caldwell E, Fan E, Camporota L, Slutsky AS. Petrucci N, De Feo C. Lung protective ventilation strategy for the acute respiratory distress syndrome. Cochrane Database Syst Rev. 2013 (2).
7. The Acute Repiratory Distress Syndrome Network. Ventilation with lower tidal volumes as compared with traditional tidal volumes for acute lung injury and the acute respiratory distress syndrome. N Engl J Med. 2000;342:1301.
8. Briel M, et al. Higher versus lower positive end-expiratory pressures in patients with acute lung injury and acute respiratory distress syndrome: systematic review and meta-analysis. JAMA. 2010;303:865.
9. Santa Cruz R, et al. High versus low positive end-expiratory pressure (PEEP) levels for mechanically ventilated adult patients with acute lung injury and acute respiratory distress syndrome. Cochrane Database Syst Rev. 2013 (6):CD009098.
10. MacIntyre NR. Evidence-based assessments in the ventilator discontinuation process. Respir Care. 2012;57(10):1611–8.
11. Thille AW, et al. Weaning from the ventilator and extubation in ICU. Curr Opin Crit Care. 2013;19:57–64.
12. Miller RL, Cole RP. Association between reduced cuff leak volume and postextubation stridor. Chest. 1996;110(4):1035–40.
13. Rivers E, et al. Early goal-directed therapy in the treatment of severe sepsis and septic shock. N Engl J Med. 2001;345:1368.

14. Elixhauser A, et al. Septicemia in U.S. Hospitals, 2009. Agency for healthcare research and quality, Rockville, MD http://www.hcup-us.ahrq.gov/reports/statbriefs/sb122.pdf.
15. Dellinger RP, et al. Surviving sepsis campaign:international guidelines for management of severe sepsis and septic shock:2012. Crit Care Med. 2013;41:580.
16. Kumar A, et al. Duration of hypotension before initiation of effective antimicrobial therapy is the critical determinant of survival in human septic shock. Crit Care Med. 2006;34:1589.
17. Havel C, Arrich J, Losert H, Gamper G, Müllner M, Herkner H. Vasopressors for hypotensive shock. Cochrane Database Syst Rev. 2011 (5). Art. No.: CD003709.
18. Dryden MS, et al. Infective complications associated with the use of the Quiton Permcath for long-term central vascular access in hemodialysis. J Hosp Infect. 1991;19:257.
19. American Society of Anesthesiology Task Force on Central Venous Access, Rupp SM, Apfelbaum JL, et al. Practice guidelines for central venous access: a report by the American Society of Anesthesiologists Task Force on Central Venous Access. Anesthesiology. 2012;116:539.
20. O'Grady NP, et al. Guidelines for the prevention of intravascular catheter-related infections. Clin Infect Dis. 2011;52(9):162–93.
21. Mermel LA, Allon M, Bouza E, et al. Clinical practice guidelines for the diagnosis and management of intravascular catheter-related infection: 2009 update by the Infectious Diseases Society of America. Clin Infect Dis. 2009;49(1):1 45.
22. Putterman C. The Swan-Ganz catheter: a decade of hemodynamic monitoring. J Crit Care. 1989;2:127–46.

Section 5
Palliative Care

Chapter 9
Palliative Care

Solomon Liao, Rosene D. Pirrello, Rebecca Liddicoat Yamarik, and Jamie Capasso

Introduction

- The World Health Organization defines palliative care as "an approach that improves the quality of life of patients and their families facing the problems associated with life-threatening illness, through the prevention and relief of suffering by means of early identification and impeccable assessment and treatment of pain and other problems [1]."
- The first half of this chapter addresses pain management including opioids and other analgesics. The rest of the chapter discusses the screening and treatment of depression,

S. Liao, M.D., F.A.A.H.P.M. (✉) • J. Capasso, D.O.
Department of Internal Medicine, Irvine Medical Center, University of California, 101 The City Drive, Bldg 26, ZC 4076H, Orange, CA 92868, USA
e-mail: ssliao@uci.edu; jcapasso@uci.edu

R.D. Pirrello, Pharm.D.
Department of Pharmacy Services, UC Irvine Health Department of Pharmacy Services, Irvine Medical Center, University of California, 101 The City Drive, Orange, CA 92868, USA
e-mail: rosene.pirrello@uci.edu

R.L. Yamarik, M.D.
Providence Trinity Care Hospice, 5315 Torrance Blvd, Torrance, CA 90503, USA
e-mail: beckyliddicoat@yahoo.com

R.N. Eskander and R.E. Bristow (eds.), *Gynecologic Oncology: A Pocketbook*, DOI 10.1007/978-1-4939-1976-5_9,

management of constipation, nausea and vomiting, bowel obstruction, ascites, and dyspnea.
- To achieve good pain and symptom management, palliative care must be patient and family centered. To achieve this centered care, the health care team must understand the patient's goals of care. A goal of care discussion involves exploring the personal values and treatment preferences of a patient in light of the diagnosis of a serious condition. The patient's goals of care frame their pain and symptom management and dictates the priority and aggressiveness of their care.
- Related to the patient's goals of care is their expectation. Complete symptom control is at times not possible or practical. Setting realistic expectations for the patient, family, and even health care professionals is important both at the outset and as their disease progresses. When pain and symptoms cannot be eliminated, the emphasis shifts to living with the symptom and managing the problems to optimize the patient's function or quality of life. The patient's survival prognosis may change their goals and expectations and therefore their pain and symptom management.

Pain Management

Commonly Used Opioids

- Table 9.1 [2] summarizes the opioid medications that are commonly used in the United States.
- Morphine remains the gold-standard opioid.
  - The benefits of morphine are:
    - It is relatively inexpensive and covered by most health plans.
    - It is available in a liquid formulation.
    - It is widely available.
    - It is well known.
  - Its familiarity translates to less medication errors compared with other opioids.

TABLE 9.1. Commonly used opioid analgesics [2].

Opioid	Dosage form	Strength	Starting doses of short-acting opioids for opioid naïve patients
Morphine	Oral solution	2, 4, 20 mg/mL	5–10 mg PO q 60 min as needed
	Tablets ER (q12 h)	15, 30, 60, 100, 200 mg	2–3 mg IV q 30 min as needed
	Tablets ER (q 24 h)	Kadian: 10, 20, 30, 50, 60, 80, 100, 150, 200 mg	
	Tablets IR	Avinza: 30, 45, 60, 75, 90, 120 mg	
	Injectable SC, IV, infusion	10, 15, 30 mg	
		Check hospital-specific concentrations	
Methadone	Oral solution	1, 2, 10 mg/mL	NA
	Tablets	5, 10 mg; 40 mg (dissolvable)	
	Injectable IV, infusion	Check hospital-specific concentrations	
Fentanyl	Transmucosal (Buccal)	Actiq:200, 400, 600, 800, 1,200, 1,600 mg	25–50 mcg IV q 30 min as needed
	Transdermal	Patches: 12 (delivers 12.5), 25, 50, 75, 100 mcg/h	
	Injectable SC, IV, infusion	Check hospital-specific concentrations	
Hydromorphone	Oral solution	1 mg/mL	2 mg PO q 60 min as needed
	Tablets ER (q 24 h)	8, 12, 24, 32 mg	0.5 mg IV q 30 min as needed
	Tablets IR	2, 4, 8 mg	
	Injectable SC, IV, infusion	Check hospital-specific concentrations	
Oxycodone	Oral solution	1, 20 mg/mL	5 mg PO q 60 min as needed
	Tablets ER (q 12 h)	10, 15, 20, 30, 40, 60, 80 mg	
	Tablets IR	5, 10, 15 mg	
Oxymorphone	Tablets ER (q 12 h)	7.5, 10, 15, 20, 30, 40 mg	5 mg PO q 60 min as needed
	Tablets IR	5, 10 mg	

The oral solutions of morphine, oxycodone and hydromorphone are useful for enteral tube administration and because they are short-acting, are usually dosed every 4 h around the clock and/or as needed

Methadone, because of its long duration of action, is an ideal "long-acting" opioid for enteral tube administration and is usually administered every 8–12 h

From Pantilet, *Hospital-Based Palliative Medicine: A Practical, Evidence-Based Approach*.

- The liquid formulation is good for people who cannot swallow pills, have a feeding tube, or have poor bowel absorption, e.g., short bowel.
- Morphine is metabolized by glucuronidation in the liver to morphine-6-glucuronide and morphine-3-glucuronide. Both metabolites are renally excreted and are known neurotoxins. Accumulation of the metabolites leads to opioid-induced neurotoxicity which manifests as myoclonus, delirium and then seizure. *Morphine should therefore be avoided in patients with moderate to severe renal impairment* but can be used cautiously and for short term in patients with mild renal impairment.

- Hydromorphone (Dilaudid) is more potent (mg to mg) than morphine but has no difference in efficacy.
  - It is available in long-acting and short acting formulations. However, the long acting formulation is extremely expensive, not covered by most insurance and is cost-prohibitive in most cases.
  - Though not as neurotoxic as morphine metabolites, hydromorphone has toxic metabolites as well and is relatively contraindicated in patients with renal failure.
  - Hydromorphone has several drawbacks in the outpatient setting:
    - It is expensive and has a high street value and therefore diversion potential.
    - It requires the use of a different long-acting opioid for maintenance pain relief.

- Oxycodone is available in long-acting (Oxycontin) and short acting formulations.
  - It is only available in oral formulations (pills and liquid) and not available parenterally.
  - The disadvantage of long-acting oxycodone is its expense as it is not yet available in a generic formulation, and therefore it is sometimes not covered by insurances. Additional drawbacks include its high potential for abuse and a high street value.
  - Like hydromorphone, its metabolites are less neurotoxic than morphine's.

TABLE 9.2. Advantages and disadvantages of transdermal fentanyl compared to oral or IV/SC opioids [2].

Transdermal fentanyl versus oral opioid	
Advantages of transdermal fentanyl	Disadvantages of transdermal fentanyl
Convenience	High cost
Continuous administration	Slower onset of action
Longer duration of action	More difficult to reverse side effects
Greater patient adherence	Slow titration
Avoids PO in patients with nausea/vomiting	Possible adhesive sensitivity
Transdermal fentanyl versus continuous IV/SC opioid infusion	
Advantages of transdermal fentanyl	Disadvantages of transdermal fentanyl
Less expensive	Slower onset of action
Easier for caregiver	More difficult to reverse side effects
Less invasive (no needles, no pumps)	Separate intermittent medication required for breakthrough pain

- Fentanyl comes in many formulations including intravenous, transdermal (TD), intranasal, sublingual and buccal.
  - It is estimated to be eighty times (80×) more potent than morphine as an analgesic.
  - Its lipid solubility, high potency and low molecular weight make it ideal for administration systemically through a relatively small area of the skin or mucosa.
  - *One of the biggest advantages of fentanyl is that its metabolites appear to be inactive*, conferring neither analgesia nor toxicity. Therefore, fentanyl does not have any neurotoxicity in the setting of renal impairment as seen in the other opioids discussed above.
  - Table 9.2 [2] summarizes the advantages and disadvantages of TD fentanyl compared to oral or injectable opioids.
  - A major disadvantage of fentanyl is its expense.
  - The FDA Black Box warns that *the transdermal patch is not intended for opioid naïve patients.*
  - Absorption into serum begins approximately 4–8 h after application; however, therapeutic blood levels are

not achieved for 12–16 h with mean time to maximum concentration between 29 and 36 h.

  - At steady state TD fentanyl produces drug levels similar to those produced by intravenous or subcutaneous infusion with the same infusion rate.
  - Levels vary between patients based on individual differences in skin absorption characteristics and fentanyl clearance rates.
  - Patients with elevated body temperature (especially >102 °F) may experience higher than expected drug absorption and must be carefully monitored.
  - Switching to an alternate oral or parenteral opioid may be required. A common myth is that fentanyl patches causing less constipation than other opioids.

- Methadone has several advantages but should be used in consultation with a palliative care or pain specialist.
  - An important advantage is that it is very inexpensive, $20 to $30 a month. Most patients can afford methadone even if it is not covered by their insurance.
  - Methadone has no known active metabolites and only needs to be dose adjusted when renal function drops below 10 %.
  - It is *the only long acting opioid that comes in a liquid formulation* and can therefore be given through feeding tubes or to patients with dysphagia who cannot swallow pills.
  - In addition to its opioid activity, methadone antagonizes the NMDA receptors, giving it a second analgesic effect.
  - Because of its very low potential for abuse and hence, low street value, Methadone is the safest option in patients with a history of drug abuse or at risk for opioid diversion.
  - Methadone metabolism differs from other opioids in that it *does not* follow first order pharmacokinetics.
    - Methadone has biphasic pharmacokinetics and therefore can be used both as a long-acting analgesic and a short-acting analgesic.

- ○ Because methadone is long acting, it is usually prescribed every 8 h in younger patients and every 12 h in older patients, when used as a maintenance analgesic.
- ○ As an as-needed, short acting analgesic, it is dosed at a minimum interval of every 3 h.
- ○ Although methadone quickly binds to the mu-opioid receptors, methadone takes 3–5 days to antagonize the NMDA-receptors and become maximally effective.
  - ■ Because of this, methadone must be titrated slowly. Increasing methadone doses more frequently than every 3–5 days is strongly discouraged given the possibility for overdose when the methadone reaches steady state.

– Opioid equivalency has only been established between oral morphine and methadone and uses a sliding scale that depends on the total amount of oral morphine equivalents required in 24 h (Table 9.3) [2].

- ○ This sliding scale is needed to account for its NMDA receptor blocking analgesic effect. The conversion ratio of oral to IV methadone is 2:1. Therefore the IV methadone dose is half of the oral dose.

– A negative side effect more common with methadone than with other opioids is the *risk for QTc-prolongation*. This risk is heightened with the addition of other QTc-prolonging medications. Although the documented cases of methadone induced QTc-prolongation have occurred only in patients taking more than 150 mg a day, EKG monitoring of patients on lower doses of methadone is prudent if they are taking other QTc-prolonging medications or if they will be taking methadone for more than 6 months. QTc-prolongation with methadone is more likely in the presence of hypokalemia and hypomagnesemia.

TABLE 9.3. Morphine to methadone conversion [2].

24 h oral morphine dose	Oral morphine:oral methadone
<100 mg	3:1
101–300 mg	5:1
301–600 mg	10:1
601–800 mg	12:1
801–1,000 mg	15:1
>1,001 mg	20:1

Please note that unlike the opioid equianalgesic equivalency chart above, given the variable metabolism of methadone, this chart can only be used left to right. Methadone should not be converted back to oral morphine equivalents using this chart. In the event the patient must stop Methadone, re-titration with an immediate-release opioid is recommended

From Pantilet, *Hospital-Based Palliative Medicine: A Practical, Evidence-Based Approach*. Copyright © 2015 by John Wiley & Sons, Inc. Reprinted by permission of John Wiley & Sons, Inc

Opioid Adverse Effects

- Since every medication has side effects, the goal of opioid therapy is to titrate to analgesia while minimizing these adverse effects as much as possible.
- These side effects can be addressed with the following approaches:
  - Use the smallest dose of opioid necessary.
  - Use of co-analgesics.
  - Treatment of the side effect, e.g., constipation.
- Table 9.4 [2] lists the most common and clinically relevant opioid side effects.
  - They can range from bothersome but benign to serious and fatal.
  - The most feared adverse effects, respiratory depression and death, are rare with good management.
    - Respiratory depression is more likely to occur in patients with impaired ventilation such as chronic lung disease, sleep apnea, or obesity.

TABLE 9.4. Management of opioid side effects [2].

Adverse effect	Management
Gastrointestinal • Constipation • Nausea/vomiting • Delayed gastric emptying • Ileus	• Prophylactic bowel regimen • PRN suppository or enema • Antiemetics, promotility agents • Opioid antagonists (methylnaltrexone) • Opioid minimizing with or without adjuvant medications
Central nervous system • Somnolence • Cognitive Impairment • Delirium • Hyperalgesia	• Psychostimulants, opioid reduction or rotation • Careful medication review and evaluation of medical scenario (for infection, neurologic or cardiac event) • Antipsychotic medication (Haldol frequently used) • Opioid reduction or rotation
Respiratory depression	• Frequent assessment and reevaluation of patient • Prescreen patients for predisposing comorbidities and medications • Supplemental oxygen or noninvasive positive pressure ventilation as appropriate • Pulse oximetry • Cautious use of dilute (1:10) naloxone if hypoxemia or respiratory rate less than or equal to 6
Cutaneous • Pruritus • Perspiration	• Trial of antihistamine, opioid rotation • Icepacks

From Pantilet, *Hospital-Based Palliative Medicine: A Practical, Evidence-Based Approach*.

- Patients with concomitantly administered sedating medications such as benzodiazepines are also at higher risk for respiratory depression.
- Pulse oximetry monitoring and supplemental oxygen are not helpful as hypoxemia typically occurs after apnea.

Opioid Conversion

- An opioid can be safely and effectively converted to another opioid using the concept of equal analgesia, i.e., opioids are equally effective but have different potencies.

- Table 9.5 [2, 3] presents an easy-to-use set of conversions.
  - While the conversion tables may give the median or the mean of that normal distribution, the user of the tables should keep in mind that a particular patient may be a fast metabolizer of one opioid and a slow metabolizer of another.
  - Since the prescriber cannot tell which patients are fast or slow metabolizers, a clinically more useful approach is direction of the patient's pain control.
    - For example, if the patient's pain is uncontrolled or anticipated to get worse, a more aggressive conversion should be used to achieve a higher dose.
    - If the patient's pain is expected to get better, then a conversion should be used to achieve a dose on the lower end of the range.
    - Similarly if a non-opioid analgesic is being added, a lower conversion dose should be used.

TABLE 9.5. Easy to use equal analgesic conversions between opioids [2, 3].

	Oral dose (mg)	IV/SC dose (mg)
Morphine	15	5
Hydromorphone	3	1
Oxycodone	10	Not available
Hydrocodone	15	Not available
Oxymorphone	5	1
Codeine	150	50
Levorphanol	2	1

Adapted from Ferris and Pirrello: *Improving Equianalgesic Dosing for Chronic Pain Management,* American Association for Cancer Education Annual Meeting Presentation, Cincinnati, OH, Sept 2005. From Pantilet, *Hospital-Based Palliative Medicine: A Practical, Evidence-Based Approach.*

This table is a *guideline sample* which attempts to account for the limitations of published tables, simplify mathematical relationships and promote consistency across practitioners. Several equianalgesic tables have been published, all of which are approximations, derived from single dose studies with small sample size and do not address cross-tolerance. The "calculated number" result should always be carefully considered in the context of the patient's clinical circumstances

- Another variation to the equal analgesia conversion is the concept of incomplete cross tolerance.
  - A patient who is taking one type of opioid may have an increased or decreased analgesia when switched to a different opioid at the "equivalent" dose.
  - To adjust for this phenomenon and to avoid over sedation when starting a new medication, the dose can be reduced 20–30 % based on the patient's pain control.
- The manufacturer's recommendation for converting from morphine to TD Fentanyl is listed in Table 9.6 [2].
  - This method requires conversion to an oral morphine equivalent and calculating the patient's 24-h oral morphine requirement.
  - This table should not be used to convert from a fentanyl patch to another opioid.
  - For patients receiving a stable dose of a fentanyl IV infusion or patient controlled analgesia (PCA), the fentanyl should be converted from IV to patch at the equivalent dose and rounding down to the nearest available fentanyl patch dose (e.g., a patient receiving a stable infusion of 60 mcg/h of fentanyl should be converted to a 50 mcg/h fentanyl patch).

Non-opioid Classes of Medications

Anti-inflammatory Drugs

- Many drug classes have direct or indirect anti-inflammatory effect. For example, antibiotics are effective anti-inflammatory medications by reducing the underlying infection while some antibiotics have direct anti-inflammatory effects as well.
- The most commonly used anti-inflammatory drugs are steroids and non-steroidal anti-inflammatory drugs (NSAIDs).

TABLE 9.6. FDA approved manufacturer's conversion from oral morphine to fentanyl patch [2].

Step 1: Sum total opioid received in 24 h and convert to oral morphine equivalents using equianalgesic table, e.g., Table 9.6	
Step 2: Using the table below, select the fentanyl patch dose that corresponds to the morphine equivalent dose range that the patient is receiving	
Daily morphine equivalent dose 24-h PO Morphine (mg/day) Equivalent	FDA approved manufacturer's conversion TD fentanyl dose (mcg/h)
60–134	25
135–224	50
225–314	75
315–404	100
405–494	125
495–584	150
585–674	175
675–764	200
765–854	225
855–944	250
945–1,034	275
1,035–1,124	300

The fentanyl patch should only be used in opioid tolerant patients, i.e., those receiving a stable dose of at least 60 mg oral morphine equivalent per day

This table should not be used to convert from a fentanyl patch to another opioid, as it will result in too high a dose of the new opioid

From Pantilet, *Hospital-Based Palliative Medicine: A Practical, Evidence-Based Approach*. Copyright © 2015 by John Wiley & Sons, Inc. Reprinted by permission of John Wiley & Sons, Inc

- They are generally thought of for musculoskeletal pain but are also effective for inflammatory visceral pain and some cancer pain, especially metastatic bone pain.

Glucocorticoids

- Due to their strong anti-inflammatory properties, glucocorticoids are one of the best and first line choices.
  - The analgesic effect of steroids begins within 24–48 h and reaches its peak in 3–4 days. After 5 days the analgesic benefit diminishes and the risks of side effect increases.

- Palliative care patients generally tolerate steroids better than NSAIDs. Steroids also have beneficial side effects for palliative care patients, such as increased appetite, weight gain, increased energy, decreased nausea, and decreased shortness of breath.
- They can reduce the effects of brain metastases and bowel obstruction.
- *Dexamethasone is the steroid of choice for most palliative care patients*, because it has a high anti-inflammatory potency compared to other steroids. Dexamethasone also has little mineralocorticoid effects and thus does not cause or increase edema/fluid retention. Since the analgesic effect is related to the dose and side effects are generally associated with duration, a short course, high dose burst of steroids is recommended for pain management.
  - Typical doses range from 12 to 20 mg per day. Even when given for only 4 or 5 days, the analgesic effect of steroids can last up to 2 weeks.

NSAIDs

- For the best results, NSAIDs should be given scheduled or around the clock.
- In the acute setting, short-acting NSAIDS such as ibuprofen are preferred, in case of adverse effects.
- Long-acting NSAIDS, such as naproxen, are easier for patients to take as an outpatient.
- For patients who are unable to take oral NSAIDs, intravenous ketoralac (Toradol) can be given.
- A proton pump inhibitor should be given with high dose NSAIDs for gastric protection.
- NSAIDs are contraindicated in patients with increased risk of bleeding, renal impairment, heart failure and/or uncontrolled hypertension.

Bisphosphonates

- Bisphosphonates reduce bone inflammation through inhibition of osteoclast function. They are particularly effective in patients with bone pain secondary to metastases.
- They are given via the intravenous route and therefore must be given in the inpatient or at an outpatient infusion center.
- These doses should be repeated monthly for continued effect and adjusted for renal function.

Neuropathic Pain Agents

Tricyclic Antidepressants (TCAs)

- Tricyclic antidepressants (TCAs) are *still the gold standard for neuropathic pain*, due to the large volume of evidence, though in practice they are not used as a first line agent.
  - The exact pain mechanism of TCAs is unknown.
  - TCAs should be dosed at night due to their sedative effects.
  - They are generally not tolerated by older patients due to their anticholinergic side effects.
  - The other major dose limiting side effect is orthostatic hypotension. Their cardiac side effects limit their use in patients with major cardiac problems.
  - Their multiple drug interactions also limit their use in patients on multiple medications.

Seratonin Norepinephrine Reuptake Inhibitors (SNRIs)

- Serotonin Norepinephrine Reuptake Inhibitors (SNRIs) are effective adjuvants for neuropathic pain. They are good choices for patients who also require treatment for depression but cannot take a TCA.
  - The doses effective for pain are often lower than those effective for depression. Just as these medications often need 2–6 weeks to reach full effect in the treatment for

depression, they also require 1–2 weeks to reach full effect in the treatment of pain.

- Duloxetine is approved by the Food and Drug Administration (FDA) for treatment of both pain and depression. It is not yet generic and therefore is expensive and often not covered by insurance companies as a first line treatment for neuropathic pain.
- Venlafaxine has the same mechanism as Duloxetine and is equally effective for both pain and depression [4]. Venlafaxine is generic and less expensive and more likely to be covered by insurance.

Gabapentin and Pregabalin

- Gabapentin is the most commonly prescribed neuropathic pain medication with a 70 % efficacy rate.
  - Built from the GABA (gamma-aminobutyric acid) molecule, its mechanism is not related to the GABA receptor, but instead it binds to the alpha-2-delta ligand receptor of the calcium channel on the cell membrane of neurons.
  - Gabapentin is started at a low and often subtherapeutic dose, because of its sedating side effect. It should be titrated over time, e.g., 2 weeks, to therapeutic effect.
  - Because of its sedating effect, gabapentin is a good choice for patients who have insomnia, a common complaint in pain patients.
  - Gabapentin is usually dosed every 8 h for seizures, but should be dosed predominately at night and at bedtime for pain to avoid daytime sedation.
    - For example, 25 % of the daily dose can be given in the morning, 25–50 % of the daily dose around 5–6 PM, and 50 % or more of the daily dose at bedtime.
  - Gabapentin is 90 % renally excreted and therefore requires dosing adjustment in patients with renal impairment.

- Pregabalin is structurally similar to Gabapentin and is thought to work in the same way for the treatment of neuropathic pain.
  - It is not yet generic and tends to be more expensive than Gabapentin. Often, insurance companies will not cover Pregabalin unless the patient has failed Gabapentin treatment.
  - A small subset of patients will respond to Pregabalin when they have not responded to Gabapentin.
  - The side effect profile of Pregabalin is the same as Gabapentin. Like Gabapentin, Pregabalin requires titration to an effective dose and should be given mostly in the evening and at bedtime.

Other Alternatives

- In patients with refractory neuropathic pain or opioid induced hyperalgesia, infusions of lidocaine, a sodium channel blocker, or administration of ketamine, an NMDA receptor antagonist, can be used for pain management, often with very good results.
- A Palliative Care or Pain Management consultation is strongly recommended for use of these medications for pain management.

Depression

Screening

- Depressive symptoms are common in women with cancer.
  - The prevalence of depressive and anxiety disorders among women with gynecologic cancers approaches 50 % [5].
- Depression is under-recognized in cancer patients and under-treated. Despite its high prevalence, depression is not a normal part of cancer.
  - The attitude of "of course she is depressed, she has cancer" needs to be eliminated. Because depression severely

decreases quality of life, routine screening for it is essential in cancer patients.

- Depression shortens the survival of cancer patients, and impacts their ability to tolerate and receive cancer therapies. The consequences of depression can be a reduction of the patient's functional status and their adherence to medical regimens. Depression can magnify a patient's perception of pain and other symptoms.
- Direct inquiry about mood is needed at every follow up visit, since its prevalence and severity have been reported to fluctuate during the patient's treatment course [5].
- An almost exhaustive number of depression assessment instruments exist for cancer patients [6]. Although these instruments are validated in and for research studies, they are not practical in a busy clinical practice.
  - Experts suggest that a single question for depressed mood during the interview provides a reliable and remarkably accurate screen.
  - The failure to identify depression is not due to the "lack of sufficiently sensitive brief screening measures" but due instead to a failure of simply asking, "Are you depressed?" [7].
  - Culturally some patients may not find the word "depression" acceptable, associating it only with "crazy" people who are locked up in psychiatric units. In these situations, a more general inquiry about their mood may be a more appropriate screening question, such as "How is your mood?", "Has your mood changed?", "Do you feel sad?" or "Have you felt more sad lately?"
- The challenge of diagnosing depression in cancer patients is differentiating "clinical" depression from a "natural reaction" to a serious and life threatening illness. The cluster of depressive symptoms is common even in cancer patients who do not have depression. This cluster includes fatigue, loss of energy, insomnia, hypersomnia, diminished

interest in sex and other previously enjoyed activities, loss of appetite, feelings of guilt, worry, restlessness, irritability, or muscle tension.

- Rather than a dichotomous distinction, these two conditions or states should be viewed as two ends of a spectrum. On one end of the spectrum is major depression. On the other end is a normal reaction to bad news. In between are minor depression, adjustment disorder, and dysfunctional grief reactions.

- The key factor to differentiate depression from an emotional reaction to cancer is hopelessness. Cancer patients with depression will express a sense of global hopelessness, while a cancer patient reacting to their illness severity can express hope, even if the hope is not for a cure.

Treatment

- The decision to treat a patient's depression is based on several factors.
- As with any medical intervention, the first and major factor is the risk to benefit analysis. The benefit analysis is based on the severity of the symptoms and what other problems the patient may have.
  - Medications are most effective in patients with the most severe symptoms of depression and anxiety disorders.
    - For example, if the patient also has pain, then the threshold for suggesting a tricyclic or an SNRI becomes lower; or if the patient has anorexia, then mirtazapine (Remeron) can help with both problems.
  - Using an antidepressant to treat other symptoms reduces polypharmacy and increases the patient's willingness to take an antidepressant, since a major barrier to depression treatment is often the patient's or family's willingness for accept treatment.
  - Non-pharmacologic support may be all that is needed for mild to moderate symptoms.
  - Non-pharmacologic modalities include:

  - Counseling.
  - Spiritual support.
  - Cognitive behavioral therapy.
  - Problem-solving therapy.
  - Relaxation and mindfulness techniques and support groups.

- Most communities have these services available.
- On the other hand, patients with the most severe form of depression may need electroconvulsive therapy (ECT).
  - ECT can be life saving for suicidal patients and patients who stopped eating because of their depression.
  - It is the most effective antidepressive therapy for severe depression and is the safest depression therapy for patients with severe illness.
  - Unfortunately many patients are reluctant to undergo ECT due to its stigmata and its amnestic effects.
- Table 9.7 lists the medications used to treat depression. Their common starting dose and dosage range, indications and additional pharmacologic actions are also included.
- All antidepressive medications are equally efficacious with approximately one third of patients having a good response, a third having a partial response, and a third having no response [8].
  - The selection of the antidepressant therefore depends on their side-effect profile, including other therapeutic benefits, and dosing convenience to improve adherence.
- The side effects of antidepressants can help with cancer-related symptoms such as neuropathic pain, fatigue, nausea, insomnia and hot flashes.
  - Many of the antidepressants are also anxiolytics.
- Atypical antipsychotics are FDA approved as adjunctive therapy when monotherapy is insufficient or when the depression is associated with psychosis or paranoia [9].

TABLE 9.7. Benefits of common medications used for depression.

Medications Starting dose/dosage range	Depression	Anxiety	Pain	Sweats/ hot flash	Sleep	Nausea	Fatigue
SNRI							
Duloxetine	+F	+F	+F	–	±	–	–
Start: 20–30 mg/day							
Range: 60–120 mg/day							
Venlafaxine XR	+F	+F	+	+	±	–	–
Start: 37.5 or 75 mg/day							
Range: 75–225 mg/day							
Tricyclics							
Amitriptyline	+F	–	+	–	+	–	–
Start: 25–50 mg/day							
Range: 100–300 mg/day							
Desipramine	+F	–	+	–	+	–	–
Start: 25–50 mg/day							
Range: 100–300 mg/day							
Nortriptyline	+F	–	+	–	+	–	–
Start: 25 mg/day							
Range: 50–200 mg							
Psychostimulants							
Methylphenidate	+	–	–	–	–	–	+
Start: 5–10 mg q day-BID							
Range: 20–60 mg/day							

Modafinil	+	–	–	–	–	–	+
Start: 100–200 mg/day							
Range: 200–400 mg/day							
Dextroamphetamine/Amphetamine	+	–	–	–	–	–	+
Start: 5–15 mg q day – TID							
Range: 20–60 mg/day							
Others							
Buspirone	+	+[F]	–	–	–	–	–
Start: 7.5 mg BID							
Range: 15–60 mg/day							
Quetiapine XR	Adjunct[F]	+	–	–	+	–	–
Start: 50 mg at bedtime							
Range: 150–300 mg/day							
Olanzapine	Adjunct[F]	–	–	–	+	+	–
Start: 5 mg at bedtime							
Range: 10–20 mg/day							
Mirtazapine	+[F]	+	–	+	+	–	–
Start: 15 mg q hs							
Range: 15–45 mg q hs							

+[F] = FDA-approved indication from Micromedex® 2.0, Truven Health Analytics 2012–2014

± = SNRIs are reported to have an approximately equal incidence of insomnia or somnolence. For those patients experiencing insomnia as a side effect, give the daily dose in the morning; for those patients experiencing somnolence as a side effect, give the daily dose at bedtime

- Psychostimulants have been used to treat symptoms of depression in cancer patients in the palliative setting because of their more rapid onset of action.
  - They are favored in patients with short survival prognosis who may not live long enough to see the benefit of other antidepressants.
  - They may be used alone or as initial therapy while longer onset medications are being titrated.
  - Psychostimulants improve the vegetative symptoms of depression and less so the patients' mood. Thus they can almost immediately improve fatigue, somnolence, anorexia, and even pain.
  - However, they can cause increased anxiety, tremors, and insomnia. Therefore stimulants should be taken first thing in the morning and not later than 1 PM in the afternoon.
  - A transdermal patch formulation of methylphenidate, called Daytrana, can be used for patients who are unable to take pills.

Constipation Management

Laxatives

- *The best laxative is the one the patient will take.* A discussion with the patient about what laxatives they have taken and are willing to take is the most effective and efficient method of selecting a laxative.
- Table 9.8 lists the common laxatives and their relative advantages and disadvantages. No head to head studies have been done to differentiate one laxative from another.
- The choice of a laxative is therefore based on practical considerations and the patients' other medical problems.
  - For example, Sorbitol's sweetness can help patients tolerate the bitterness of other liquid medications, such as opioids, when mixed with them (the Mary Poppins's Principle).

TABLE 9.8. Classes of common laxatives.

Mechanism class	Name	Advantages	Disadvantages
Stimulant	Senna	• Easy to take pill • Inexpensive, over the counter	• Mild • Causes cramping
	Bisacodyl	• Easy to take pill • Inexpensive, over the counter	• Mild • Causes cramping
	Milk of magnesia	• Easy to take • Liquid • Inexpensive, over the counter	• Mild • Not for dialysis patients
	Magnesium citrate	• Stronger: more effective • Liquid	• Not for dialysis patients • Can cause dehydration and electrolyte abnormalities
Osmotic	Sorbitol	• Sweetness can overcome bitterness of other medications • Stronger: more effective • Liquid	• Too sweet for some, esp. elderly • Mild cramping • Bloating • Risk of fecal incontinence
	Lactulose	• Helps with encephalopathy in liver patients • Liquid • Stronger: more effective	• Too sweet for some, esp. elderly • Expensive • Bloating • Risk of fecal incontinence
	Polyethylene glycol: PEG, miralax golytely	• Inexpensive, over the counter • Stronger: more effective • Well tolerated	• Can cause dehydration and electrolyte abnormalities • Risk of fecal incontinence
Fiber	Psyllium: metamucil	• Good for irritable bowel • Inexpensive, over the counter • Treats fecal incontinence	• Should not take with opioids and diuretics • "Gritty" taste
	Guar gum: benefiber	• Good for irritable bowel • Inexpensive, over the counter • Treats fecal incontinence	• Should not take with opioids and diuretics
	Methyl cellulose: citrucel	• Good for irritable bowel • Inexpensive, over the counter • Treats fecal incontinence	• Should not take with opioids and diuretics

- Patients with end-stage renal disease should not be given magnesium based laxatives or laxatives with phosphate, since dialysis patients have difficulty eliminating these electrolytes from their systems.
- Lactulose is preferred in patients with advance liver disease to also aid in their encephalopathy management.

- Recent randomized comparison trials show that stool softeners, such as docusate (Colace), add nothing to a laxative regimen, such as senna, and therefore need not be given [10].
- Fiber laxatives should not be given to patients on opioids or other medications that slow the bowel, because of the increase risk of fecal impaction.
  - For the same reason they should not be given to patients who are on diuretics or who cannot consume sufficient fluids.

Enema

- The effectiveness of an enema is dependent upon two related factors: how high up it will go and how long the patient can retain it.
  - *Enemas are highly operator dependent*. The person administering the enema must constantly reposition the patient in order for the enema to make all the turns in the colon.
  - The most basic enema is sodium phosphate (Fleets), which is over the counter.
  - Other enemas in escalating effectiveness are:
    - Mineral oil.
    - Tap water.
    - Retention enemas, such as lactulose or barium.
  - For home patients, the home health or hospice nurse can administer a milk and molasses enema as the retention enema.
  - *For patients with fecal impactions, the rule of thumb is to "pull from below before pushing from above,"* i.e., an enema should be given first. .

After the patient starts moving their bowel, no matter how small the stool, an aggressive oral laxative regiment can then be given

Alternate Options

- For patients with refractory constipation or fecal impaction, several options are now available.
  - Traditionally a Harris flush would be the next step for a fecal impaction that has not responded to enemas.
  - If a Harris flush is ineffective, then *the final resort is a flushing colonoscopy*.
  - For opioid-induced constipation, subcutaneous methylnaltrexone, a peripheral opioid antagonist can be effective without precipitating a central opioid withdrawal [11]. It is also an option for patients who refuse enemas.
  - Finally the new, selective chloride channel agonist, Lubiprostone (Amitiza), promotes stool passage by increasing intestinal fluid secretion and motility.

Nausea/Vomiting

- Like any symptom management, the management of nausea and vomiting should be approached through targeting of the underlying mechanism. Understanding of the neurotransmitters and mechanisms involved allows for focused therapy that minimizes side effects and cost, rather than giving ondansetron (Zofran) to everyone.
- Figure 9.1 outlines a systematic approach to the causes of nausea that feed into the vomiting center of the brain. A systematic approach reduces the likelihood of missing the underlying diagnosis or cause.
- Though most physicians think of the gastrointestinal (GI) track as the most common cause of nausea, many other organs also send input to the vomiting center. If, however,

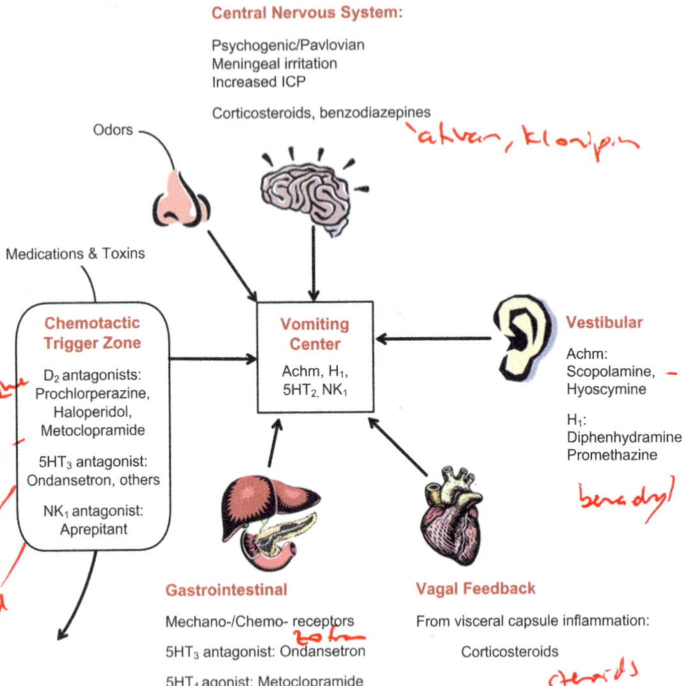

FIG. 9.1. Mechanisms of nausea and vomiting and associated treatment.

the GI track is the most likely source of the nausea and vomiting, metoclopramide (Reglan) is the best empiric therapy, because of its multiple effects on the GI track.

- Psychogenic nausea does not mean that the patient's symptom is fabricated or that the patient is "crazy." Rather this nausea is a Pavlovian response, a subconsciously learned behavior. The nausea and vomiting persists even after the initial cause has been removed and becomes chronic.
  - That initial cause is now replaced with an associated trigger, and exposure to that trigger produces the Pavlovian response.
  - Classically a patient may vomit upon seeing the cancer center or infusion center or even seeing a bag of chemotherapy before it is hung.

- Typically these patients do not lose much weight or hydration.
- Treatment is around the clock benzodiazepine for a few days to break the cortical association, since trigger avoidance is usually not practical or possible.

- Any brain metastasis, including leptomeningeal disease, can cause nausea and vomiting.
  - Persistent "intractable" nausea and vomiting should prompt a workup for brain metastasis.
    - A short course of high dose steroids, such as dexamethasone for 5 days, provides temporary relief by reducing the associated edema and inflammation until more permanent treatment of the brain lesion is provided.

- The chemotactic trigger zone (CTZ) is the most common site through which medications cause nausea and vomiting.
  - The physiological role of the CTZ is to protect us from food poisoning by monitoring our blood stream for toxins and inducing emesis.
  - It is a dopaminergic center, and many antiemetics work through the CTZ as a dopamine blocker, e.g., prochlorperazine (Compazine) and haloperidol (Haldol).
  - Other antiemetics are mixed dopamine blockers and anticholinergics, such as promethazine (Phenergan) and Trimethobenzamide (Tigan).
  - The addition of the anticholinergic activity, reduces the side effects of the dopamine blockade (such as dystonia) while adding a second antiemetic effect on the vestibular system.

- Asking about vestibular triggers should be part of every nausea and vomiting history. The olfactory nerve feeds directly to the vomiting center.
  - Unfortunately there is no treatment for odor-induced nausea other than avoidance and covering up the smell.

Bowel Obstruction

- Malignant bowel obstruction (MBO) occurs in 25–50 % of patients with ovarian cancer and can occur at any stage of disease [12].
- Several different mechanisms are often at play:
  - External compression of intestinal lumen by tumor or edema.
  - Infiltration of intestinal mesentery serosa and muscle by tumor leading to decreased motility and pseudo-obstruction.
  - Intraluminal obstruction by tumor.
  - Fibrosis from radiation or previous surgery [13].
- Figure 9.2 shows the mechanisms of the symptoms from a bowel obstruction [14].
- Symptoms vary depending on the site of obstruction, whether proximal small bowel versus colon. Often there are multiple sites of obstruction. Pain is the most common feature, present in over 90 % (Table 9.9) [15].

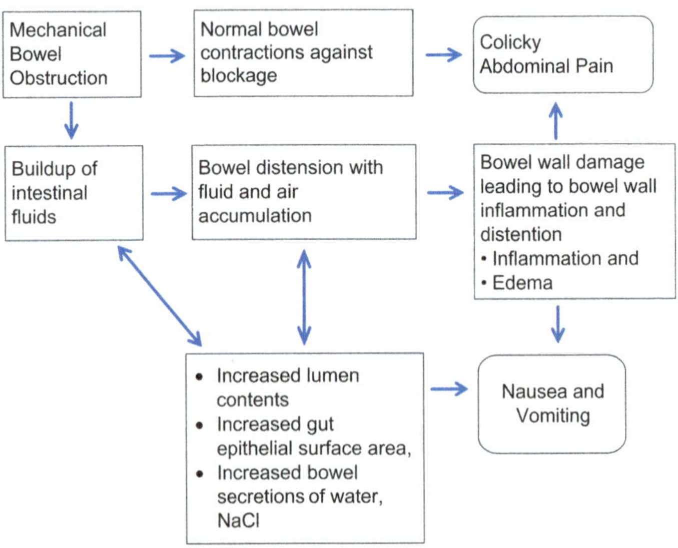

FIG. 9.2. Mechanism of bowel obstruction symptoms.

TABLE 9.9. Symptoms of bowel obstruction based on location.

Symptom	Gastric/small bowel	Colon
Vomiting	Large volume, undigested food, or watery	Small amount, fecund
Pain	Severe, short intermittent, peri-umbilical, occurs at start of symptoms	Late symptom, crampy, longer intervals between episodes
Abdominal distension	May be absent if gastric	Present
Anorexia	Always	May not be present

- Unlike non-malignant causes of obstruction, MBO often occurs slowly over time. It can be intermittent and partial and progress over time to complete obstruction.
- Typically MBO is not an emergency in ovarian cancer and bowel strangulation or perforation is uncommon. Therefore, time can be taken to perform the proper radiological tests and decide on the best treatment.

Diagnostic Evaluation

- Abdominal X-ray series in the supine and standing positions are the best first investigation when small bowel obstruction is suspected, in order to document dilated loops of bowel with air fluid levels.
  - If no evidence of obstruction is present, functional ileus is more likely.
- CT scan can help to evaluate disease extent, localize the site of obstruction, and assist in treatment decision making.
  - It is more sensitive and specific in determining the cause of malignant bowel obstruction compared to plain film.
  - Carcinomatosis, however, may be missed on a CT scan. For example, ovarian cancer deposits of less than 0.5 cm are seen only 20 % of the time on CT [16, 17].
- Endoscopy should be performed if gastric outlet, proximal duodenal obstruction or colonic obstruction is suspected and stenting is a potential treatment.

Management

- Options for management of MBO include:
  - Surgical bypass.
  - Stomal formation for distal small bowel or large bowel obstruction.
  - Endoscopic stenting of duodenum or colon.
  - Pharmacologic management.
  - A venting gastrostomy.
- The decision about whether to take patients to palliative surgery is difficult, and the data upon which to base decisions is limited.
  - Factors associated with poor outcomes for surgery are:
    - Older age.
    - ECOG 3–4 performance status.
    - Generalized carcinomatosis as the cause of the MBO.
    - Multiple sites of obstruction.
    - Large volume ascites.
    - Poor nutritional status.
    - Bowel motility disorder.
- Laparotomy to surgically correct a MBO is best undertaken in patients with:
  - Good performance status.
  - A minimum life expectancy of at least several months.
  - A single site of obstruction.
  - Absence of ascites.
    - The possibility of a stoma should be discussed prior to surgery.
- For patients who are not candidates for surgery, pharmacological therapy can be given with the goal of reducing pain and colic and reducing nausea and vomiting to acceptable levels without the use of a nasogastric tube.
  - For pain relief, opioids should be given subcutaneously or intravenously and preferably through a PCA.

- Medications to reduce gastrointestinal secretions to alleviate nausea and pain (Table 9.10).
  - Octreotide is superior to Scopolamine for resolving MBO symptoms and is well tolerated with minimal side effects.
  - A long acting octreotide injection can be given in the form of an intramuscular depo shot, but subcutaneous injections must be continued for an overlap of 1 week after first depo injection. Intramuscular injections can then be given monthly [13].
  - Dexamethasone should be given along with Octreotide to reduce tumor inflammation and speed up the resolution of the MBO.
    - High doses of 16 of 20 mg a day need to be given for 5 days, initially parenterally then enterally if and when the patient tolerates liquids. An anti-emetic should be given around the clock to prevent nausea.

- The indications for a venting gastrostomy are:
  - Failure of pharmacologic treatment in a non-operative patient.
  - High likelihood to re-obstruct.
  - The benefits of a gastrostomy tube are:
    - It is more comfortable than a nasogastric tube.
    - It allows patients to eat food by mouth for oral gratification.
    - It allows relief of nausea and vomiting at home using a suction machine or large syringe to decompress the stomach.
  - Gastrostomy tubes can be placed even in patients with diffuse carcinomatosis, tumor encasing the stomach, and ascites.
  - If the patient has ascites, a pre-procedure paracentesis should be performed to reduce the risk of leakage.
  - More than 90 % of patients have relief of their nausea and vomiting with a venting gastrostomy.

TABLE 9.10. Drugs to reduce gastrointestinal secretions in bowel obstruction.

Medication	Category	Route	Dose	Side effects/issues
Scopolamine	Anticholinergic	SQ, IV, or IM	0.6–1 mg TID-QID	Dry mouth, confusion, urinary retention, constipation
Scopolamine (transderm scop)	Anticholinergic	Transdermal	1.5 mg patch q 72 h	Dry mouth, confusion, urinary retention, constipation
Glycopyrrolate (robinul)	Anticholinergic	SQ or IV	0.2 mg q 4–6 h	Dry mouth, urinary retention, constipation
Octreotide (sandostatin)	Somatostatin analogue	SQ or IV	400–1,200 mcg/day, continuous infusion or intermittent BID to TID	Expensive, long acting IM monthly injection available for long term use

- Complications occur in 15–25 % of patients and include (in order of frequency) leakage, peristomal infection, obstruction of the tube, tube migration, catheter malfunction, hemorrhage, and peritonitis.
- Chemotherapy can be safely given after gastrostomy tube placement [18].

Ascites

- Malignant ascites is the abnormal accumulation of fluid in the peritoneal cavity due to cancer.
- In ovarian cancer, it is present at approximately one third of patients at the time of diagnosis and two thirds at the time of death [19].
- The symptoms resulting from malignant ascites are myriad and difficult for patients to tolerate.
  - The most difficult symptoms include abdominal pain, abdominal distension, early satiety, nausea/vomiting, dyspnea, orthopnea, difficulty ambulating, and difficulty bending over [20, 21].
- Mechanisms of malignant ascites from cancer could be due to any of the following:
  - Increased vascular permeability.
  - Increased fluid production.
  - Lymphatic obstruction.
  - Renin-angiotensin activation.
  - Portal hypertension from hepatic metastases.
- Under normal conditions, peritoneal fluid is produced by capillary membranes of the peritoneal cavity, and the fluid is reabsorbed through lymphatic channels. Cancer disrupts this through multiple mechanisms.
  - Firstly, tumor microvasculature is leakier, causing increased fluid with high protein concentrations to flow into the peritoneal cavity.
  - Tumor cells, endothelial cells, and vascular endothelial growth factor produce excess fluid.

- Lymphatic channels are often obstructed by tumor, preventing fluid reabsorption and fluid return to the venous system.
- Decreased blood volume from inadequate lymphatic return causes activation of the renin-angiotensin system and resultant sodium and fluid retention by the kidney.
- Lastly, hepatic metastases can cause portal hypertension and ascites [21, 22].

Treatment

- The overall data for *diuretic use* in malignant ascites is weak. Trials comparing diuretic use to paracentesis do not exist.
  - Approximately 40 % of patients may respond to diuretic use [20]. Diuretic response can best be expected in ascites caused by massive hepatic metastases with portal hypertension and serum-ascites albumin gradient of >1.1.
  - Spironolactone, an aldosterone antagonist that decreases reabsorption of water and sodium in the kidney, is most often cited as the first line treatment for malignant ascites.
    - The starting dose is 100 mg/day and doses up to 400 mg/day have been reported.
  - Furosemide in a starting dose of 20 mg/day can be added and increased to 40–80 mg/day to balance the serum potassium.
  - In liver cirrhosis, a ratio of 100:40 for spironolactone and furosemide results in normokalemia. Spironolactone can cause hyperkalemia, and electrolytes should be monitored during therapy.
  - A goal weight loss of 0.5 kg/day to not more than 1 kg/day is optimal. Over diuresis increases the risks of hypotension from intravascular volume depletion and subsequent renal injury.
  - Starting at lower doses of diuretics and increasing gradually is thought to decrease these risks.

- Furosemide is more likely to cause hypotension and can be given in two divided doses.
- Spironolactone should be dosed once per day due to its long half-life [23].

• *Paracentesis* is the most common treatment for malignant ascites and is very successful in improving symptoms.

- Removal of up to 9 L at a time have been reported without complications of hypotension or renal dysfunction [19]. Drainage of up to 5 L without use of IVF or albumin replacement is generally safe and will not cause hypotension.
- Complications of the procedure include:
  - Hypoproteinemia.
  - Hypotension.
  - Secondary peritonitis.
  - Significant hemorrhage, bowel perforation, and pulmonary embolism are rare [24].
- Paracentesis should be performed under ultrasound guidance when possible. Re-accumulation is common. Therefore, limiting parenteral fluid administration is optimal to prevent rapid re-accumulation.
  Using the same exact site repeatedly is safe, and performing paracentesis in an office setting is common. Paracentesis can be done even in the home, e.g., with hospice patients.
- Paracentesis and diuretics are often used in combination to manage ascites. There is no limit to how often patients may have the procedure.

• For patients requiring frequent paracenteses, more often than weekly, interventional radiologists can insert *tunneled peritoneal catheters*.

- The patient is left with approximately 12 in. of a drain which can be taped to their abdomen and is not visible underneath clothing.
  - Ascites fluid can then be drained at home, into bags which attach to the catheter.

  - Published rates of infection and occlusion are reported to be approximately 4–6 % [20].
  - This procedure should be considered for patients with a life expectancy of at least 30 days.
  - It should also be performed prior to discharge to hospice in patients needing more than weekly paracentesis or to hospices without a physician to perform paracentesis in the home.

- More recently, chemotherapeutic interventions for the treatment of malignant ascites have been examined.
  - Given the apparent dependence of ascites formation on abnormal tumor vascularity and permeability, it was hypothesized that VEGF inhibitors would show efficacy in the treatment of ovarian cancer associated ascites.
  - Clinical trial exploring the antiangiogenic agent bevacizumab have shown success in the management of malignant ascites.
    - Numnum et al. described four patients with recurrent ovarian cancer and ascites requiring frequent paracentesis who were treated with intravenous bevacizumab at a dose of 15 mg/kg IV every 3 weeks.
  - All four patients demonstrated symptomatic relief of ascites, with manageable toxicities.
  - No therapeutic paracenteses were required after initiation of therapy with bevacizumab (follow up of up to 6 months) [25].
    - Hamilton et al. described a case report detailing the impact of intraperitoneal bevacizumab (5 mg/kg) on severe symptomatic ascites in an elderly patient with advanced, recurrent, ovarian cancer and a very poor functional status [26].
      - The authors reported a dramatic improvement in ascites and quality of life parameters following two doses.

- Additionally, *VEGF-trap*, a fusion protein that prevents VEGF receptor binding, has also been studied in the treatment of refractory ascites.
- VEGF-trap, or aflibercept, incorporates the second binding domain of the VEGFR-1 receptor and the third domain of the VEGFR-2 receptor [27].
  - By fusing these extracellular protein sequences to the Fc segment of a human IgG backbone, developers created a chimeric protein with a very high VEGF binding affinity, binding all isomers of the VEGF-A family [27, 28].
- Several single agent and combination phase II clinical trials have explored the safety and efficacy of VEFG-trap (aflibercept) in the treatment of ascites associated with advanced stage solid tumors, including ovarian cancer [29, 30].
  - Two published trials investigated the use of VEGF-trap in the treatment of advanced stage epithelial ovarian cancer and symptomatic malignant ascites.
    - Colombo et al. enrolled 16 patients with advanced chemo-resistant epithelial ovarian cancer and symptomatic malignant ascites onto an open-label, phase II trial assessing the efficacy and safety of aflibercept [31].
      - The primary endpoint was repeat paracentesis response rate (RPRR), with response defined as at least a twofold increase in time to repeat paracentesis compared with the baseline interval.
        - Aflibercept was considered effective based on a hypothesis that the RPRR was ≥60 %. Median time to repeat paracentesis was 76.0 days (95 % CI 64.0–178.0), which was 4.5 times longer than the baseline interval (16.8 days).

- Gotlieb et al. specifically explored treatment of malignant ascites in patients with advanced stage epithelial ovarian cancer using aflibercept [32].
  - Mean time to repeat paracentesis was significantly longer with aflibercept than with placebo (55.1 vs. 23.3 days; difference 31.8 days, 95 % CI 10.6–53.1; $p=0.0019$). Notably, in the aflibercept group, two patients did not need a repeat paracentesis during 6 months of double-blind treatment.

Dyspnea

- Dyspnea is the subjective sensation of “air hunger” or “breathlessness.” Its objective counterpart is shortness of breath. Though the two are usually related, they do not necessarily correlate. For example, patients with panic attacks may have a lot of dyspnea leading to hyperventilation but their respiratory status is otherwise objectively normal. On the other side of the coin, many patients with chronic cardiopulmonary diseases may appear short of breath and have very abnormal objective respiratory numbers but subjectively have very mild symptoms.
- *The causes of dyspnea range from head to pelvis*. Though most physicians tend to think of the cardiopulmonary systems first, the other anatomical areas should be systematically consider, so as not to miss a diagnosis or contributing factor.
- Since dyspnea is a subjective perception, the final common pathway for dyspnea is the cortex of the brain. Thus even when the cause of the dyspnea originates somewhere else, anxiety is often associated, and benzodiazepines may help.
  - Brain lesions, e.g., metastases or infarctions, in the cortex or in the respiratory centers of the brain, can rarely be the primary cause of dyspnea.
  - Nasal lesions can cause subjective dyspnea even when airways are still patent.

- For example, epistaxis may lead to significant anxiety and dyspnea, even when the hemorrhage does not have significant systemic impact.

– Metastases to the head and neck can lead to airway obstruction.

  - Short term palliation of the obstruction can be achieved with steroids, since most of the acute obstruction is due to edema.
  - Long term palliation may require radiation or surgery.

- Cardiopulmonary causes of dyspnea are myriad.

  – The most common cause seen in women with gynecological malignancies is pulmonary emboli.
  – In the last days of life, the most common cause is an aspiration pneumonia.
  – Pleural effusions from the cancer are frequent causes that can be alleviated with repeat thoracenteses or placement of a pleural drain.
  – Pulmonary metastases and lymphangitic carcinomatosis are rare as are pericardial involvement.
  – Airway obstructions can be treated with bronchoscopic stent placement with or without laser therapy.
  – Pulmonary lymphagitic spread can be palliated with high dose steroids and portents a survival prognosis of days to weeks.
  – Pericardiocentesis can provide temporary relief from malignant pericardial effusions until a pericardial window can be placed.

- Spinal metastases can cause dyspnea through two potential mechanisms.

  – Spinal cord compression or nerve root impingement at or above the C5 level can lead to paralysis of the diaphragm.

    - Again high dose steroids can provide short term palliation until more definitive therapy with radiation or surgery is performed.

– Multiple spinal metastases may lead to vertebral compression fractures, causing kyphosis.
  - Thoracic kyphosis if sufficiently severe causes a restrictive lung disease. Diaphragmatic expansion can also be impaired by tense malignant ascites.

Treatment

- Non-specific, first line pharmacological therapy for dyspnea is an opioid.
  – All opioids have this effect. However, despite their demonstrated safety, opioids are still underutilized for dyspnea symptom management [33, 34].
- Bronchodilator, mucolytic or saline nebulizer therapy is beneficial if wheezes are audible or if a mucous plug is suspected.
- Non-pharmacological therapy, such as a fan blowing on the face or cool compresses to the face, take advantage of the diving reflex.
- The administration of oxygen has no benefit compared to medical air in patients without hypoxemia [35].

Conclusion

Many therapies are available to provide pain and symptom management to women with gynecological malignancies. Good symptom management requires a systematic approach based on the mechanism of the symptom. Palliative care can improve the quality of life for cancer patients throughout the entire course of their illness. Physicians who care for these women should have a basic competency in palliative care and be able to refer more complex or complicated cases to their palliative medicine colleagues.

References

1. WHO Definition of Palliative Care. http://www.who.int/cancer/palliative/definition/en/. Accessed 5 June 2014.
2. Pantilet S, Anderson W, Gonzales M, et al. Hospital-based palliative medicine: a practical, evidence-based approach. Copyright © 2015 by John Wiley & Sons, Inc. Pre-publication.
3. Ferris and Pirrello. Improving equianalgesic dosing for chronic pain management. American Association for Cancer Education Annual Meeting Presentation, Cincinnati, OH, Sept 2005.
4. Attal N, Cruccu G, Baron R, Haanpää M, et al. EFNS guidelines on the pharmacological treatment of neuropathic pain: 2010 revision. Eur J Neurol. 2010;17(9):1113–e88.
5. Chase DM, Monk BJ, et al. Supportive care for women with gynecologic cancers. Expert Rev Anticancer Ther. 2008;8(2):227–41.
6. Kirkova J, Davis MP, et al. Cancer symptom assessment instruments: a systematic review. J Clin Oncol. 2006;24:1459–73.
7. Chochinov HM, Wilson KG, et al. Are you depressed? screening for depression in the terminally ill. Am J Psychiatry. 1997;154:674–6.
8. Li M, Fitzgerald P, Rodin G. Evidence based treatment of depression in patients with cancer. J Clin Oncol. 2012;30:1187–96.
9. Gao K, Sheehan DV, Calabrese JR. Atypical antipsychotics in primary general anxiety disorders or comorbid with mood disorders. Expert Rev Neurother. 2009;9(8):1147–58.
10. Tarumi Y, Wilson MP, Szafran O, Spooner GR. Randomized, double-blind, placebo-controlled trial of oral docusate in the management of constipation in hospice patients. J Pain Symptom Manage. 2013;45(1):2–13.
11. Thomas J, Karver S, Cooney GA, Chamberlain BH, et al. Methylnaltrexone for opioid-induced constipation in advanced illness. N Engl J Med. 2008;358(22):2332–43.
12. Pothuri B, Montemarano M, Gerardi M, Shike M, et al. Percutaneous endoscopic gastrostomy tube placement in patients with malignant bowel obstruction due to ovarian carcinoma. Gynecol Oncol. 2005;96(2):330–4.
13. Matulonis UA, Seiden MV, Roche M, Krasner C, et al. Long-acting octreotide for the treatment and symptomatic relief of bowel obstruction in advanced ovarian cancer. J Pain Symptom Manage. 2005;30(6):563–9.

14. Ripamonti CI, Easson AM, Gerdes H. Management of malignant bowel obstruction. Eur J Cancer. 2008;44(8):1105–15.
15. Ripamonti C, Twycross R, Baines M, Bozzetti F, et al. Clinical-practice recommendations for the management of bowel obstruction in patients with end-stage cancer. Support Care Cancer. 2001;9(4):223–33.
16. de Bree E, Koops W, Kröger R, van Ruth S, et al. Peritoneal carcinomatosis from colorectal or appendiceal origin: correlation of preoperative CT with intraoperative findings and evaluation of interobserver agreement. J Surg Oncol. 2004;86(2):64–73.
17. Jacquet P, Jelinek JS, Steves MA, Sugarbaker PH. Evaluation of computed tomography in patients with peritoneal carcinomatosis. Cancer. 1993;72(5):1631–6.
18. Rath KS, Loseth D, Muscarella P, Phillips GS, et al. Outcomes following percutaneous upper gastrointestinal decompressive tube placement for malignant bowel obstruction in ovarian cancer. Gynecol Oncol. 2013;129(1):103–6.
19. Harding V, Fenu E, Medani H, Shaboodien R, et al. Safety, cost-effectiveness and feasibility of daycase paracentesis in the management of malignant ascites with a focus on ovarian cancer. Br J Cancer. 2012;107(6):925–30.
20. Fleming ND, Alvarez-Secord A, Von Gruenigen V, Miller MJ, Abernethy AP. Indwelling catheters for the management of refractory malignant ascites: a systematic literature overview and retrospective chart review. J Pain Symptom Manage. 2009;38(3):341–9.
21. Becker G, Galandi D, Blum HE. Malignant ascites: systematic review and guideline for treatment. Eur J Cancer. 2006;42(5):589–97.
22. Woopen H, Sehouli J. Current and future options in the treatment of malignant ascites in ovarian cancer. Anticancer Res. 2009;29(8):3353–9.
23. Runyon BA. Management of adult patients with ascites due to cirrhosis: update. 2012. http://www.aasld.org/practiceguidelines/Documents/ascitesupdate2013.pdf. Accessed 11/12/13.
24. Sangisetty SL, Miner TJ. Malignant ascites: a review of prognostic factors, pathophysiology and therapeutic measures. World J Gastrointest Surg. 2012;4(4):87–95.
25. Numnum TM, Rocconi RP, Whitworth J, Barnes MN. The use of bevacizumab to palliate symptomatic ascites in patients with refractory ovarian carcinoma. Gynecol Oncol. 2006;102(3):425–8.

26. Hamilton CA, Maxwell GL, Chernofsky MR, Bernstein SA, Farley JH, Rose GS. Intraperitoneal bevacizumab for the palliation of malignant ascites in refractory ovarian cancer. Gynecol Oncol. 2008;111(3):530–2.
27. Stewart MW, Grippon S, Kirkpatrick P. Aflibercept. Nat Rev Drug Discov. 2012;11(4):269–70.
28. Stewart MW. Aflibercept (VEGF Trap-eye): the newest anti-VEGF drug. Br J Ophthalmol. 2012;96(9):1157–8.
29. Gaya A, Tse V. A preclinical and clinical review of aflibercept for the management of cancer. Cancer Treat Rev. 2012;38(5):484–93.
30. Teng LS, Jin KT, He KF, Zhang J, Wang HH, Cao J. Clinical applications of VEGF-trap (aflibercept) in cancer treatment. J Chin Med Assoc. 2010;73(9):449–56.
31. Colombo N, Mangili G, Mammoliti S, et al. A phase II study of aflibercept in patients with advanced epithelial ovarian cancer and symptomatic malignant ascites. Gynecol Oncol. 2012;125(1):42–7.
32. Gotlieb WH, Amant F, Advani S, et al. Intravenous aflibercept for treatment of recurrent symptomatic malignant ascites in patients with advanced ovarian cancer: a phase 2, randomised, double-blind, placebo-controlled study. Lancet Oncol. 2012;13(2):154–62.
33. Clemens KE, Quednau I, Klaschik E. Is there a higher risk of respiratory depression in opioid-naïve palliative care patients during symptomatic therapy of dyspnea with strong opioids? J Palliat Med. 2008;11(2):204–16.
34. Gomutbutra P, O'Riordan DL, Pantilat SZ. Management of moderate-to-severedyspnea in hospitalized patients receiving palliative care. J Pain Symptom Manage. 2013;45(5):885–91.
35. Davidson PM, Johnson MJ. Update on the role of palliative oxygen. Curr Opin Support Palliat Care. 2011;5(2):87–91.

Index

A

Acid–base disorders
  arterial sample values, 361
  bicarbonate–carbon dioxide buffer system, 360
  definitions, 361
  Henderson-Hasselbach equation, 360
  management, 364
  metabolic acidosis, 362, 364–365
  metabolic alkalosis, 363, 365
  mixed acid–base disorders, 364
  respiratory acidosis, 363
  respiratory alkalosis, 364
Acute respiratory distress syndrome (ARDS), 341–343
Adenocarcinoma, 11, 86, 97, 116, 120, 125
Adjuvant Chemotherapy Trial in Ovarian Neoplasia (ACTION), 20–21
Adjuvant therapy
  ASTEC and EN.5 pooled trial 1, 150–151
  GOG 99, 148, 149
  GOG 249, 151
  high intermediate-risk, 147–148
  low intermediate risk, 150
  PORTEC I trial, 148, 149
American Joint Committee on Cancer (AJCC) TNM staging, 95, 96
American Society for Colposcopy and Cervical Pathology (ASCCP), 62, 63
Ascites
  chemotherapy, 406–408
  diuretics use, 404–405
  mechanisms, 403–404
  paracentesis, 405
  symptoms, 403
  tunneled peritoneal catheters, 405–406

B

Bartholin's gland carcinomas, 94–95
Basal cell carcinoma (BCC), 94
Bilateral salpingo-oophorectomy (BSO), 139, 163
Bleomycin, etoposide and cisplatin (BEP), 43

C

Cancer antigen 125 (CA 125), 4, 5
Carcinosarcoma
  management
    advanced stage III and IV, 162
    early stage I and II, 161–162
    sentinel assessments, 162, 163
    surgery, 160–161
  type II lesions, 135

R.N. Eskander and R.E. Bristow (eds.), *Gynecologic Oncology: A Pocketbook*, DOI 10.1007/978-1-4939-1976-5,

Central venous access (CVA)
  catheter infection
    aseptic technique, 353, 354
    catheters and sites
      selection, 353, 354
    CVC and PICC
      replacement, 353, 354
    hemodialysis catheters,
      353, 354
    origin of, 354–355
  device placement
    PAWP waveform, 359–360
    pressure waveforms and
      interpretation, 356–357
    pulmonary artery catheter
      insertion, 356
    pulmonary artery
      waveform, 358, 359
    right atrium pressure
      waveform, 358
    RV pressure waveform,
      358, 359
    Seldinger technique, 355
    Swan–Ganz catheter,
      356, 357
  device selection, 352–353
  indications, 352
  site selection, 353
CERVARIX vaccine, 60
Cervical cancer
  anatomy, 55
  angiogenesis, 78–79
  CA4 and CA4P, 79
  clinical stage, 65, 66
  diagnosis, 61
  DMXAA, 79
  genetics, 67
  HPV genome, 56–58
  incidence, 56, 58
  indications
    complications, 67, 69
    pelvic spaces, 67, 69
    Piver and Rutledge
      classification, 67, 68
    postoperative adjuvant
      therapy, 71
    treatment, 67, 68
  metastatic cervical cancer
    GOG 110, 73, 74
    GOG 149, 73, 74
    GOG 169, 74
    GOG 179, 74, 75
    GOG 204, 74, 75
    GOG 240, 74, 76–77
  mortality rate, 56
  neoadjuvant chemotherapy, 80
  ovarian transposition, 70
  pathology
    histologic types, 65, 66
    paracervical and parametrial
      lymphatics, 64
    stage and mode of
      treatment, 65
  pelvic exenteration, 80
  PET/CT staging, 65, 67
  in pregnancy, 80–81
  prevention, 59–60
  radiation therapy
    clinical trials, 316–319
    early bulky stage IB2
      and IIA, 315
    early non-bulky stage IB1
      and IIA, 313–314
    GOG 120, 316
    GOG 123, 316, 317
    locally advanced stage
      IIB–IVA, 71–73, 315
    microinvasive stage IA, 312
    NCCN guidelines, 321
    NCI Canada study, 316, 320
    RTOG 90-01, 316
  risk factors, 59
  robotic-assisted surgery, 70
  screening, 61–63
  sexually transmitted oncogenic
      virus, 56
  squamo columnar junction, 58
  VDA, 79
Chemotactic trigger zone
      (CTZ), 397
Chemotherapy
  CINV (*see* Chemotherapy-
      induced nausea and
      vomiting (CINV))

diarrhea (*see* Chemotherapy-induced diarrhea (CID))
drugs, dosage, and frequency, 206, 218–227
extravasation
agents and management protocol, 257–259
antidotes, 260–262
causes, 256
cold protocol, 260
irritants and vesicants, 256
prevention, 257
risk factors, 256–257
warm protocol, 260
febrile neutropenia
antibiotic treatments, 249–251
antifungal treatments, 249, 252–253
clinical assessment, 254
definitions, 246
diagnosis and workup, 247–248
follow-up, 254–255
high and low risk patients, 248, 249
indications, 254
MASCC scoring index, 248, 249
microbiological infection, 247
primary prophylaxis, 248
risk factors, 246
treatment duration, 255
HSR
desensitization, 266
grading, 264, 265
incidence, 262
mechanism, 262–264
platinum hypersensitivity, 264
prevention, 264
taxane hypersensitivity, 264
peripheral neuropathy
chemotherapy selection, 241
clinical manifestations, 240–241
definitions, 239–240
evaluation, 241, 242
nonpharmacologic treatment, 245
pharmacologic prevention, 243–244
pharmacologic treatment, 244–245
principles, 244
risk factors, 239, 240
pharmacological agents and clinical pearls, 206–217
Chemotherapy-induced diarrhea (CID)
complicated diarrhea, 238–239
evaluation, 235–236
nonpharmacologic treatment, 236
pathogenesis, 235
pharmacologic treatment
diphenoxylate and atropine, 237
loperamide, 237
octreotide, 238
opium tincture, 237
paregoric, 238
principles, 236
signs and symptoms, 235
uncomplicated diarrhea, 238
Chemotherapy-induced nausea and vomiting (CINV)
complications, 228
definitions, 206, 227
etiology, 228
high therapeutic index agents
corticosteroids, 230
5HT3 receptor antagonists, 206, 230
neurokinin-1 receptor antagonists, 231
low therapeutic index agents
benzodiazepines, 232
butyrophenones, 232
cannabinoids, 232
metoclopramide, 231
olanzapine, 232
phenothiazines, 231
principles, 232
rescue medication, 234

Chemotherapy-induced nausea and vomiting (CINV) (*cont.*)
  risk factors, 228–229, 232–233
  treatment regimens, 233–234
Choriocarcinoma (CCA), 12, 177, 178
CID. *See* Chemotherapy-induced diarrhea (CID)
CINV. *See* Chemotherapy-induced nausea and vomiting (CINV)
Clark's and Breslow systems, 95
Clear cell carcinoma, 11, 147, 151, 153
Clinical target volume (CTV), 299
Combretastatin A-4 (CA4), 79
Combretastatin A-4 phosphate (CA4P), 79
Controlled mechanical ventilation (CMV), 340
Cowden syndrome, 138
Critical care
  acid–base disorders
    bicarbonate–carbon dioxide buffer system, 360
    definitions, 361
    Henderson-Hasselbach equation, 360
    management, 364
    metabolic acidosis, 362, 364–365
    metabolic alkalosis, 363, 365
    mixed acid–base disorders, 364
    respiratory acidosis, 363
    respiratory alkalosis, 364
  CVA (*see* Central venous access (CVA))
  fluid resuscitation
    bolus, 349
    crystalloids, 349
    inotropes, 349–350
    vasopressors, 349–352
  mechanical ventilation (*see* Mechanical ventilation (MV))
  sepsis (*see* Sepsis)

D
Depression
  antidepressive medications, 388, 389
  atypical antipsychotics, 389
  benefits, 389–391
  ECT, 389
  non-pharmacologic modalities, 388–389
  psychostimulants, 392
  respiratory depression, 378, 379
  screening, 386–388
  side effects, 389
Drug 5,6-dimethylxanthenone-4-acetic acid (DMXAA), 79
Dyspnea
  air hunger/breathlessness, 408
  brain lesions, 408
  cardiopulmonary, 409
  nasal lesions, 408–409
  spinal metastases, 409–410
  treatment, 410

E
Embryonal rhabdomyosarcoma, 121
Endometrial cancer
  clinical trials, 301–305
  early stage I–II
    chemotherapy, 308, 309
    EBRT, 302, 306, 309
    GOG-99 trial, 307
    JGOG-2033 trial, 308
    PORTEC-2, 307–308
    PORTEC-1 trial, 306–307
  locally advanced stage III–IV
    GOG 122 trial, 310–311
    GOG 184 trial, 310
    GOG-0249 trial, 311
    GOG 0258 trial, 312
    MaNGO ILIADE-III, 309–310
    NSGO-EC-9501/EORTC-55991, 309–310
    PORTEC-3, 312
    sandwich trials, 311

uterine corpus cancers
  adjuvant therapy (*see* Adjuvant therapy)
  chemotherapy, 153–155
  combinatorial therapy, 156
  da Vinci robotic surgical system, 141
  diagnosis, 134
  FIGO surgical staging, 139
  GOG Lap 2 trial, 139–141
  lymphadenectomy (*see* Lymphadenectomy)
  management, 138–139
  meta analysis, 140
  origin, 134
  risk assessment, 146–147
  SEER, 141
  type II lesions, 135
  type 1 lesions, 134–135
  vaginal brachytherapy, 151–152

Endometrioid carcinoma, 11

Epithelial cancer
  adjuvant chemotherapy
    advanced stage, 21–23
    early stage high-risk cancer, 19–21
    HIPEC (*see* Hyperthermic intraperitoneal chemotherapy (HIPEC))
    intraperitoneal chemotherapy, 23–25
  antiangiogenesis therapy
    angiogenic pathway and targeted inhibitors, 28, 29
    bevacizumab, 28
    endothelial cells, 28
    indications, 34, 35
    phase 3 randomized trials, 29–33
    preclinical animal models, 28
    pro-angiogenic mediators, 28
    vasculature, 28
  cytoreductive surgery, 15–17
  genetics and hereditary ovarian cancer
    BRCA1 and BRCA2 mutations, 6–7
    HBOC, 6
  neoadjuvant chemotherapy, 17–19
  ovarian germ cell tumors
    management, 41–42
    VAC, 42
    VBP *vs.* BEP, 42–43
  PARP inhibition and synthetic lethality
    germline BRCA1 and BRCA2 mutations, 34
    NHEJ, 34
    PARP-1 deficiency, 34, 37
    phase 3 trials, 36, 39, 40
  pathological considerations
    clear cell carcinoma, 11
    endometrioid carcinoma, 11
    germ cell tumors, 12
    high grade serous carcinoma, 10
    LMP neoplasms, 12
    low grade serous carcinoma, 10
    mucinous carcinoma, 10
    serous and mucinous LMP, 12
    tumor markers, 12
  risk factors, 3–4
  screening and diagnostic methods
    BRCA mutation, 6
    cancer antigen 125, 4, 5
    Lynch syndrome, 6, 8
    pelvic examination, 4
    PLCO cancer screening trial, 5
    ROCA, 5
    TVUS, 4, 5
    UKFOCSS phase 2 study, 5
  signs and symptoms, 9
  surgical management

Epithelial cancer (*cont.*)
diagnostic and therapeutic methods, 13
FIGO staging system, 13–15
External beam radiation (EBRT), 123, 152, 294, 296, 302, 306
Extramammary paget's disease, 97
Extravasation
agents and management protocol, 257–259
antidotes
dexrazoxane, 261
doses, 261–262
hyaluronidase, 260–261
sodium thiosulfate, 260
causes, 256
cold protocol, 260
irritants and vesicants, 256
prevention, 257
risk factors, 256–257
warm protocol, 260

F

Febrile neutropenia (FN)
antibiotic treatments, 249–251
antifungal treatments, 249, 252–253
clinical assessment, 254
definitions, 246
diagnosis and workup, 247–248
follow-up, 254–255
high and low risk patients, 248, 249
indications, 254
MASCC scoring index, 248, 249
microbiological infection, 247
primary prophylaxis, 248
risk factors, 246
treatment duration, 255

G

GARDASIL vaccine, 59–60
Germ cell tumors, 12, 41–43
Gestational trophoblastic disease
algorithm, 190–191
clinical trials
Brazil trial, 190
GOG 57, 188
GOG 69, 189
GOG 79, 189
GOG 174, 189
GOG 275, 189
GOG 26U, 189
Northwestern trial, 190
Thailand trial, 190
diagnosis
blood work, 183
chest imaging, 184
complete hydatidiform moles, 181
HCG levels, 182–183
partial moles, 181
pelvic imaging, 184
ultrasound, 181
epidemiology, 175–176
FIGO staging system, 184–185
genetics, 179–180
pathology
CCA, 177, 178
cytotrophoblast, 176
hydatidiform mole, 176–177
intermediate trophoblast, 176
MMP, 178
PSTT, 178, 179
syncytiotrophoblast, 176
survival, 195–196
treatment
chemoresistant/recurrent GTN, 195
GOG protocol 242, 187
high risk GTN, 187–188, 193–194
low risk GTN, 187, 192–193
metastatic lesions, 194–195
Gracilis myocutaneous (GM) flaps, 107, 110
Gynecologic Oncology Group (GOG)
GOG 57, 188

GOG 69, 189
GOG 79, 189
GOG 110, 73, 74
GOG 149, 73, 74
GOG 169, 74
GOG 173, 102
GOG 174, 189
GOG 179, 74, 75
GOG 204, 74, 75
GOG 240, 74, 76–77
GOG 270, 104
GOG 275, 189
GOG 122 trial, 310–311
GOG 184 trial, 310
GOG-0249 trial, 311
GOG 0258 trial, 312
GOG 26U, 189

H

Henderson-Hasselbach equation, 360
Hereditary breast and ovarian cancer (HBOC), 6, 7
Hereditary non-polyposis colon cancer (HNPCC) syndrome, 8, 137, 138
High grade serous carcinoma, 10
HIPEC. *See* Hyperthermic intraperitoneal chemotherapy (HIPEC)
HSR. *See* Hypersensitivity reactions (HSR)
Human papillomavirus (HPV), 56–58, 86, 117
Hypersensitivity reactions (HSR)
  desensitization, 266
  incidence, 262
  mechanism, 262–264
  platinum hypersensitivity, 264, 265
  prevention, 264
  taxane hypersensitivity, 264, 265
Hyperthermic intraperitoneal chemotherapy (HIPEC)
  cytoreductive surgery, 25, 27
  GI malignancies, 25
  multi-institutional phase 2 study, 28
  peritoneal mesothelioma, 25
  phase 2 clinical trial, 26, 27
  pseudo-myxoma peritonei, 25
  uses, 25, 26

I

Intensity modulated radiation therapy (IMRT), 123
International Collaborative Ovarian Neoplasm Trial 1 (ICON1), 20

J

Japanese Clinical Oncology Group (JCOG), 19

L

Leiomyosarcoma
  adjuvant therapy, 164–165
  advanced/recurrent disease, 165–167
  BSO, 163
  bulky nodes removal, 164
LMP. *See* Low malignant potential (LMP)
Low grade serous carcinoma, 10
Low malignant potential (LMP)
  adjuvant chemotherapy, 36
  advanced-stage and recurrent disease, 36
  early-stage disease, 36
  GOG, 37, 40
  platinum-based chemotherapy, 40–41
  serous and mucinous LMP, 12
Low tidal volume ventilation (LTVV), 343
Lymphadenectomy
  GOG, 145

Lymphadenectomy (*cont.*)
 intraoperative risk assessment, 142
 Panici and ASTEC trial, 143, 144
 pelvic and para-aortic lymphadenectomy, 142
 staging and dissection, 143
Lymphoscintigraphy (LSG), 102
Lynch syndrome, 6, 8, 138

M
Malignant bowel obstruction (MBO)
 CT scan, 399
 endoscopy, 399
 management
  laparotomy, 400
  pharmacological therapy, 400–402
  surgical bypass, 400
  venting gastrostomy, 401, 403
 mechanisms, 398
 symptoms, 398–399
 X-ray, 399
Malignant melanoma, 95–96
Malignant mixed mullerian tumors (MMMT). *See* Carcinosarcoma
Matrix metalloproteinases (MMPs), 178
MBO. *See* Malignant bowel obstruction (MBO)
Mechanical ventilation (MV)
 ARDS, 342–343
 assist controlled mode, 340
 CMV, 340
 endotracheal cuff leak, 338, 339
 IMV, 341–342
 mechanism, 337
 plateau pressure, 338
 SIMV, 341
 volume-cycled ventilation, 339
 weaning technique
  endotracheal tube and trachea, 345
  extubation, 343
  SBT, 344–345
  ventilation, 344
Mucinous carcinoma, 10–11

N
Nonhomologous end joining (NHEJ), 34, 35

O
Opioids
 adverse effects, 378–379
 anti-inflammatory drugs
  bisphosphonates, 384
  glucocorticoids, 382–383
  NSAIDs, 383
 easy-to-use equal analgesia, 380–381
 fentanyl, 375–376
 hydromorphone, 374
 ketamine administration, 386
 lidocaine infusions, 386
 methadone, 376–378
 morphine, 372, 374, 381–382
 neuropathic pain agents, 386
  gabapentin, 385
  pregabalin, 386
  SNRIs, 384–385
  TCAs, 384
 NMDA receptor antagonist, 386
 opioid induced hyperalgesia, 386
 oxycodone, 374
 refractory neuropathic pain, 386
Ovary
 epithelial ovarian cancer (*see* Epithelial cancer)
 LMP
  adjuvant chemotherapy, 36
  advanced-stage and recurrent disease, 36
  early-stage disease, 36
  GOG, 37, 40
  platinum-based chemotherapy, 40–41

serous and mucinous LMP, 12
sex-cord-stromal tumors, 44

P

Palliative care
ascites (*see* Ascites)
constipation management
enema, 393–394
flushing colonoscopy, 395
laxatives, 392–394
depression (*see* Depression)
dyspnea
air hunger/breathlessness, 408
brain lesions, 408
cardiopulmonary, 409
nasal lesions, 408–409
spinal metastases, 409–410
treatment, 410
MBO (*see* Malignant bowel obstruction (MBO))
nausea/vomiting
brain metastasis, 397
CTZ, 397
gastrointestinal track, 395–396
mechanisms, 395, 396
pavlovian response, 396–397
vestibular triggers, 397
pain management (*see* Opioids)
prognosis, 372
World Health Organization, 371
Papillary serous carcinoma (UPSC)
adjuvant therapy, 159–160
optimal cytoreduction, 158
surgical staging, 158
Papilloma TRIal against Cancer In young Adults (PATRICIA), 60
Peripheral neuropathy
chemotherapy selection, 241
clinical manifestations, 240–241
definitions, 239–240
evaluation, 241, 242
nonpharmacologic treatment, 245
pharmacologic prevention
amifostine, 243
erythropoietin, 243
glutamine and acetyl-l-carnitine, 244
glutathione, 243
IV calcium and magnesium, 244
serotonin-norepinephrine reuptake inhibitors, 244
vitamin E, 243
pharmacologic treatment, 244–245
principles, 244
risk factors, 239, 240
Placental site trophoblastic tumor (PSTT), 178, 179, 182, 183, 188
Pulmonary artery wedge pressure (PAWP), 359–360

R

Radiation therapy
bony anatomy-based planning, 300
brachytherapy
dose and organ tolerance, 298–299
interstitial radiation, 296
intracavitary, 296, 297
landmarks, 301
LDR/HDR system, 296, 298
cervical cancer
clinical trials, 316–319
early bulky stage IB2 and IIA, 315
early non-bulky stage IB1 and IIA, 313–314
GOG 120, 316
GOG 123, 316, 317
locally advanced stage IIB–IVA, 315

Radiation therapy (*cont.*)
microinvasive stage IA, 312
NCCN guidelines, 321
NCI Canada study, 316, 320
RTOG 90-01, 316
compton effect, 289
cycling cells, 292
3D CT-based planning, 299
definitions, 289
EBRT
cervical and vulvar cancers, 294, 295
cyber knife, 296
gamma knife, 296
proton therapy, 294
stereotactic radiotherapy, 294
fallopian tube carcinoma, 327
inguinal radiation, 300–301
inverse square law, 293–294
ovarian cancer, 326
oxygen, 291–292
palliative radiation, 327–328
para-aortic radiation, 300
photoelectric effect, 290
primary peritoneal carcinoma, 326–327
radiobiology, 290
radiocurability, 292
radioprotectors, 293
radiosensitivity, 290–291
radiosensitizers, 293
therapeutic ratio, 292–293
vaginal cancer
brachytherapy, 324
HPV infection, 323–324
late-stage disease, 324
retrospective study, 324–326
vulvar cancer
advanced stage II–IV, 322–323
incidence, 321
limited stage I, 321–322
Risk of ovarian cancer algorithm (ROCA), 5

S
SCC. *See* Squamous cell carcinomas (SCC)
Sentinel lymph node biopsy (SLNB)
GOG 173, 102
GOG 270, 104
GROINSS V, 103
GROINSS VII, 104
inguinofemoral lymphadenectomy technique, 104
lateral and midline tumors, 103
LSG, 102
metastases, 102
risk, 104
Sepsis
diagnostic criteria, 346, 347
Escherichia coli and *MRSA* infections, 345–346
landmark signs, 345
management
broad-spectrum antibiotics, 346–347
parameters, 348–349
surviving sepsis campaign care bundle, 347–348
MODS, 345, 346
severe sepsis, 346, 348
SIRS, 346
Seratonin norepinephrine reuptake inhibitors (SNRIs), 384–385, 388
Single-strand annealing (SSA), 34
Squamous cell carcinomas (SCC)
epidemiology, 116
histology, 86, 87, 93
pathology, 93, 120
survival rates, 126
Surveillance Epidemiology and End Result database (SEER), 141
Synchronized intermittent mandatory ventilation (SIMV), 340, 341

Systemic inflammatory response syndrome (SIRS), 346

T

Transvaginal ultrasound (TVUS), 4, 5
Tricyclic antidepressants (TCAs), 384

U

Uterine corpus cancers
  carcinosarcoma
    advanced stage III and IV, 162
    early stage I and II, 161–162
    sentinel assessments, 162, 163
    surgery, 160–161
  diagnosis/screening, 136
  endometrial cancer
    adjuvant therapy (*see* Adjuvant therapy)
    chemotherapy, 153–155
    combinatorial therapy, 156
    da Vinci robotic surgical system, 141
    diagnosis, 134
    FIGO surgical staging, 139
    GOG Lap 2 trial, 139–141
    lymphadenectomy (*see* Lymphadenectomy)
    management, 138–139
    meta analysis, 140
    risk assessment, 146–147
    risk factor, 134
    SEER, 141
    type II lesions, 135
    type 1 lesions, 134–135
    vaginal brachytherapy, 151–152
  epidemiology, 133
  genetics, 137–138
  leiomyosarcoma
    adjuvant therapy, 164–165
    advanced/recurrent disease, 165–167
    BSO, 163
    bulky nodes removal, 164
  recurrent/metastatic disease, 157
  staging, 137
  UPSC
    adjuvant therapy, 159–160
    optimal cytoreduction, 158
    surgical staging, 158
  uterine sarcomas, 135–136

V

Vaginal brachytherapy (VBT), 151–152
Vaginal cancer
  clinical presentation, 118
  diagnosis, 118
  epidemiology, 116–117
  pathology
    adenocarcinoma, 120
    embryonal rhabdomyosarcoma, 121
    melanoma, 121
    SCC, 120
  post-treatment, 126
  pretreatment evaluation, 118
  prognosis/survival, 126–127
  radiation therapy
    brachytherapy, 324
    HPV infection, 323–324
    late-stage disease, 324
    retrospective study, 324–326
  risk factors, 117
  screening, 117
  staging
    direct extension, 119
    FIGO staging classification, 118–119
    hematogenous spread, 120
    lymphatic dissemination, 120

Vaginal cancer (*cont.*)
treatment
adenocarcinoma, 125
melanoma, 125–126
neoadjuvant chemotherapy, 122
pediatric embryonal rhabdomyosarcoma, 126
radiation, 123–124
stage I disease surgery, 122
stage II–IV disease radical surgery, 122
stereotactic radiosurgery, 124
Vaginal intraepithelial neoplasia (VAIN)
5-FU cream, 115
imiquimod, 115–116
laser ablation, 115
petroleum jelly and zinc oxide cream, 116
surgical excision, 115
VAIN. *See* Vaginal intraepithelial neoplasia (VAIN)
Vascular disrupting agents (VDAs), 79
Verrucous carcinoma, 94
VIN. *See* Vulva intraepithelial neoplasia (VIN)
Vinblastine, bleomycin and cisplatin (VBP), 42–43
Vincristine, actinomycin-D and cyclophosphamide (VAC), 42, 43, 126
Vulva intraepithelial neoplasia (VIN), 88
Co_2 laser ablation, 113
imiquimod, 113–114
topical 5-fluorouracil (5-FU), 114
vulvectomy, 113
wide local excision, 113
Vulvar cancer
advanced stage III and IVA
GOG 101, 106
GOG 205, 106
myocutaneous flaps, 107, 110
preoperative imaging, 105–106
skin flaps, 107–109
skin grafts, 107
surgical excision, 105
advanced-stage II–IV, 322–323
clinical presentation, 89
complications, 111–112
early stage I and II
groin lymph nodes, 100–101
positive/narrow margins, 98, 99
primary groin radiation, 101
primary tumor, 98, 99
SLNB (*see* Sentinel lymph node biopsy (SLNB))
superficial lymphadenectomy, 101
epidemiology, 86–87
FIGO staging classification, 90–92
incidence, 93, 321
limited-stage I, 321–322
mode of spread, 89–90
pathology/histology
Bartholin's gland carcinomas, 94–95
basal cell carcinoma, 94
extramammary paget's disease, 97
malignant melanoma, 95–96
SCC, 93
verrucous carcinoma, 94
postoperative management
IFLND, 107, 109
preventative measures, 109, 110
radical vulvectomy, 107, 109
pretreatment evaluation, 89
recurrent and distant metastatic disease, 111
screening, 87
survival, 112

VAIN
5-FU cream, 115
imiquimod, 115–116
laser ablation, 115
petroleum jelly and zinc oxide cream, 116
surgical excision, 115
VIN, 88
Co_2 laser ablation, 113
imiquimod, 113–114
topical 5-fluorouracil (5-FU), 114
vulvectomy, 113
wide local excision, 113
Vulvar reconstruction
myocutaneous flaps, 107, 110
skin flaps, 107–109
skin grafts, 107

CPSIA information can be obtained at www.ICGtesting.com
Printed in the USA
LVOW01s1115211114

414933LV00009B/20/P

9 781493 919758